Edward Bruce Bynum, PhD

Transcending Psychoneurotic Disturbances: New Approaches in Psychospirituality and Personality Development

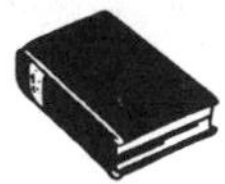

Pre-publication REVIEWS, COMMENTARIES, EVALUATIONS . . .

"In a daring leap involving new conceptual models, Bynum portrays the human being as an energetic system in search of both balance and growth. This book discusses both the anxieties and the stresses of our time, while it provides readers the tools by which anxieties and stresses can be addressed."

Stanley Krippner, PhD
Distinguished Professor of Psychology,
California Institute of Integral Studies

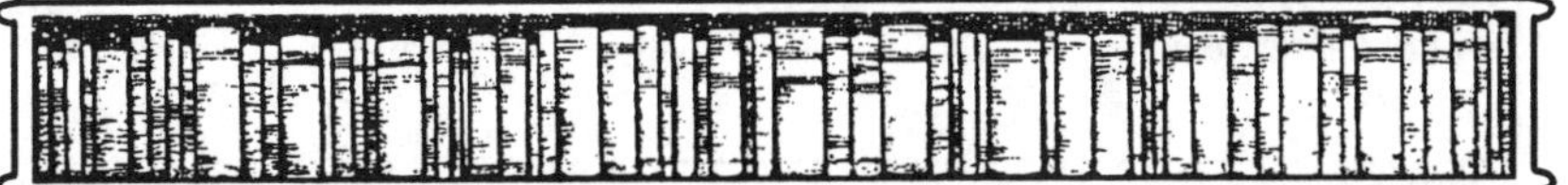

More pre-publication
REVIEWS, COMMENTARIES, EVALUATIONS . . .

"A MIGHTY SYNTHESIS OF KNOWLEDGE AND FEELING, SCIENCE AND POETRY, CLINICAL OBSERVATION AND SPIRITUAL INSIGHT. E. Bruce Bynum is both a practicing clinical psychologist and a person involved with various sacred traditions. He brings together these aspects of his life experience in a work that speaks powerfully to lay and professional people alike. His theme is the evolution of consciousness to enlightenment and the psychoneurotic distortions that can occur as people seek to express the divine life-force in various ways. In examining his topic, Bynum takes us on an awesome journey through time and space, reliving the history of our species from its beginnings in the African savanna to its highest expression so far in the sages and spiritual giants of recent centuries. He describes our journey in a narrative style that is sensitive, powerful and at times even breathtakingly beautiful. I regard this book as an important contribution to our understanding of the mind and its operation in the world."

John White, MAT
Author, *Future Science,*
and *Kundalini, Evolution and Enlightenment*

"THIS IS A PIONEERING BOOK IN TRANSEGO PSYCHOLOGY. Bynum, while being appreciative of the major contributions of various schools of object relation-based ego-psychology of Freud, Piaget, Mahler, Sullivan, and Kohut, envisions the next step in the development of human psychology. This is a progression from object relations to field relations. Dr. Bynum raises the 'new' question that the 'self' is not localized in the mind, but is 'non-local,' a field of interconnected relations. The self was seen as an event experienced as a luminous substructure, self-regulating of a radiant transcendental life-force, which itself was the bedrock of the material world, mind, and attention. Earlier concepts of object relations were based upon a world view founded upon presubatomic physics that defined relationships between separate objects or atoms. Whereas, modern subatomic physics has redefined reality as the relatedness of interacting fields without boundaries, symmetry breaking processes, fluctuating subsystems, transient states of order, and non-linear processes.

More pre-publication
REVIEWS, COMMENTARIES, EVALUATIONS . . .

It is with such an orientation that the author has revisited both Western psychological clinical reports and the historical academic texts of India, China, and Africa. A valuable model was presented to define psychological diagnostic issues and therapeutic treatment issues. TRULY WONDERFUL."

Richard D. King, MD
From the Preface; Author, *African Origin of Biological Psychiatry*

Harrington Park Press
An Imprint of The Haworth Press, Inc.

NOTES FOR PROFESSIONAL LIBRARIANS AND LIBRARY USERS

This is an original book title published by Harrington Park Press, an imprint of The Haworth Press, Inc. Unless otherwise noted in specific chapters with attribution, materials in this book have not been previously published elsewhere in any format or language.

CONSERVATION AND PRESERVATION NOTES

The paper used in this publication meets the minimum requirements of American National Standard for Information Sciences–Permanence of Paper for Printed Material, ANSI Z39.48-1984.

Transcending Psychoneurotic Disturbances

New Approaches in Psychospirituality and Personality Development

HAWORTH Psychotherapy
E. Mark Stern, PhD
Senior Editor

New, Recent, and Forthcoming Titles:

Families and the Interpretation of Dreams: Awakening the Intimate Web by Edward Bruce Bynum

Transcending Psychoneurotic Disturbances: New Approaches in Psychospirituality and Personality Development by Edward Bruce Bynum

Transcending Psychoneurotic Disturbances

New Approaches in Psychospirituality and Personality Development

Edward Bruce Bynum, PhD

Foreword by Molefi Kete Asante, PhD
Preface by Richard D. King, MD

The Harrington Park Press
An Imprint of The Haworth Press, Inc.
New York • London • Norwood (Australia)

Published by

Harrington Park Press, an imprint of The Haworth Press, Inc., 10 Alice Street, Binghamton, NY 13904-1580

Library of Congress Cataloging-in-Publication Data

Bynum, Edward Bruce, 1948-
Transcending psychoneurotic disturbances : new approaches in psychospirituality and personality development / Edward Bruce Bynum.
p. cm.
Published simultaneously by The Haworth Press, Inc.
Includes bibliographical references and index.
ISBN 1-56023-028-2 (alk. paper)
1. Neuroses–Miscellanea. 2. Vital force. 3. Transcendence (Philosophy) I. Title.
[DNLM: 1. Personality Development. 2. Personality Disorders. 3. Spiritualism. WM 190 B994t]
RC530.B86 1993b
616.89–dc20
DNLM/DLC
for Library of Congress 92-1578
CIP

To my Living Teachers of the Three Worlds:

My beloved wife Alyse,
whose edgeless strength and guidance
has helped me to recapture
the subtle terrain of my own heart;

My mother, through
whose body I entered
the ocean of this life;

and to She-who-has-no-name,
the first Avatar still Living in our blood,
who Ages ago on the African savannas
wove our genes and Lineages together . . .

ABOUT THE AUTHOR

Edward Bruce Bynum, PhD, is a clinical psychologist and Director of the Behavioral Medicine Program at the University of Massachusetts Health Services. He is the author of *The Family Unconscious* and *Families and the Interpretation of Dreams*. He has published widely in both popular and professional journals. Some of his work has been translated into German, Japanese, and Russian. He is a student and practitioner of Kundalini Yoga.

CONTENTS

Foreword

Edward Bruce Bynum's work *Transcending Psychoneurotic Disturbances* is a continuation of his quest for the sustenance of eternal light in human personality. Gifted with a broad intelligence which has allowed him to access the numerous publications and research of others, he has demonstrated in this volume that singular quality a close a scholarly reading makes necessary for the material in this area, depth.

Following the concepts and ideas that have stood as keys to understanding the psychoneurotic distortions of the life force, Dr. Bynum examines in detail–as a scientist should–the fundamental nature of these distortions. His grasp of the human personality is equal to his understanding of the basis of our search for the transcendent. His quest for the light is the same one as that seen by the early African thinkers such as Kagemni, Ptahhotep, and Khunanup; the Chinese thinkers such as Kung-Futzi and Lao-Tzu; the Hebrew thinkers Jeremiah, Isaiah, and Ezekiel; the Greek thinkers Thales, Isocrates, Democritus, and Plato.

During the great and long reign of the African king Tuthmoses III, the incessant search for the nature of life after death was undertaken by the greatest minds of the day. They wrote their ideas in what became known as the *Book of What Is in the Netherworld*. But in all of their searching and questing for that one final word, the priests and scholars had to admit that they could not know for certain what was in the netherworld. Thus, they prepared deceased persons for the journey by making sure that the various attributes of their lives, tokens of material possessions, favorite foods and most honored fabrics and clothing went with them to the netherworld. After all, the deceased might need some of those things. In this wonderful book, Dr. Bynum tells us that there are some things that are more precious than gold, more luxurious than the richest fabrics, and more spiritual than amulets. He finds in the questing human consciousness the answer to the imponderables of life and gives us the insight necessary to chart our own pathways towards the light, however great or however small. Light is light.

Human beings have always sought ways to touch the groundedness in their own personalities, to encounter the invisible and yet to reach the light which would explain the nature of human existence. In the *Myth of Sisyphus* Albert Camus asks the question, "Who is the absurd man?" He answers by saying that the absurd one is "He who does nothing for the eternal." Dr. Bynum's aim is to post markers on the track of life so that those who quest will be able to see their way from the roots to the top. And the reader is fortunate because there are good signs on the track.

This is a powerful book. Its power is not simply in the amount of information the author has amassed though he has given us an incredible amount of information about human personality and the quest for the light. Even in the midst of darkness, this man envisions the light. He is an optimistic writer whose sense of the possible permeates the entire book. Actually this is part of the strength of the volume because the author's enormous capability in understanding the nature of our existence gives him the upper hand in providing the markers along the way. There is evidence throughout this book of the wealth of his knowledge about the nature of science, physics, human personality, and the perennial search for fulfillment and joy. One reads this book with the clear idea that here is a writer who enjoys living.

What he has given us is a true picture of the great cross-fertilization of human history and culture. Our indebtedness to the philosophers of every culture and every region is stated clearly and unequivocally. Indeed we are made to see the inevitability of growing toward the same pathways of our inner natures. Since the cycles of nature, the seeds of renewal, and the seasons of our quests come together in our own mature selves we are subjects of the most elemental and fundamental powers of the universe. Dr. Bynum's work is an excursion into ourselves. We are better for the work that he has done. We are more knowledgeable about ourselves and we know the way to the light. Now it is our choice to journey toward the light but we, at least, have some real idea about how to proceed.

The twentieth century has been a century of searching. It is proper that *Transcending Psychoneurotic Disturbances* by an outstanding thinker concerned with the human search for light, the essence, the generative quality of life, become a major book, one of the signposts of the time. I believe that this volume will have a significant impact on the way we imagine ourselves in terms of the past, present, and future because the seeds of light that it spreads in our minds will bring forth numerous products of the spirit.

Molefi Kete Asante, PhD

Preface

This is a pioneering text in Transego Psychology. The author, while being appreciative of the major contributions of various schools of the object relations-based ego psychology of Freud, Piaget, Mahler, Sullivan, and Kohut, boldly envisions the next step in the development of human psychology. For this book illuminates the progression from object relations to field relations. Dr. Bynum raises the "new" question that the "self" is not localized in the mind or mental process, but rather is "non-local" in nature, a field of interconnected relations. The self is seen as an event experienced as a luminous substructure, self-regulating of a radiant transcendental life-force, which itself is the bedrock of the material world, mind and attention. Earlier concepts of object relations were based upon a world view founded upon presubatomic physics that defined relationships between separate objects or atoms. Whereas modern subatomic physics has now redefined reality as the relatedness of interacting fields without boundaries, symmetry breaking processes, fluctuating subsystems, transient states of order, and nonlinear processes.

It is with such an emergent new orientation that the author has revisited both Western psychology clinical reports and the historical academic texts of India, China, and Africa for the human experience of the life-force in particular nonboundary phenomena. A valuable model was presented to define psychopathological diagnostic issues and therapeutic treatment issues. Truly wonderful.

Richard D. King, MD
President, Km-Wr Science Consortium, Inc.
Los Angeles, CA

Introduction

All is light; light, the substratum and matrix of all that exists. All that exists is a relative of light. A vast, stellar, interpenetrating witness looks out through the lens of analysis at the flux and foment that passes for the material universe. Boundless emptiness graced with a few spasms of light fill the expanding, timeless sight. Focused attention on just a tissue of light reveals galaxies and nebulae spiralling through the abyss. Further scrutiny unfolds a more local solar system of stars, planets, and scattered debris. An even deeper attention to the material expanse of just one planet among many reveals geology, history, the whole spectral analysis of minerals. Minerals break down into elements and elements reveal atoms. Soon these objects and atoms give way to sub-atomic spaces and these then open to sub-quantum fluctuations, shifting matrixes. Without word, breath, or sound soon only emptiness and fleeting intimacies of light again fill the sight of this vast, inter-penetrating witness. Yet in all this analysis and abstraction of the dynamic and eternal, a crucial movement has been missed.

The life-force, evolution and all its forms are curiously absent. The bias of dissection, analysis, and reductionism completely bypass a most obvious production. For reasons and causes that mysteriously escape the materialist bias of order, somehow life and consciousness emerged on the scene. Call it what you will, negative-entropy, or some strangely irreversible process of increasing complexity, or simply the life-force.

This negative entropy of the life-force contradicts the second law of thermodynamics which compels all systems to ultimate dissolution and heat death. It is held to operate on the material plane. However, it is obvious that life evolves in this plane. This negative entropy parallels increasing complexity and this complexity of information, it seems, increasingly reflects the dynamics of light. The material world with its "discrete objects" and the world of organic process evolving into progressively more differentiated forms would appear at first to operate on contradictory or conflicting laws. We need a new principle of organization, a principle of science and space-time that is deeper than, or subsumes, these other two great and obvious principles, that is to say, principles and laws that give rise to or unfold the others. Some of these requirements may be satisfied by principles of "self-organization" of systems, principles of unfoldment and enfoldment. We may even find at some point that this self is light itself.

These principles provide breathing space for the obvious theatrics of the everyday material world and the inner drama of the life-force with its close energies and functions. Everything is involved.

All are reflections of a process that appears to move from simple to complex in an immeasurably intelligent and luminous way. The life-force, in all its colors, contours, and subtle expressions, must be taken into account in this unfoldment and saga. This marvelous play of forms and forces cannot be reduced to random chemical combinations or the final work of a long disintegrated star. It is permeated by, and permeates, the whole material array; its expansion and contraction mirror the cosmic expanse. It is in all and aspects of all are in it.

So above us in the distant constellations known and still to be known energies thunder and ride. Below the atom dance worlds in process and shifting vibration, their meaning, as Bohr showed, intimately involved in the whole context. This is not poetry or a sorcerer's dream. This is the vision of modern science. Indeed, Einstein unraveled the equivalence of matter and energy showing matter to be a form of energy and light. Later DeBroglie formulated the other side of the insight and showed that even matter itself was composed of waves, "matter waves" that propagate through space. Therein every object is an expression of light!

We are an expression of light! In a strange sort of way "matter" has been magically de-materialized in modern science. With this comes a new understanding of any "object" as a condensation or localization of these vast interconnected energies. This deeply affects any notion of objects-in-relation to other objects as we shall see in our perspective on "object-relations." The life-force, in particular, manifests dynamics and processes that do not reflect the notion of discrete objects in interaction with other discrete objects. A new perspective emerges in the sea of energy and light that is not so much object relations, object splitting and all their fleetingly conditioned states, but rather field and energetic relations in an enfolded and ultimately interconnected matrix. This is the perspective taken here and throughout this book. It is to recognize a freer sea of energy, intelligence, and luminosity in which we as consciousness fluctuate and have our cohesion.

It would seem that the linear lens of abstraction and analysis, of "inner" and "outer" gives way to a more spherical vision, of all in each and each in all. A holonomic universe appears before us as an undivided whole in flowing movement. In this more inclusive way, life, matter, and death, even time itself and therein movement, are all interconnected through intelligence on innumerable levels.

Through it all runs the life-force in its illimitable forms, a radiant, intelligent, transcendental force. It is an energetic process that breeds increasing complexity, that for whatever reasons manifests an expanding mystery, consciousness. This essay is of and about this luminous, conscious, transcendental force and equation in our human adventure, the five-fingered form. It is a tangible, body-felt and well-traveled ancient route rooted in the biochemistry and embryology of our nervous system. It is as intimate as our breathing, more personal than the inner corridors of our sleep. Indeed, it may be the very root of our deeply *personalizing* tendency in the living universe. For this and other reasons, a primordial figure of ourselves must be contacted and traced through the whole evolutionary escapade, from primitive gatherer and seer to the more modern form. Thus "She" is born in the ancestral past and her vibrant memory is felt each beet-red morning. Like all life we know of, it begins near water.

Civilization is a distant dream to her, an unimaginable future. Between her rising on the African savanna/foothills of her ancestors untold millenniums ago, through the age of early civilization on to our present, she and her progeny have witnessed the interplay and spell of the life-force. Every archeological excavation is a testimony to her preoccupation and love-affair with its innumerable forms. The earliest intuition of the Divine is always female. Each great upheaval of land and climate or cultural unrest disturbed the hard won equilibrium. It intimately altered her perception of the earth and made evolution and consciousness integrate in a higher, more inclusive, order.

This early one we call She-who-has-no-name. She is the offshoot, the progeny of "Lucy," the ancient female unearthed at Olduvai Gorge near the great lakes in east Africa. "Lucy" rested there for perhaps three or four million years. She-who-has-no-name is a more recent ancestor, somewhere in the orbit of 200,000 years ago. Her peculiar strength and destiny is that all our known human gene pools as deciphered by mitochondrial DNA studies are crisscrossed streams that flowed through her ocean. She-who-has-no-name runs through the blood of each of us today. She is implicated genetically and physically in each one of us; each of us is implicated in each other. Humanity met there in her and greatly still arches upwards toward a still unmet civilization. In this sense She-who-has-no-name was the first Avatar moving us collectively between the Australopithecus Africanus and the stars. From her eventually came primordial religion and technology which married in unique patterns in the river mouths of valleys all over the earth. Similar ideas and transformations also emerged everywhere from the human quest. The life-force was discovered before the conquest of land, animals, and all the rest. It sustained her progeny through thousands of generations.

There is on-going debate about the specifically African origin of She-who-has-no-name, some arguing an African origin (Vigilant et al., 1991), some claiming to refute it on statistical grounds (Templeton, 1991). The technical debate on the DNA analysis goes back and forth (Hedges, Kumar, and Tamura, 1991). However the overwhelming preponderance of evidence from fossil records, morphological data, and anatomical correlations plus other molecular data strongly imply an African genesis. By Gloger's law of necessity warm-blooded mammals in a hot and humid climate required dark skins to survive. We are all the children of an ancient, dark-skinned African woman and our tribes have criss-crossed the globe numerous times.

Upheavals of many kinds lead to new integrations, new insights and twists on the perennial quest, a quest nourished in the nervework and cells of her kind. By the sixth and seventh centuries B.C.E., a great new dawn of religious and noetic temperament arose *all* over the earth. It integrated technology and the noetic in a radically new net.

It was the time, this new age of Axis, when the diverse regions of the earth saw new beginnings, fusions, and higher equilibriums in human cultural, cognitive, and noetic life (Hutchison, 1969). From Greece to Israel, to India and China, not to mention the Upper African Nile and the world of the Mesoamericans, men and women, progeny of the ancient one, emerged into a new noetic consciousness. In some curious way they were all interconnected in the shared ocean of human consciousness.

Israel produced its age of God-intoxicated prophetic voices; Jeremiah (650-580 B.C.), Ezekiel (625-570 B.C.) and Deutero-Isaiah (550 B.C.). They brought a more personal, moral, and intimately subjective God into the world. The vast Persian empire produced the new seer/prophet Zoroaster, whose notions of God, and good and evil were so similar to the Hebrews. In India of the Axis age emerged the Buddha and Mahavira of the Jains. In China emerged Lao-Tzu and Confucius. And in ancient Greece, drawing its scholarship from even older Kemetic Egypt and the upper Nile, arose the early philosophers and scientists of what was later to be called Western civilization; Thales, Xenophanes, and the celestial, harmonically intoxicated Pythagoras. The later Western philosophers, Socrates, Plato, and Aristotle, built their edifice on these (Bernal, 1987) Many of the other Greek luminaries also studied the mysteries in the libraries and temples of the Egyptian "Houses of Life."

These Kemetic Egyptian Houses of Life were well aware of the life-force, the dynamic unconscious, and the methods for awakening and guiding the forces of evolution. They had three levels of initiation, the neophyte, the nous, and the awakened ones, the "sons of light." Their methodologies guided the initiate through the psychoneurotic distortions of the life-force to the goals of illumination. Their esoteric medical and spiritual technology was literally designed for transcending psychoneurotic disturbances. Their philosophy was really the foundation of later Greek philosophy and science (James, 1954).

What is common to all of the above from the Kemetic Egyptians to the Age of Axis, is the peering past and beyond the material mirage to the enfolding-unfolding substratum and undercurrent of the world process, the great undivided whole of life, matter, intelligence and design. In the Greek poetry of the Axis Age one can see the rise and stabilization of the individual, subjective consciousness and the uniquely intimate philosophical issues that therein arise (Jaynes, 1976). All these came at a time of great fluctuation from the norm, of a new synthesis of matter, man, and mind. The primordial one of this essay lived in an even earlier time of such vast change and upheaval that profoundly affected consciousness. We, her progeny, also live in such a period. The current of the life-force and evolution, however, flows in the nervework and blood cells of every era we live in.

In that direction, this study will look at the human adventure with and in this current of living energy and consciousness which we will call the life-force. It is a radiant, interpenetrating, and transcendental current or force that has arisen in "dead" matter. *Out* of this life-force consciousness has emerged and *into* this life-force consciousness has descended. Evolution it seems is not only the <u>upward push</u> toward greater complexity, but when a so-called "natural selection" works, it represents a greater "neatness of fit", an expression and <u>pull toward</u> a more subtle and inclusive manifestation of order in the universe. These play out in all the personality styles of this book. This essay is about the peculiar dynamics of this radiant, intelligent, transcendental force in its human adventure. Each chapter is a different expression and approach to how we, her progeny, deal with this reality in our unique psychological ways. For that very reason alone we are pulled to go beyond the normal boundaries of "modern psychological" insight and touch the whole undivided range of human consciousness. This entails not only an analysis of unconscious dynamics, but also of subtle, causal, and what are termed superconscious or transcendental states. This will allow room for the psychic, the transpersonal, and the noetic, areas largely selectively unattended to in this age of intellectual domination by scientific materialism. We will not repress the sublime, nor blindly embrace the reductionist bias of contemporary Western science. Rather, as in other upheavals, we will seek to assimilate it and then move beyond.

The perspective taken is an energetic one, in which both consciousness and energy are all pervasive. Objects, of all varieties, are seen to unfold and localize or concentrate out of the more primary matrix of nonlocal process that itself gives rise to objects, space, and time. The intuition or notion of "objects" is functional but held in parenthesis. This is to accept, from the very beginning, the ancient Abhidhamma notion of Samkhara-dukkha, or the recognition of "suffering as conditioned states" in which *all* object seeking is illusory and the reflection of a contracting tendency in the body-mind from that all pervasive life-force.

We are not throwing the baby out with the bath water. Not at all. Instead, we are simply pointing out that the life-force, by its very nature, is an expansive, unfolding process whose essence will elude a purely reductionist lens and instead requires a constructivist lens, such that its tendency toward greater and greater complexities and more inclusive wholes can be recognized. In this sea "objects" are functional and yet not absolute and eternal. In this digest, indeed, we are all only transitional objects!

But there is another more sequestered purpose for taking this perspective openly and at this point. By consciously doing so, it subtly cultivates the expectation and goals outlined in the later methodology section of this story. At a certain juncture in the methodology section, or in any deeper meditative practice, space and time and the actual "object" of attention begins to dissolve or deconstruct into percept, pattern, and form within and against, and apparently unfolding out of, a background of boundaryless, interconnected energy, light, and intelligence. This "light" begins to permeate and unfold the perceptual field at a certain level. This can be realized by you, the reader, at the level of direct experience. By cultivating this ground, or sea, of intelligent light, from the onset it becomes easier to recognize its unfoldment in your own intimate process.

Sometimes the patterns are seen as external to ourselves, sometimes internal to ourselves. Occasionally, we recognize the patterns to be ourselves in transformation. This is not only poetry, but the bedrock of both modern science and the ancient introspective sciences:

> The views of space and time which I wish to lay before you have sprung from the soil of experimental physics, and therein lies their strength. They are radical. Henceforth space by itself, and time by itself, are doomed to fade away into mere shadows, and only a kind of union of the two will preserve an independent reality.
>
> –Hermann Minkowski, 1908
> on *Space-Time*

> . . . Once [we] . . . experience . . . a state of complete dissolution where there is no more distinction between mind and body, subject and object . . . we look around and perceive that . . . every object is related to every other object . . . not only spatially, but temporally. . . . As a fact of pure experience, there is no space without time, no time without space; they are interpenetrating.
>
> –D. T. Suzuki
> on the *Avatamsaka Sutra*
> of Mahayana Buddhism

Our species has carried on this intimate affair with the all pervasive long before evolution in us became conscious of itself. Now this drama is played out daily in most of us. It was the drama of the ancient one, despite the pressures for survival, food and whatever else composed the texture of everyday life. It lives and works through us at this very moment. Each of us, in our own personality style and way, has our own take on its heartbeat. If we were, in an Afrocentric sense, to "personalize" this process that implicates light and intelligence on all levels, from birth to death and perhaps back again, we would choose the ancient and more inclusive Kemetic myth and dynamic of Osiris. His reach was greater than Oedipus, and he knew the Gods, resurrection, and the bardo or underworlds beyond. This process is rooted in ourselves. This we hope to understand, even from its ancient beginnings.

To that end the first chapter opens in our shared, primordial past. Here the life-force, humanity, and consciousness are first seen to *consciously* interpenetrate. In many ways it is her story painted on the canvas of shared mind. Here we will locate in the body-mind and nervous system the very root of this living luminosity and evolutionary force. We will trace it from its roots in the human embryo as it interacts with light and suggest its connection with the dynamics of neuromelanin and the central nervous system's unfoldment in embryogenesis. Just as we must study the "cold dark matter" of the stellar abyss that seems to account for much of the energy of the external universe, we must study the warm dark matter of our own inner universe. The inner world reflects the outer world, both scientifically and metaphorically. Chapter 2 focuses on the different threads of human development, particularly cognitive, affective, and noetic development, the roots of human transcendence. This will be a triple assent, intricate and long. Please forgive shortsightedness here wherever you find it.

Chapter 3 peers into the intimate, subjective world of the modern borderline personality. It includes both clinical and contemporary aspects much of which we can easily locate within ourselves. Chapter 4 dwells on that modern character of bureaucracies and rituals, the obsessive-compulsive personality. Here we see intellect, creativity, and the will to novelty frozen in the world of fear and tension. Chapter 5 presents the offshoot of fear, devastation, and the failure of higher insight. Unfortunately, this paranoid style takes hold in the world of social and political violence more each day.

Chapter 6 introduces that exotic, panicked creature of the shattered self, the multiple personality. Here also are embedded glimpses of our greater nature and involvement with planes of consciousness rarely seen by the normative mind. Each in his/her own way must come to real terms with the paradoxically empty and transcendental nature of the current of living energy we call the life-force. The chapter on embodiment or the psychosomatic journey is one we all share. The subtle effects of the mind on the body at innumerable levels reflect the stabilization of consciousness in living matter and afford the most intimate laboratory of all for the human experiment in the cosmos. Chapter 8, on the psychospiritual dynamics of forgiveness, opens this web of interconnecting consciousness such that we transform our deepest motivations through its trials and expanses. The family unconscious system of shared reflections is profoundly implicated in all of this.

Each personality style or syndrome will be presented and explored as a localization or even condensation of consciousness and energy in confluence with the evolutionary principle of the life-force. As a matter of organization, each chapter will present the contemporary formulation of each personality style, then highlight its limitations, and finally, hopefully, extend where appropriate to a wider model. The ego arises here as only one in the latest processes of stabilization in the mentalized or psychological dimension of the human adventure in consciousness. This drama of the stabilization of increasingly more complex and subtle processes is again a reflection of teleos, or the evolutionary impulse, seeking wider and wider expression in and through our species. When the ego itself becomes the ossifying principle or level of development, then crisis occurs. At present each personality style presented engages in this awesome and exquisitely intimate struggle.

Each personality style can be seen as *both* an opening to what is "below" it and the classical unconscious "regression dynamics" that are associated with it, *and* an opening to what is "above" it, including the transpersonal dynamics implicated in it. Psychoanalysis and psychodynamic perspective, emerging largely from Freud and the genius of the Jewish intellectual tradition, have brought the lower, subterranean consciousness into the waking state. Freud had available to him as a working intellectual practice not only the exegetical methodology of the Torah and Talmudic studies, which seek out *the hidden levels of meaning,* the *original intention* of passages and provide *extensive commentary* on them, but he also *drew* from other currents of Jewish mysticism (Bakan, 1958). These currents influenced the psychoanalytic method of dream interpretation, play on words, and the free association technique. Freud was aware of some of this lineage and even older Kemetic Egyptian influences and had the courage to say so despite the prejudices of his scientifically Eurocentric age (Freud, 1939). We see Freud as a great liberator, and psychoanalysis as a kind of "special theory of relativity" in need of a "general theory" that opens to both the unconscious and the transconscious. We seek only to bring the higher and paradoxically ancient lineage into the waking state. This "higher" is not confined to only "Eastern" traditions, but to practices and methods of peoples of diverse cultures and traditions, all of whom are inextricably linked by shared roots to the ancient one, She-who-has-no-name. This will be especially true of the ancient Kemetic Egyptian lineages established perhaps around 6,000 B.C.E. (Diop, 1974) in which we have our first clear references to this biogenetic and psychospiritual life-force, that is later to see its full technical elaboration by their close cousins, the mysterious dark Dravidians of southern India. Hopefully, in some small way, we can help exchange the psychology of mechanisms and matter for process and light.

Finally, because we are scientists and require replications, observation and "maps" of the area, we present the actual methods of observation out of which the whole arch of personality syndrome development arises. It is to be put to the test by actual experiment and practice in order to move from faith in the arguments and statements to realization of their ground nature. This perspective is a transpersonal one and as such draws heavily from previous experiment and observation of this radiant current in its play in the human condition. It goes well beyond the normative boundaries of "modern psychodynamic" interpretation, and yet does not present itself as a fully transformative discipline. That is left to other systems. What it does is point, invite a trial test, and ask for a decision in the laboratory of your own experience.

When this is done, even if only sporadically practiced, any reader over time will come to directly experience an aspect of that radiant, intelligent, transcendental force first intuited by that ancient one on the shores of some vanished lake, moonlit and distant, untold millenniums ago.

REFERENCES

Bakan, D. *Sigmund Freud and the Jewish Mystical Tradition*, Van Nostrand, Princeton, NJ, 1958.

Bernal, M. *Black Athena: The Afroasiatic Roots of Classical Civilization. Vol. 1. The Fabrication of Ancient Greece 1785-1985*. Rutgers University Press, New Brunswick, NJ, 1987.

Diop, A.C. *The African Origin of Civilization* (trans. by M. Cook), Lawrence Hill and Co., Westport, CT (1955), 1974.

Freud, S. *Moses and Monotheism*, Vintage Books, New York (1939), 1967.

Hedges, S.B., Kumar, S. and Tamura, K. "Human Origins and Analysis of Mitochondrial DNA Sequences," *Science*, Vol. 255, February 1991, 737-739.

Hutchison, J.A. *Paths of Faith*, McGraw-Hill, New York, 1969.

James, G.G.M. *Stolen Legacy*, United Brothers Communications Systems, Newport News, VA (1954), 1989.

Jaynes, J. *The Origin of Consciousness in the Breakdown of the Bicameral Mind*, Houghton Mifflin, Boston, 1976.

Minkowski, H., In A. Einstein et al. *The Principle of Relativity*, Dover, New York, 1923.

Suzuki, D. T., Preface to B. L. Suzuki. *Mahayana Buddhism*, Allen and Unwin, London, 1959.

Templeton, A.R. "Human Origins and Analysis of Mitochondrial DNA Sequences," *Science*, Vol. 255, February 1991, 737.

Vigilant, L., Stoneking, M., Harpending, H., Hawkes, K., Wilson, A.C. "African Populations and the Evolution of Human Mitochondrial DNA," *Science*, Vol. 253, September 1991, 1503-1507.

SECTION I.
GENESIS, INTELLIGENCE, AND LIGHT

The eternal primordial matter, without beginning or end, is engaged in an evolution, a perpetual becoming, thanks to its intrinsic property which is the law of transformation, elevated to the level of a divinity. Matter, together with the evolutionary movement that always pushes it to change its form, to evolve, are both eternal principles.

–Cheikh Anta Diop
Civilization or Barbarism:
An Authentic Anthropology

Chapter 1

The Ageless Journey

THE ROOTS OF LUMINOSITY IN SCIENCE AND RELIGION

> . . . mankind is slowly evolving towards a sublime state of consciousness of which fleeting glimpses have been afforded to us by all great seers and mystics of the past and present. There is no doubt that some of the leading intellectuals of this era accept the existence of an evolutionary impulse in the race, but the ultimate goal and the modus operandi of the impulse, according to them, are still shrouded in mystery.
>
> –G. Krishna
> *The Biological Basis of Religion and Genius*

From Ancient Savanna to the First Temples

She stretched her eyes over endless savannas looking for her tribefolk, family, and home. Her senses took root in the world of soil, danger, and survival. Beyond the faint smells in the air, the play of wind and sand between the grasses, she learned to decipher the meaning in footprints left weeks ago. Between the dung and early flowers her small dark frame reflected itself in ancient ponds and lakes where quick deer and animals watered themselves for a million years before her arrival. Her survival was inextricably linked to sensing how all she saw was organic, connected, on knowing the right move at the right time that would ransom her life. Perhaps it was only a fleeting thought bursting up from a sea of instinct and dim intuition that occasionally spoke to her that all of this drama, both her waking and dreaming, issued from a great but common living source. To her, everything moved and was alive.

Direct perception, not intellect, unreeled a current of living energy pervading all things; herself, her clan, the air, the trees, the changling earth she walked upon. The water she drank was the clear blood of the world. These many things were part of some living One, an awesome and dark power that cajoled, illuminated, nurtured, and punished all that she saw, heard and felt. In her primordial sense, she saw life immanent in all things; intuitively, her reflection transcended even that. This she knew, She-who-has-no-name. Into each morning she rose and arched like an angel, groaned like an ape.

She, and every life, had a carbon base and form. Evolution had worked the pulse up and through her line for perhaps 14 million years since the beginning of crude Ramapithecus in the middle of the Miocene age, the "age of the ape." She and her kind had unfolded along the instinctual way like the other primates in the vast inhabited African continent shaped like a skull. Along her spine and into the brain could be traced the lineage of the reptile, then the mammalian and then the superimposed but wider neocortex or modern brain (MacLean, 1970). Part of her legacy was ingrained in the grey and black neuromelanin nerve tract that captured sunlight and perhaps held the primal memories of the old ways. In a subtle way it was a luminous tract using neuromelanin to point itself from the coccyx to the crown.

She was everyone's mother in the blood cells, DNA and human chains that crisscrossed the sub-Sahara with the herds and beasts and tribes perhaps 200,000 years and 10,000 generations ago (Lemonick, 1987; Schmeck, 1986; Wright and Tierney, 1988). She is implicated in each of us today, and by extension, each of us is implicated in each other. There are no known human bones found outside of Africa over 500,000 years old. Before her even then were 3 or so million years of proto-human beings wandering the mother continent before the great migration to everywhere except Antarctica. All roots of all her kind are collective and ultimately African (Ardrey, 1967). This is true both psychologically and genetically. In other words, the vast human collective unconscious at its root is really the African unconscious and we all partake in its process daily despite different cultural, linguistic, and localized coloring. This is the recent treasure of "Lucy" unearthed in the rocky lower beds of Olduvai Gorge near the great lake.

Even the ancients were aware of this! Dynastic Egypt spelled out in scrolls in the "Houses of Life" and painted on walls the legends of their upper Nile birth. The upper Nile is of course Nubia, its many pyramids and later Meroe. The papyrus of Hunefer traces this lore to the foothills of the Nile around Mount Kilimanjaro and the Rwenzori mountains. Their oldest God of all was "Bes," a tiny dark pygmy or diminutive Africoid Twa person. There is this in our collective memory, this, and so much more. In the carbon base of evolution and life there is a darkness and mystery that is partially hidden, yet full of light. It reaches into the generative order of things.

In years of wandering and settling and then wandering again, she and her offspring saw the patterns and cycles of the seasons. From duration and repetition came time and memory. Her family and clan gathered seeds and then grew them. Eventually wild capricious nature showed habit and prediction. Control, even in this small way, over the world of nature and matter, subtly drew out of her a sense of world pattern and a growing control of inner nature. They cross-fertilized; they reflected each other. In time the cycles of nature were seen in herself. Then came to consciousness ideas of the life-force, a fear/worship of greater powers in life, then the burial of the dead, their renewed seed and, in the area where cultivation of crops arose came finally, perhaps, reincarnation. The notion of reincarnation seems to have invaginated into every religion. Who knows? Perhaps the notion of life unfolding from the seed gave rise to the intuition of vaster life and consciousness enfolding us all. In any event, it was obvious that all the drama, the inner and the outer, was a vast, interconnected living organism and force. Her monthly blood cycle and the moon were on the same course. She was the object and origin of early religion. Moment to moment, like all the other animals in unison, her breathing sounds, her inhalation and exhalation, repeated the soft murmur "ham sa, ham sa." In time, this became the sacred words AHUM, AMEN, AMENTA and AUM.

In this wildly pre-rational, pre-personal collage of fear, hope, and survival, the great majority of her tribe would live and grow. The powers and forces of the unseen world were obvious and everywhere present. The trees and great beasts, even the winds were slowly personified, a reflection of her own still developing inner state. The world, tribe, dreams and medicine were a boundless unity, an undivided whole. All healing ceremonies were accompanied by rhythm, pattern, and music. There was a wild card to play each day in the gamble for water or the trip far away from the group of others. When something went awry, she looked for "who" was the matter, not "what" caused it. Behind and through this river of images and events was the immanent and luminous current of life in the spine. It all seemed to breathe a natural balance, harmony, and order. In her would breed the first approximation of what later progeny would call Maat, or Tao, or the Way.

This balance, or cooperation and harmony, was a central aspect of her tribal/clan life. She survived through cooperation. It was extremely functional. Mimicked and innate sounds were recognized by those who lived together. Certain sounds in the forest meant death or life-giving water. Sound and smell were on an even keel with vision. The power of vocal sound, however, enriched communication and spun a web of local community. This power of sound became the power of the word, of rhythm and vibration. Eventually the generative power of the word, the amma and the nommo (Jahn, 1961) were established. It was a cornerstone of early civilization that spread through all other groups. This will to higher and more inclusive order and harmony, this movement toward finer and more abstract rhythms in action and cognition, is repeated in the deepest life-course of all her descendants. It is another face of evolution.

As the ages accumulated and her many tribes and branches sprawled and multiplied all over the planet, each one developed myths, collective dreams, and other ways of living in the world. Certain times the tribes came together, cross-fertilized, then split apart. Development was constantly unpredictable, uneven. Groups bifurcated at crucial moments leading to death, or more growth, and much greater organization.

Long before the arrival of She-who-has-no-name, perhaps by the morning of the Pleistocene age, some two million or so years ago, there had arisen in east central and south Africa at least two large branches of *Australopithecus*, the family of Hominidae, the early family of her kind. One, the larger of frame, *Australopithecus boisei*, surprisingly burned out. The more supple one, *Australopithecus Africanus*, survived.

By the afternoon of the Pleistocene, several branches of *Homo erectus*, her direct lineage, wandered the planet. Her remains are found in China, in Europe, in Java, and of course, in Africa. Cataclysms and migrations threw the world into flux, stimulated the instinct and memory of survival. Feedback nourished culture. A stressful environment, both inner and outer, created novel situations that were far from equilibrium stimulating the creative on all levels. Still deeper similarities remained. Every culture known to her progeny humankind before and after her in some way, in some fashion, rediscovered and kept alive the sense of energy pervading the world of the senses, the world of objects, the world of the forms.

Even in our own age, a child's early intuition is that everything is alive. The seer and poet have not forgotten this. Her kind had discovered the elemental smoke and fire and then noticed that same fire seemed to come out of the mouth of humans on a cold day. Something rhythmic and life-giving was rooted in the breath. That intuition of the inner fire was soon frozen in primitive paleological thought. The wandering tribes noticed that certain animals–the birds–could fly through the air freely, uncontrolled. Some of her descendants also discovered that in some strange way when they slept at night they too could fly in a different kind of air and land, a land as real and powerful as when they woke and walked about. They etched their discoveries on cave walls, carvings, small repetitive movements and behaviors that later became the outward rituals that eventually matured into psychocultural religions. These gave some measure of control over the worlds.

She used tools and her descendants multiplied them. Death became more personal, grew alongside an uncommon capacity to recognize order. Yes death, the body's sleep of final silence and decay. Different and distant relatives had other solutions to this emergent problem of death and loss. Some buried tools with their sleep-crouched relations, added food, flowers, and potions. Our burial of the dead is a universal and unmistakable sign of death-awareness and the concomitant sense of self-awareness in the universe. Even the crude Neanderthal, who had no roots in Africa, buried its dead. It is the dawn of finitude, self, and the intuition of infinity. This quantum leap in evolution and the transcendental impulse of her kind began about 1,700,000 to 200,000 years ago (see Chart 1.1).

These old ones carried these even more ancient voices within

CHART 1.1. Paleolithic Age.

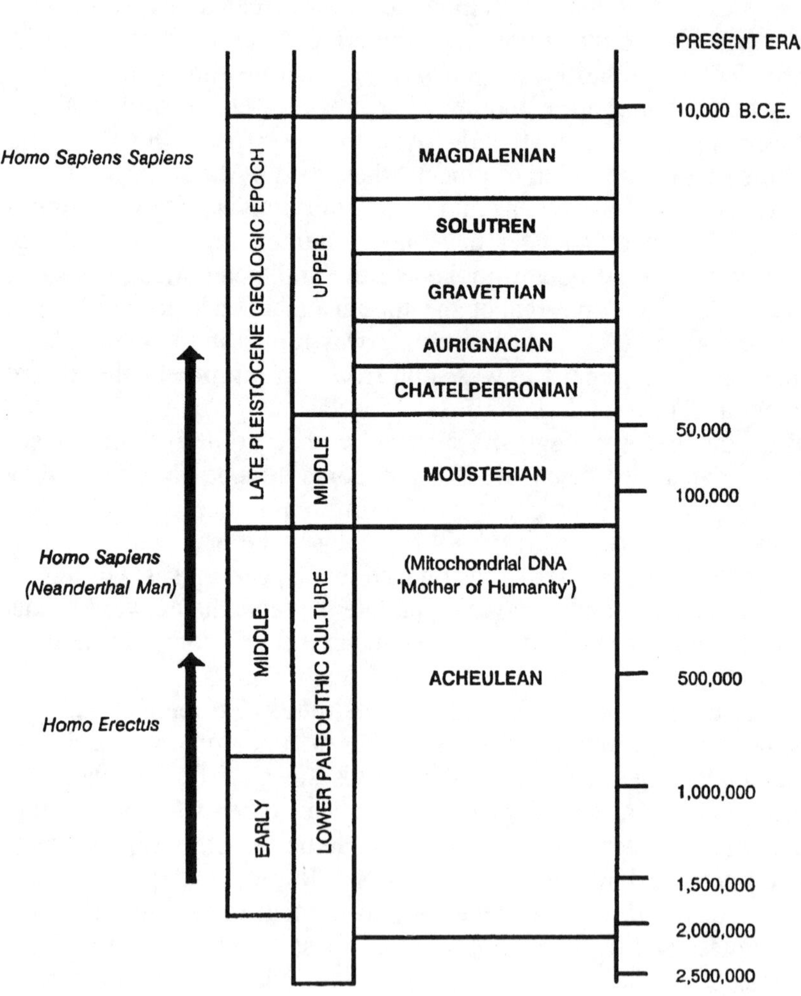

themselves afterward for years, sometimes for generations. No doubt in times of stress and massive upheaval, the voices came up from silence to warn, help, and guide the tribes of humans. Each family had voices, each tribe had its leaders. Time and death had a different status, and thus so did memory, with its power, reach, and influence (Jaynes, 1976).

Some of her descendants ate the dead, dreamed of sucking the life-force out of their brains and bones gathering magical and sacramental powers for use as their own. This was not only in the larger bone deposit areas and caves at Choukoutien, but all over the globe in smaller places where the new *Homo erectus* gathered, hunted, and arched toward sustained thought. Our early mother of the lakes, caves, and flowers searched the skies for earthly clues. She felt only the vaguest intuition that the force that held her down to earth was the same one that locked the tiny fires in the sky together and held tight the vast worlds in the stellar abyss.

All these different forms, animals, and events were threaded by her primitive sense of a universal personality, of a seamless, pervasive, and absolute force and life-energy suffusing all things. This feeling and intuition or Personalism is our common inheritance regardless of where later on the planet our more local tribe and coloring called home. In the diversification of tribal customs and the explosive effect of language and symbols that began perhaps 50,000 years ago, different orders of knowledge in her kind arose. With a finer expansion in language and observations, and its even greater development in symbol and integrative thinking, eventually matured organized magic. This later became the basis of systematized religion, seeking to order and navigate the seen and unseen currents of the world. This development later became science, which inexorably brings us back to that Oneness in all this diversity. Underlying all the multiplicities of expression in these ancient cultures about a universal energy is the sense of an expansive, intelligent living force. This is the testament and legacy of innumerable temples and doctrines scattered over the stretches of earth her kind has touched.

Before we go much further, let us quickly recap her lineage prior to her arrival and follow her footsteps briefly after her age had passed. This will help place her in perspective before the rise of her progeny's pyramids, temples and luminous dreams. As stated earlier her kind's first descendants arose in the Miocene age, the "age of the apes," that dawned some 25 million years ago. Many species shared the earth at the same time. *Ramapithecus*, the first great ground dwelling ape to wander deeper into the open savannas, arose perhaps 14 million years ago. His remains have been found not only in Olduvai Gorge in Tanzania, but also in Asia and Europe.

The chimpanzee-hominid divergence began perhaps 4 to 7 million years ago and this intermediate phase saw the rise of the "proto-hominid" phase. The *Australopithecus* genus then emerged around 4 million years ago. The most famous of this line is "Lucy," unearthed by Donald Johanson in the Hadar region of Ethiopia in 1974 (Johanson and Edey, 1981). Lucy lived some 3 1/2 million years ago. Mary Leakey, the wife and lifelong colleague of Louis B. Leakey, unearthed another in the genus *Australopithecus afarensis* at Laetoli in Kenya. This genus is considered to be ancestral to *all* later hominids, including other *Australopithecine* species and Homo genus, including modern humans (Leakey and Lewin, 1979). This is really the dawn of humanity. This family member was a considerable improvement over those before her. She was a more efficient bi-pedal walker; lived in hunting and gathering societies, which by the way reflected an essentially cooperative spirit and was reinforced by evolutionary forces; and was perhaps 3 1/2 to 5 feet tall. It is also significant that she had less and less body hair than her progenitors which lead to both more sweat glands for better heat loss and an increase in skin melanin in order to protect her from the sun's ultraviolet radiation. This means her skin was dark as an adaptation and harmonious reaction to her environment. This she passed on to her own progeny.

About 2 million years ago a new hominid genus arose in east Africa, *Homo habilis*, also unearthed by Louis and Mary Leakey. She had a larger brain case then her earlier cousin *Australopithicus*, 750-800 cc versus 600 cc. She was also the first to make and use stone tools. This fact was later confirmed by their son Richard E. Leakey with the now famous skull #1460 found in the Omo region of northern Kenya in 1972. *Homo habilis* fossils, like those of *Australopithicus*, are so far confined to the continent of Africa. She was not only a toolmaker and author of the first real human culture, but her warm dark hands may have been the first to use fire!

Also the bones of another toolmaking Homo are known that are perhaps 2.4 million years old who may have been neither *Homo habilis* or *Homo erectus*. She arose when the world's climate changed and made the earth drier and colder by 5-10 degrees Celsius, leading to a massive change in vegetation growth and possibly a change in species behavior and the "death" of *Australopithicus*.

Homo habilis continued to evolve, adapting to the changing environment until a new species of Homo arose around 1.75 million years ago called *Homo erectus*. Her brain case was approximately 800-1200 cc, which overlaps with our own of 1200-2000 cc. She was some 4 1/2-5 feet tall, an excellent toolmaker, melanin rich in skin tone, and apparently migrated at times to Europe and Asia even though the vast majority of her kind remained in Africa. Somewhere around a million years ago she was the only hominid group on earth until the appearance of both Neanderthal man and our own genus *Homo sapiens sapiens* some 200-150,000 years ago. *Homo sapiens sapiens* and Neanderthal were on the earth during the same period for about 50,000 years. For unknown reasons Neanderthal died out 40-30,000 years ago. He was an evolutionary dead-in.

The earliest *Homo sapiens sapiens* are found in Africa from 200,000 years ago. None are known outside of Africa over 150,000 years ago. There are presently no known fossil remains of *Homo sapiens sapiens* in Europe before 50,000 years ago. She was quite adept at changing her environment as a function of living in it. *All* humans today are from this family lineage. This is attested to by not only the preponderance of fossil remains, but also morphological, and mitochondrial DNA studies. In all likelihood our own DNA mother arose in Africa and passed on to us her increasing brain size and complexity, tool making genius, dark skin protection and affinity for cooperative group living. She also bequeathed to us in her travels and reflections the seeds of transcendence. From crude but courageous *Ramapithecus* to *Homo sapiens sapiens* the drama of human evolution unfolded itself out in Africa. Perhaps each branch, each new species quickened the spiritual impulse toward light and civilization. After generation upon generation this luminous seed finally took root.

Somewhere between perhaps 17,000 and 10,000 B.C.E. an organized group of her progeny migrated from the upper Nile to the lower Nile in the area that today covers Egypt, Nubia, and the Sudan. This was the first sustained civilization that we have any definite evidence of in which society, religion, and science were integrated and passed on from generation to generation (Diop, 1974). The history (her-story) of this region is replete with references to the cross-fertilization, retreat, advance, and retreat again of the peoples of Egypt, Nubia, Ethiopia (Kush), and Sudan (Fairservis, 1962).

The fulcrum of this culture was a balance between the rule of the pharaohs, their religions and their technology–a technology that eventually raised the first pyramids and established the first writing. It was the time of Imhotep (5345-5307 B.C.E.), the "father" of scientific medicine, master architect and special advisor to King Zoser of Egypt. He knew the pyramids of Giza and the earlier step pyramid with its vast surrounding structures at Saqqara. Indeed, it is not too much to point out that the core of luminaries that much *later* laid the foundation for Greek science and philosophy were students and initiates of the mystery schools of ancient Egypt. It is generally ignored that Plato, Empedocles, Thales, Pythagoras and others studied in the Kemetic African civilizations. Indeed the grand lodge at Luxor was internationally known and recognized as the largest and greatest library in the ancient world. It housed not only texts on mathematics, medicine, and engineering, but also the writings and practices in their religion and science of the life-force. That science made an intimate connection between knowledge, light, and the deeper recesses of the mind and brain core, our common inheritance.

There is considerable evidence to suggest that these ancients were aware of a connection between light, the pineal gland, and the subtle rhythms or wavefronts of the brain. In other words, biological psychiatry seems to have arisen back then (King, 1990). Here we see the earliest true "science" focusing on mind, matter, and light.

Whatever the relationship may have been there is certainly ample evidence to suggest that the ancient Egyptians and Nubians knew of the life-current and its course through the body and brain. Somewhere between 6000 and 3000 B.C.E. a more sophisticated conception and awareness of the current became widespread in these cultures and "peoples of the sun." This may have been due to a yet unclear relationship between melanin in the brain and spinal cord, sunlight, and the availability of long periods of stability in the open, climatically hospitable land. Clearly the early sciences of medicine, material technology, and high religion were integrated into a functional and vibrant world view in this earliest of true human civilizations (Diop, 1991, 1985; Pappademos, 1985; Lumpkin, 1985). By 5000 B.C.E. the progeny of She-who-has-no-name had consciously awakened the light of the mind by the knowledge of light and energy in the world.

On the later routes between Egypt, East Africa, and the Indian subcontinent the mystery schools were active in the laboratory of the mind's inner states. The luminous current in the spine had been discovered by accident, luck, or sacred herbs and translated into the Earth Mother fertility religions. Practices of many kinds flourished to investigate its subtle but observable workings in the very body they inhabited. The ancient world is replete with paintings, records, and excavation sites of temples to these forgotten sanctuaries of the first human glimpse into the inner light (Mookerjee, 1982). Egypt's upper Nile people and their genetic cousins, the dark Dravidians of southern India, are the ones who first called this mother and serpent of powers Kundalini. This was known and practiced at least 2000 years before the Aryan invasions of northern India. The later Eastern or Oriental systems of Tantra were based on the earlier Draconian or Typhonian cults of ancient Egypt and the upper Nile, especially the Ophidian cults (Grant, 1979).

At the very least this intuition of inner radiance and directionality is an archetype of the human mind, rooted in its very operation. When directly perceived it initially feels like a dim seamless adumbration of some vast unutterable nature. The Gold Coast Africans called this force Wang; the Cabalists called it Yesod. Plato called it Nous; the Hebrews called it Rauach. The Asians, in their many different ways, called it Ki or Ch'i. In Yoga it is known as the Prana-Shakti and Kundalini Shakti, the current that is felt as "basic aliveness" and energy in the universe (White and Krippner, 1977). Children naturally see it but soon join the conspiracy and forget. Others stumble upon or recognize it again and follow it back to its source in the Absolute.

Some of her progeny, like the !Kung people of southern Africa, continue to this day to use the energy to heal their community and themselves, perhaps employing the same deep rhythmic incantation devices and shared images to operationalize the autonomic nervous system and those other aspects of our nature as we have done from the earliest of dawns (Katz, 1982). These practices touch upon pathways of energy and structures in the human body that are still shrouded in mystery to contemporary, orthodox medicine and science. As one indigenous healer put it, "In your backbone you feel a pointed something, and it works its way up. Then the base of your spine is tingling, tingling, tingling, tingling . . . and then it makes your thoughts nothing in your head."

Some of these so called "primitive" peoples evolved elaborate symbol written languages, possessed an extricate and extensive physiological and anatomical knowledge, and were able to chart the course of distant stars that only recently became known to Western telescopes and computers. I am referring to the invisible white dwarf and dwarf nova companions of Sirius known to the Dogon people of West Africa for a thousand years (Griaule and Dieterlen, 1986). These people trace their origin to the Nile valley before they left and expanded westward. Their knowledge of Sirius was held to be intimately interconnected with their knowledge of their own bodies! In fact, many of the ancient "technologies" that direct and navigate these subtle bodily energies are at the foundation of many nearly forgotten African practices, practices severely repressed by Christian and Islamic religions for political, theological, and yes, epistemological reasons.

It is clear that the ancients and others were well aware of this subtle anatomy of humanity and its enormous potential to innervate the body-mind with a luminous, living, and intelligent energy (Avalon, 1974). Not all, however, used this radiant, life-sustaining current to the full potential and instead focused on its by-products in fallen forms of pseudo-science and witchcraft. Some of this continues today despite the fact that this potential source is embedded in a healing/medical system that is partly modern and practiced in the treatment of medical and psychological problems (Edgerton, 1971).

Its most common and intensified expression is in the form of a current or serpent curling along inside the hollow of the spine. No doubt that ancient one sensed this luminous current, this implicit and still unfolded somatopsychic route around her spine and projected its inner expression outward into the environment in the form of the snake. It should be noted here that early on in the human embryo fetal cells form a long tube. This neural crest later becomes the brain. Those living cells along its full length evolve into the light interacting melanocytes and the roll of endocrine glands, i.e., pineal, pituitary, thyroid, and all the rest. It is the inner trajectory of the embryo and evolution, of light and fire and intelligence as we know it. It is a most basic process, representing in itself the forms of life-force, power, and intuition/wisdom. Her progeny in diverse ways expressed this development and symbolism, from Haitian voodoo to Tibetan forms, from the modern medical caduceus to the Nagas of the Buddhists, to even the Avatar of Judea and his eternal gospel "therefore be ye wise as serpents and harmless as doves."

The medical caduceus may actually be an external reference or symbol of this common internal pathway of light and energy. We can only suggest the process that unfolds when this criss-crossing pattern is opened or flooded with the life-current, the life-current that first manifests itself in the endocrine and melanocyte places along the embryonic spine. This symbol associated with medicine first arose in Egypt, then later in Greece, and finally Rome.

The criss-crossing lines intersect at critical places–places referred to as chakras in Yogic terminology. They reflect the *movement* of this energy in the body of most people. Psychologists refer to this form of bodily experience as "organismic perception." It is not too far a conjecture to say that the Egyptian "Life" sign, or ankh, with its full loop at the top may represent the full awakening of this energy in the body-mind! The energy has fully flooded the head or brain and made single the formerly double-helix lines of the caduceus. One has only to note the "current" felt in the brief awakening of this energy as it circulates through the somatosensory areas of the brain and its reverberation on the walls of the lateral and third ventricles of the brain (Sannella, 1987). Much of this may seem new or overly technical speculation, but most of it was known in the Nile valley 2,000 years before the birth of Christ (see Chart 1.2). These traditions must be verified ultimately by experiments in our body/minds! My own experience here has witnessed three lev-

CHART 1.2. Ancient Symbols of the Dormant Awakened and Fulfilled Life Current.

Awakened

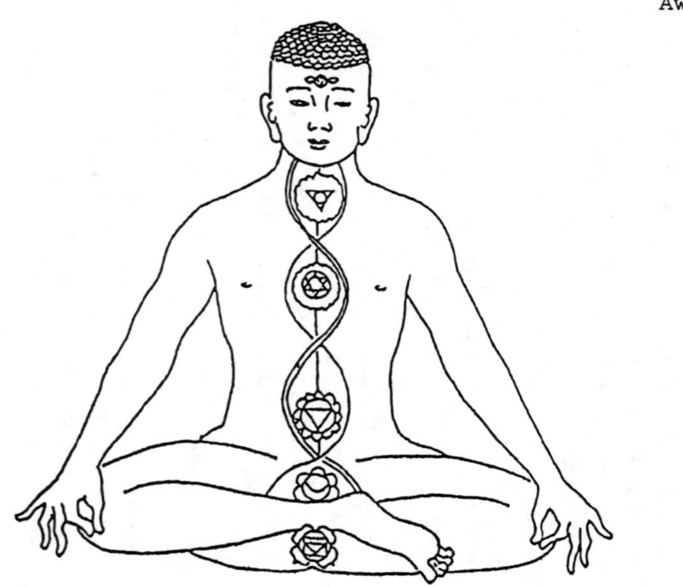

The Yogic seven chakras each associated with a plexus and a level of consciousness. This is the symbol of the awakened current moving to the brain.

The flow of the Life current awakened and fulfilled in the braincore.

The Mysterious Serpent

Dormant

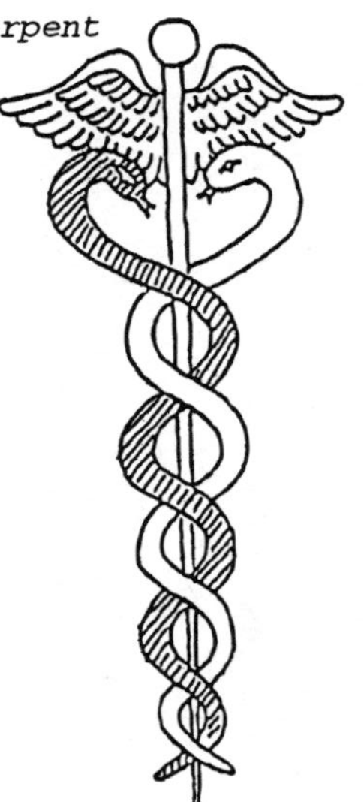

The Medical caduceus and its seven centers each associated with a specific homonal and endocrine function. The current in its dormant state.

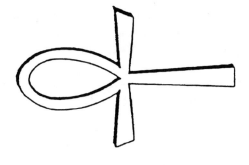

The Egyptian Ankyh or symbol of Life and the life current in its potential state.

els to this life-current. The first is the basic life-energy and is associated with the classical libido. The second and deeper is associated with a blissful and sometimes extremely intense movement along the spinal line and into the brain. The third level is perhaps the deepest, in my experience, and is associated with a luminous movement from the right side of the heart, up through the throat to the brain and back down again. The methodology chapter will probe this more deeply.

We will return to this specific process in our later chapters on psychosomatic process and methodology. For now we only mention it in the context of embryology and energy to lay a foundation for what is to come. In many ways the early embryonic pathway of evolution, intelligence and, yes, light, is the template for the second evolution of the body-mind, the full awakening of this luminous current of living energy.

The ancient one's progeny developed elaborate sects and culture bound "mystery schools" for this secret knowledge acquired over time and expansion. As we stated before, these early ideas of the later Yogas are seen in the description of ancient Egyptian rites and methods of the upper Nile practiced at least 4,000 years before even the Arab jihads swept out of Arabia swallowing northern Africa (Asante, 1984). References to the higher refinement of the primeval contact and formulation of this energy and its mysteries can be found today in the *Coming Forth by Day and the Going Forth by Night*, also known as the *Egyptian Book of the Dead*. Trade routes by land and sea connected the east coast of Africa with southern India such that the ideas of union, of yoga and the life-current, were open to experimentation in religion, health, cosmology, and medicine (Thakkur, 1977).

Our ancient mother could sense this energy immanent and immediate in her state of being fused with nature. Attention and reflection were not sustained enough yet to transcend this world of energy and forces by recognizing it's source in that nameless condition of unconditioned free consciousness. In the modern-day West this energy is called bioplasma. Indeed, it seems that those early religions, those early sciences of experience, were the first systematic attempts by the human mind to harness this all-pervasive energy and the intuition of a radiant unity or life-force prior to and innervating all experience. Certainly as "primitives" our perception was different. Perhaps as we have differentiated and grown deeply into civilization we have lost contact with some of our more basic senses that may spill over occasionally in the esp or psi episode, in the dream, or in the uncanny experience. Eventually it finds its way into the finer sciences of the mind and mysticism.

So much has been done before us! In the childhood of our race it took thousands and thousands of dawns, literally millions of hours of experimentation, yet all our different tribes of humanity became aware of and attempted to yoke this tangible sense of universal energy. In the external world, yoking, harnessing and understanding this energy grew into our materialistic science. Yet was not technology there at the birth of religion? The increasing knowledge of the external world reflected the increasing knowledge of the inner world. In the inner world this subtle energy became systematized in various sciences especially acupuncture and certain schools of profound inner and outer transformation, through the methodologies of meditation. For the first time in a very long period of our collective history we are beginning to go beyond our adolescent separation of inner and outer experience, of race and region, and to reemerge in a more highly differentiated unity that brings inner and outer together in one "undivided whole" movement.

The innumerable sciences and religions of the day are now meeting in a common world, a common "global village." Now that some degree of communication between the highest developed sciences and some of the perennial truths of oneness behind multiplicity in the earth's religions are getting a chance to communicate with each other, a profound and soothing realization is emerging. The realization is that through all the intricate displays, paths, and different ways that science and religion have worked out their methodologies, they are both seeking the source of that absolute, that One behind the multiplicities that we experienced when intelligent thought first made its appearance in our minds.

It is a perennial urge embedded in the nervework of our kind. In each age, each religion had a different perspective and a different meaning of the One. These manifold perceptions of the One and the problem of the One and the Many have been analyzed from Asian perspectives with enumerable subtleties (Chan et al., 1969). There are historical and Western perspectives and cross-currents (Hutchison, 1969; Schuon, 1984). However, the intuition of radiant Oneness is the substratum of them all. This is our common inheritance.

The One and the Many

How our ancient mother dealt with the first notions of Oneness and many is an endless story. Nearly all the early gods were female (Stone, 1976). No doubt her reflection in the water that sustained life, her observations of the female in *all* forms being the gateway into this life, all these must have naturally suggested to her and her kind that the life giver was female. Yet that body, that giver of life, could also give birth to many. The Many and the One came naturally together, like the seasons that follow the seasons and the deaths that follow the births. There was no problem in the perception of the One in the Many and the Many in the One. Perhaps the "problem" only arose later when her kind lost that primeval embeddedness in nature in the upward arch toward stable mind and thought.

A deeper look at this notion, however, reveals the One in the Many and the Many in the One to exist, or oscillate, as psychospiritual principles, side by side. The many gods of ancient Hinduism have a formless God at the source. Prior to that development in human thought the family of gods usually had a leading figure who was most powerful of the gods. The pantheons of ancient Egypt, Greece, Meso America, and Africa abound with such references in scattered temples and ruins of nearly forgotten races. Her future progeny would continue to experiment with this primal notion of the One and the Many until they arrived at the manifest Many in the unmanifest One. To this day that notion dominates the spiritual vision of the East. The Western tribes have taken a different route and arrived at the One god without another in Judaism, Christianity, Islam, and many forgotten, unsuccessful others.

Whatever be their expressions of this notion of the One, her progeny have found it to be the wellspring of their deepest intuition, the literal light and background of their most sublime vision. Perhaps in some future fluctuation like those of the past a greater synthesis will emerge. In any event, she saw the first rise of her kind into the boundless light, felt within her sex future radiant beings on the evolutionary step.

At this point in our development it is irrelevant whether some of these religions teach that the highest Oneness is unity with God in some separate "personal" relationship or whether they reach a samadhi or other transcendental state. It does not matter. What we are dealing with on an *empirical* basis is the fact that all the religions do seek in their own way, from their own perspective, that One without another, that absolute and transcendental radiance.[1] It is the sea of light and living feeling in which all matter and creatures are swimming; it is the literal light and ocean of process in which mind and meaning are all moving. Many are those, perhaps only fleetingly, who have realized the fourth state and to this day dwell amongst us to testify and verify that realization. That testimony is that the Absolute is light, that the highest state for a human being is to regain the body of pure life, the material and the unmanifest energy that pervades the whole universe in various forms. By material we mean here not solid material necessarily but the very stuff of existence. Beyond this realm of phenomena, and yet giving rise to this phenomena, is "That," the root source of the real "I." It is the source towards which the "I" sense points, pure consciousness beyond form. It is luminosity, intelligence, and profound peace. It is also our common inheritance.

How Science Embraces the One and the Many

In the last section we saw how intuitions of oneness and "I-ness," even the early and dim intuitions of She-who-has-no-name, were intimately associated with light. In the first section we traced how the earliest known human civilizations, i.e., the Egyptians and Nubians, focused their religion and science on the union of man, mind, and light. It would seem that nearly all human science tacitly accepts the intimacy of mind, matter, and light. Our "modern" science has revealed to us, particularly in the studies of modern physics, that the world is truly intimately interconnected, is One.

1. There are traditionally considered to be four states of human consciousness in most world systems of scientific introspection dating from the earliest of eras. They are the waking state, the dream state, the condition of deep, dreamless sleep, and the transcendental fourth state of Turyia. The fourth state enfolds and is simultaneously conscious of the three other states yet pervades and transcends them in a radically boundless, luminous, and intelligent way.

Through the mirage of particle physics a basic unity or Oneness emerges (Capra, 1976). The coordination of distant systems in the universe, through what is termed quantum interconnectedness and Bell's theorem, shows that in a real sense we are all One and deeply embedded in a supraluminal reality! Bell's theorem, which suggests that distant systems can coordinate and communicate with each other at a "speed" faster than known light speed, is an established fact and as such does not even require quantum theory as its support. The world process is indeed intimately interconnected, intelligent, and non-local. Even so, $E = mc^2$ is common knowledge and shows clearly that this solid matter is condensed energy, that this very object that you look upon right now is a form of localized, even frozen energy and light.

The implication of what most high school students already know, namely that that $E = mc^2$ is really true, has not entirely sunk in yet. To have it street knowledge that all matter, including this physical body of mine and yours, is a form of light, ultimately having no boundaries and *employing* space and time to manifest itself, is a radical notion. In this vast sea of light or free energy of even the known universe, all kinds of unknown and unseen currents, life-forms, and non-local relations of matter, energy and consciousness abound. This implicates generative orders infinitely beyond the presently conceived quantum-relativistic field. Indeed above and below a certain level of our observation, all is radiance! The distant quasars receding from us at 90 percent of the speed of light are registered as pulsating forms of radiation, light, and energy. They stretch our eyes over the seemingly limitless expanding universe. Present day tools reach down to the sub-atomic level of particle interaction where there are no finally distinct, unchanging objects, but rather a pulsating, shifting web of energy relationships, a mirage of movements and "resonances." In this nearly inconceivably subtle and expansive space-time-continuum of energy and radiance, our perception of our unchanging body-mind existence is an abstraction! We are *in, of* and *about* this sea of light. Religion was first to conceptually and experientially elaborate this luminosity. For 500 years in the West it has been eclipsed by science in its search into more locally stable matter. Now science takes up the beacon's light of method to explore this luminosity that is prior to both science and religion.

In present day physics, although there are different ways of approaching this absolute Oneness, just as there are in religions, clearly this intuition of subtle, intelligent life and energy in the universe emerges. In the present day Gauge Symmetry theories of quantum field theory, all the different forces or energetic interactions of the universe are drawn together and held to be balanced, uniform, and permutations of one field or process. There are different so-called coupling strengths of the four fundamental forces or interactions but all of these appear at different levels to enfold back into one. The implications of Bell's theorem, which indicates that the universe is non-local, or in other words, is in intimate contact with itself over immense distances seemingly instantaneously; the possibility of a radical marriage between the subatomically rooted quantum field theory and the galactically embracing theory of relativity, the micro and macro universes; and the quantum interconnectedness of things in the universe, all suggest that a new synthesis is emerging.

Finally, there is the deeply holistic approach of physicist David Bohm (1980). This is the vision of the implicate order and what is termed the holonomic universe. Here the reality of nonlocality and the essential interconnectedness of the universe of matter, energy, and consciousness itself is shown to emerge in a system that is at root a manifestation of the absolute One. Indeed, given these new principles of matter, energy, and nonlocal interactions, the status of matter itself is now transtemporal and transpatial, or in other words, transcendental!

This sense of a unified and interconnected universe, with each part affecting every other part, is also emerging in other areas of science. In the neuro-sciences, there is the very powerful, heuristic approach of the holographic theory of memory and brain function by Karl Pribram (1981). Here, memory is implicated in a total brain process whose functions may reflect the operations of a holographic universe. It is not merely one voice crying out by itself, but has much empirical and theoretical support from other neurologists, experimental psychologists, and other disciplines. In biology there is a reflection of this Oneness in the theories, approaches, and observations of Sheldrake in his thesis of morphogenetic fields. In this theory, the actual form of influence on the structure of intricate biological forms is seen to be interconnected to all other forms of influence of these biological systems across great distances. These distances cross our conventional understanding of space and time; Again the notion of interconnectedness and non-locality arises. Also from biology are the observations of Lydell Watson (1980). Here the phenomenon of watching a generation of monkeys discover something and then having other monkeys at great distances almost simultaneously discover it, indicates, again, a unified order and intelligence in the world of known life forms.

Each example above has been empirically observed and supported. Some have gone even further and identified what appears to be the intelligent force of evolution itself which is latent and sleeps in the biology of each of us (Krishna, 1971). Its awakening and development is the goal of Yoga science and appears to be the fountainhead of genius and profound religious experience. Some of the medical and clinical repercussions of the emergence of this dynamism or psychogenetic force are already being clinically treated in the community (Sannella, 1987). The progeny of the small framed woman who spent so many nights beside the ancient lakes of our history have brought us, in many ways, a deeper insight into her original intuitive gaze.

In the world of clinical psychology, a new vision of wholeness is taking place. Experimentation in the often underfunded and neglected science of Psi is occurring and data is accumulating, especially in the former Soviet Union! What is quite clear is that for all the different experiments, for all the different approaches, a consensus emerges that there is an immanent, transcendental energy that is intelligent, and that in some way we interact with in all our different states of consciousness, waking, dreaming, and deep sleep. We add the exploration of the *Family Unconscious* (Taub-Bynum, 1984) in which many of these observations of biology and interconnection within family systems occurs. In the system of the family, that ancient, perennial, and constantly shifting web of intimate thoughts, information, and relationships, unusual channels of communication are seen. Some is seen in the shared imagery of the dream. Some is even seen in episodes of psi information events. All of these, from the startling findings of the new physics, through the powerful exploration in neurology and biology, over to the living observational science of psychology, and particularly family processes, we see that a sense of interconnectedness pervades all the fields of knowledge. Several recent books written by family members about their family and intimate thought experiences testify to the increasing awareness and acceptance of these phenomena by the general public (Dillion and Dillion, 1984; Schwarz, 1980).

Because of the above and so much more, the paradigm of scientific materialism, in which the world is reduced to innumerable lifeless objects bouncing off of each other in a random way, with its built-in limitations for the human consciousness, is finally dying. Because of pervasive non-local causality in some physical processes, the implicate order enfolding us all, the recognition of new developments is psi, family field theory, supplanted by new developments in neurology and biology, for this and so many more reasons, scientific materialism appears to be in its twilight. It is the end of that implicit doctrine of "epistemological loneliness" in modern science so that our root sense of isolation and inherent alienation from nature is recognized to be a myth. We are the offspring of that root gatherer, that primal singer and harvester by the lake who would have no grasp of our present day dissociation from the alive nature all around us. This change is very powerful, for it bodes well about our changes and our perceptions of not only human development, but the actual *goal* of human development and the various functional aspects of human development which we will explore in the next chapter. We are beginning to see that our present *perception* of being an isolated but logical and scientific ego, an island of awareness in a sea of ignorance and separation from nature and other human beings, is at the bottom of this alienated condition. Indeed, it may be the sense of collective isolation shared by the vast majority of us on this planet that has found expression in our perpetual cultural symbols and memories of "slavery in Babylon" and similar references found in other cultures.

The recognition that science is changing from scientific materialism to some new form of science, yet still remaining science, is a difficult process but a necessary one. Every age sees its science change and this is the way we see ours changing, in the very assumptions of itself. Science as a way of viewing the so-called natural world, in which we the observers are somehow ultimately excluded or abstracted from the process of observation, is seen to be coming to its end. Science can no longer persist in this way, otherwise it becomes a dehumanizing experience perpetually reducing the human to bits and pieces and ignoring the radiant transcendental energy that we have intuitively known from the dawn of our intelligent experience. Either science adapts in its particular way to recognizing that or science may become a trivial tool appropriate only for the external world. The observer can no longer be extracted from the process but, indeed, may actually be the substratum of it. Much as the protohuman mothers of our ancient mother had to discover that the animals of the day world gave rise to the animals of the dream, we must *reverse* and *elevate* this insight so that we may see how the outer world correlates with and reflects the deepest structures of our inner world. Then we can go further.

THE RISE OF THE NOETIC

This search, this seeking in various ways for the Absolute, appears to be rooted in our very biology and Being as much as in our need for survival, sex, food, the experience of love, and the inevitable mix of them all with fear and power in the family matrix. In any combination of these, in any matrix of the influences of these dynamisms, the search for the Absolute matures. Rooted in our biology, the urge toward the Absolute is not culturally determined, for it appears in every culture, in every time, in every age. It is more akin to the "generative grammar" that is rooted in both our surface and deep structure experience of mind itself.

Science and religion often serve different passions, but both have a common root. While contemporary science, as an endeavor, proclaims no ultimate values, its followers have always been imbued with the search for the Absolute hidden in diversity and law. Newton sought to write the speech of God in his great universal laws of celestial gravitation. Earlier, Galileo had also proclaimed mathematics to be the speech of God. Descartes' dualism implied the existence of supra-rational intelligence and force, for while the world was taken to be independent of the human observer, its very objectivity was based on it constantly being witnessed by God!

Both Pascal and Leibnitz, the discoverer of the calculus, stated the same impetus as these others in their deepest motivations for science. The fabled twentieth century's Einstein, Heisenberg, Schroedinger, Bohr, Bohm, and Oppenheimer had no conflict with reputedly "mystical" world views and may even have entered that realm from time to time in the pursuit of science. And this is to name only the mathematicians and physicists! Much earlier, of course, when there was no real perceived split between these two arms of knowledge, Pythagoras of Greece and the Egyptian mystery schools sought the lost variants of life in a theology of divine numbers and their relationships, thereby continuing and extending the Western scientific branch of mathematics (Jaynes, 1976). Finally the great physicist Maupertuis saw God in the pure abstractions of the great laws of nature which human reason could discern behind natural phenomena. In all other areas in the world that which passed for science and religion always enjoyed a better marriage.

Perhaps to differentiate from religion was necessary at first and so the new international scientific enterprise voted for "no values," etc. It is a renaissance value that needs refocusing today. The roots of the scientific movement, however, are nourished by such noetic motivation. The same is true in every field of "creative" science. The deep motivation is to understand the real or ultimate laws of Nature, to grasp the Absolute by reason and method. This is always a mysterious process, this intuition and knowledge of a world still in the process of creation. Dostoevsky said "Man needs the unfathomable and the infinite just as much as he does the small planet which he inhabits." Einstein remarked that "The greatest experience we can have is the experience of the mysterious. It is the source of all true beauty and insight." As such, we must agree with geneticist Dobzhansky (1971) about this deep impetus for knowing the "unfathomable and the infinite" that is the goal of science and nourishes all its independent roots and creators among humankind. Indeed it seems "indisputable that the potentiality to experience such hungers is biologically, genetically, implanted in human nature." It is the ground of our ultimate concerns, a process we bring into this world and begin unfolding shortly after birth.

This intuition of the Absolute and the apparent interconnectedness of all intelligent living forms can be found even in the earliest emotional affective expressions of the infant. Empathy as fellow feeling and unity, even among infants and children, is noted in scientific studies reported even in the mass media (*Newsweek*, March 10, 1984). This is the origin of the spiritual life of children. These new findings challenge our basic psychological assumptions about isolation, psychological theory built upon these notions of isolation, the present day bias toward causal reductionism in science, and therein potentially the *misinterpretation* of what is called primary narcissism. The supposed primacy of gross matter in psychic development, and therein the limits of the development of the ego, are also called into question. It will be pointed out at this juncture that such theories, commonly called psychodynamic theories, are in truth based on the assumptions of atomism and determinism, relics from the temples and age of logical positivism, and erected upon the dying empire of scientific materialism. We will explore more of this in Chapter 2.

Given that this intuition and urge toward the Absolute is the testimony of the mystics of all times, and because it is rooted in all cultural histories being the trajectory of what the child in his earliest "sustained mental experiences" arches up toward, it seems only natural for us to recognize that this is an intimate aspect of human biology, organization, and aspiration. Indeed it is an intuition and urge that is directly in-formed by the life-force itself. Therein, this seeking for the Absolute must be treated accordingly with all other powerful developmental patterns known to science. We are, therefore, in need of new assumptions relative to the unfolding psycho-spiritual trajectory of human beings. The reductionism of contemporary science, be it expressed in physics or psychoanalysis, must be expanded to include teleology and purpose, intelligence and unfoldment. Nestled in all of this are the roots of transcendence.

With the increasing development in unity, not only hierarchically, but also in terms of enfoldment and unfoldment, it appears that consciousness not only arises, but also descends. In other words, consciousness for the human being occurs not only as the human being develops outwardly and upwardly but also as a human being develops inwardly, consciousness also descends from more subtle, inclusive unmanifest and sublime levels. If we accept the undivided wholeness of all life and intelligence, that the world is truly one vast sea of light and energy, then our assumption of exclusive rising up through the evolution of consciousness must be taken as that, as an assumption, and cannot therein exclude the possibility of a consciousness force descending! Freud and his followers saw consciousness rising upward and outward in development. Aurobindo and his followers saw that also, as well as that consciousness descends (Satprem, 1968). The noetic appears to be embedded in our nature and unfolds through development. When the search for the noetic, the Absolute, the transcendental, is thwarted or frustrated, we fall into the central focus of this book, the psychopathology based on the frustration of the human need to experience and transcend what is deeper than verbal language for him because he knew it before the rise of verbal language. Indeed, the human may move beyond all experiences conditioned by physical, mental, and biological states. That is the realization of the radiant, intelligent, and transcendent energy, the source of his own inner and outer experiences, his own self-illuminated Self.

To us it would seem that in addition to the well-known and well-established sources of neurosis, psychosis and psychopathology, that we also should note the human aspiration for the Absolute. In many individuals the development of neurosis and/or psychosis in various forms can be seen as a failure in the process of development. This is a failure to develop into Wholeness and yet a continual longing for that biologically embedded need. We will begin to look at neurotic and psychotic development with this added dimension, a dimension that opens a way out of reductionist dogma and allows purpose, intelligence and teleology to breathe. This is not in any way to invalidate, but rather to expand, the vision of the first great wave of modern psychological insight in the West. Thus, looking at the development of the psyche of the individual is necessary, and this, of necessity, includes the ego.

Notice how a fish can live in the water, experience and dwell there, and never notice, or see, the water. Notice how the hawk flies through the air, knows the air very well, but never sees it. Both fish and hawk exist in their element, see it in the sense of feeling it, but never actually visually see it. They know its effects and their effects upon it and they learn mastery and flight. Where humans live is a world of consciousness primarily, of thought, form, and experiences.

We do not see consciousness, as the bird does not see air, and the fish does not see water, yet we live within its constraints, within our understandings of space and time generated by our experience of mental constructions. We do not see within the mental operation embedded in consciousness the radiant, intelligent, interconnected energy that breathes life and is a substratum of all of these experiences. The great pulse of consciousness and light is a fleeting noetic experience and is obscured or frozen in the modifying conditions of mind and matter. Remember that material objects are actually patterns of trapped light according to modern physics and that mind has somehow been found and develops in matter. It is quite possible that mind, in all its permutations and subtle manifestations, and matter, with all its objects and its matter-energy manifestations, may be both unfolded from a deeper, unmanifest order, and that deeper order may indeed be consciousness itself. Clearly we must learn from sensation and this adventure in matter and energy but we must recognize our inherent press and structure for transcendence and development embedded in our nature. If you do not already feel that this is the case, execute this simple psychological experiment. Simply say whatever comes to your mind in answer to the ancient question, "What Am I?" After each response you will note that the "I" experience is always *separate* from the answer! It is always an "object," be the response a name, or race, or other conventional label. The "I" is never directly observable and yet *all* observations arise in it.

We cannot and will not attempt to restructure all of what is termed psychopathology or psychobehavioral dysfunction in the light of these new assumptions and ancient insights. This is much too large a task. Instead we will look at the "major syndromes," including the process of ego development and other psychological developments, recognizing that at the root of all of these, buried in the blood and nervework of humankind, is the schema for transcendence.

PSYCHOSIS VS. "SPIRITUAL EMERGENCE OF EMERGENCY"

Arising from the assumptions and data advanced earlier concerning the startling findings of the new physics, the emergent latticework of biology and neurology, and also the curious insights derived from working in family systems in regard to the interconnectedness of dreamscapes, psi, and emotional/empathic relations, there comes the need to differentiate here between levels in this vast, alive "undivided wholeness." It must be done because too often in psychopathological states there also arise experiences of transcendent illuminated states of consciousness and vice versa. A great deal of madness that is seen is just that, simply madness. However, a significant percentage of what is seen clinically as a form of illness or pathology appear to be failed attempts at higher and wider integration and transcendence of previously limiting conditions. Therein we must differentiate between "a spiritual emergency" and true psychosis. One of these clearly involves what is called classical ego *regression* to some earlier, partially fused, pre-personal condition, or even in some cases, ego disintegration without concomitant greater ego integration afterwards. This is classical psychosis or madness, and psychodynamic theory is particularly good in understanding this truly regressive process.

From this perspective we can possibly avoid the common error in both theory and clinical technique of reducing the sublime to the infantile and neurotic as Freud often did, and the opposite of elevating the regressive and infantile to the mystical as Jung was inclined occasionally to do. The catatonic is not in nirvana; the schizophrenic is not a shaman or a mystic, and the person falling apart in his/her psychotic hallucinations is not having an epiphany.

In the case of a spiritual emergency, a person may experience some forms of ego regression, but embedded in this experience are always insights into the nature of reality that can be substantiated by other persons. Also in "awakening" experiences that, with our Western materialistic prejudice against altered states of awareness we would call psychological dysfunctions, there are many well-known patterns and styles reminiscent of awakenings in cultures in which the spiritual emergence into a greater, more inclusive reality is accepted by that culture. Thus, in the cases of genuine psychosis there is indeed *regression*–or falling back–to what can be termed a pre-ego state in which there is a lack of real differentiation between the person and the environment, with its associated fears of destruction, hostile dissolution and ego death.

Our primeval mother by the Lake and silent places was largely pre-personal and fused with her world. However, she adjusted to it, knowing nothing else. She was deeply embedded in the earthly consciousness, sensed and knew its moist, vernal rhythms such that the life-force, the current of living energy, was diffused and immanent in all things. She gave birth to the early gods as she did to her human offspring. Yet it was knowledge of objects and forms, of collages and necessity. As yet there only fleetingly arose the intuition of the current itself out of which all the objects, forms, and occasions were arising. It was not yet transcendental, not yet going beyond the mirage of descriptions and thoughts where consciousness is seen everywhere in the universe, in matter and objects, even in the consciousness of conscious beings. She could not yet sustain that intuition beyond objects and forms, however, where consciousness takes on all the attributes of things yet is ultimately transcendent and without attributes. The fall into madness consists in the ego's wild grasping for steady objects and names while all the while searching for the current itself.

In the other state or series of conditions, which we would call mystical or transegoic, the person integrates in a harmonious way this same grasping ego, accepts the levels and the ultimate illusory quality of the ego, and in the expansive process experiences a greater sense of identification with the Absolute and the unmanifest beyond form and name. This expansive, emergent identification far transcends the capacity of the person to translate this into the world of objects, forms, words, and ideas that most of us are limited to and familiar with. A ship or methodology is needed to navigate this current. Hopefully, what will emerge out of this study is a clearer recognition of the strategic influence of meditation in psychotherapy and also working with the body itself as is done in hypnosis and behavioral medicine in order to navigate these luminous waters. These methods loosen the tight, frozen conditions of the body-mind such that the substratum and energy matrix so often alluded to in this journey will be freed to embrace its source and innately transcendent and unconditioned condition.

Sporadically in meditation, one may experience some psychological states of ego regression, oceanic feeling, and the intuition of Oneness. If this process occurs too quickly there arises what is referred to here as a psychospiritual crisis with mixed noetic and clinical aspects (Lukoff, 1985). When experiences of this nature arise and are at odds with an established institution of beliefs such as a church, it is termed a *psychoreligious problem*. When the experience involves conflict with a relationship to a transcendent force or being, it is referred to as a *psychospiritual problem*. Neither is inherently pathological yet goes very deep. Sustained meditation, however, will greatly unfold and guide this biologically and ontologically rooted, unfolding potentiality of the human being. This unfolding potentiality will help and guide the human being to realize the earliest aspiration, which is transcendence of, not dissociation from, the body and the material world, to ultimately transcend even the play of mind and form itself, to go beyond the theater of multiplicity into the absolute radiant Oneness intuited by our ancestors millennia ago. To trace this trajectory we begin with the exploration of our own body-mind and the ego's development in and through this body-mind. The influence of the ego's attempt to control or contract upon experience and therein freeze attention will be pivotal in our exploration. Out of this will gradually come the planes of the mind as they differentiate from their undercurrent and substratum, which is consciousness.

The actual behavioral situations and psychological/psychiatric syndromes we will deal with out of the wealth of possibilities may at first seem arbitrary. It is not. These syndromes and behavioral patterns can be seen as progressive levels of attempts to deal with psychological and noetic anxiety on the surface/void of the Absolute, that Absolute which is void yet paradoxically full of radiant and intelligent life energy! The anxiety within this ripple on the void will be seen to be translated eventually back into that radiant void which is the fate of all anxiety.

Before that, however, let us look again at exactly what the ancient inheritance is in the body-mind that we have to work with.

HER PSYCHIC LEGACY: THE LUMINOUS CURRENT

So what have we in our possession right now that might convey some sense of progression or movement of complexity and intelligence in nature and yet is intimately associated with our own individual development? To answer this question requires some technical exploration but, it is necessary and grounding on our way. The world's cultures are rich with references to "life-force" movement, of a certain evolutionary impetus and trajectory up along the spine. The deep brain core runs down and out the brain-stem down to near the base of the spine. The spinal cord itself is an extension of the original embryonic neural crest. It is a longish white cylinder, oval in cross section. The inner matter is dark grey and the outer surface is white. In the brain itself this is reversed and the outer surface is grey while the inner bulk is white. In the brain itself this is reversed and the outer surface is grey while the inner bulk is white. The brain has 12 presently known areas of high neuromelanin concentration; however melanin is not only found in the brain, spinal system and skin surface. It is also located in the gastrointestinal tract, all the major internal organs of the body, and also the white blood cells.

Modern neuroscientists have shown that this light-interacting melanin is present in the brain of all animals with the degree of its pigmentation clearly increasing as creatures progress up the evolutionary path (Marsden, 1961; Scherer, 1939). Mammals have the highest intensity of this; primates have the highest among the mammals (Cotzias, 1974). Finally, even among the primates the higher the evolutionary form of brain complexity and organization or similarity to the human type, the richer the light-interacting biochemistry of the brain and its root, the spine. It is a luminous current, a life propagating line and force.

We are focusing on melanin and neuromelanin in human development for several reasons beyond those already mentioned above because it appears to be intimately associated with the process of evolution. It is a unique biopolymer! It can transduce *both* acoustic and electric energy fields and apparently generate enough heat to effect metabolic processes. This is quite significant and we will return to this in a moment.

It is present in each stage of embryological development from oocyte to mature adult organism. In vertebrates, it grossly condenses during embryological development of the highly pigmented neural crest system which coincides with the formation of the neural tube and then disperses to many strategic homeostatic locations throughout the entire organism (Barr, 1983). Thus individually and collectively it is intimately involved in the process of evolution and the development of the human brain. This brings us to the evolutionary schema of brain researcher P.D. MacLean.

Some time ago MacLean (1970) pointed out how the human brain had a tri-part or "triune" structure to it that reflected the evolutionary unfoldment from the earliest creatures with primitive brain structures all the way "up" to man. The early reptilian lineage has superimposed on it the later mammalian brain structures. Then in the course of evolution this mammalian brain itself was superseded by the higher cortical process of the cortex. Still higher up the mammalian line is a more evolved and subtle neocortex eventuating in the self-conscious and the potentially self-transcending human brain. Again melanin is present in the brain of all animals with the degree of its pigmentation steadily increasing as one rises up the evolutionary arch.

This process, as mentioned above, begins early for the human species. Even in the earliest stages of embryonic development we can observe an unfolding neural crest system which produces a significant quantity of melanin and other pigments. This neural crest is the precursor of the spinal column and brain core. Yet even before this fine neural crest or neural tube formation there are organizationally active melanized cells available to the unfolding system. This embryological melanin system, both prior to and actually during the unfoldment of the neural crest, may actually organize the entire neuroendocrine system, including the GI tract and elongating neural crest (Barr, 1983)! Melanin, it seems, is active and directional prior even to the first heartbeat.

Melanin brings with it a most sensitive and highly specialized molecular process that is intimately associated with light itself and life in all carbon based life forms. Melanin is photoactive; it absorbs light. It will orient itself toward light in both diffuse and direct environments. This light current we believe is a most essential dynamic in the human life process.

There is in all likelihood a *sustained current* that guides embryological patters in development. It is clearly not the on/off variety of current we are more accustomed to seeing in the traditional physical sciences. This current seems to be organized or localized innately around this light-sensitive melanin and neuromelanin system (Barr, 1983). We are reminded here of neuroscientist Lashly's early idea of "lines of force" in embryological development guiding the organism's growth from the earliest of days (Pribram, 1991). Embedded here is the notion of brain processes and wave-fronts in interference patterns in the deep structure of our neural matrix and the potentially *holographic dynamics* of their communication and operation.

Indeed, given the very high degree of internal cellular organization or coherence and the somewhat elastic or flexible and charged structure or lattice work of this system, a certain flow or bio-current or life-force if you will, can be seen to literally conduct itself through this biosystem along certain lines of force. It is already established that melanin has semiconductive properties (Barr, 1983). Melanin responds to a critical applied electrical field by *changing its conductivity.* It can be seen as high as ten degrees of magnitude! This response is in two areas, threshold level and memory switching. The first, the threshold switching, occurs when a low conductivity is elevated to a high conductivity state in a critical electric field. The second, the memory switching, occurs when a sample of melanin remains in a high conduction state when the critical field is removed but can return to a lower state by the application of even larger electrical fields or current (Filatous, 1976).

Interestingly enough this current, informed by certain particular polymer characteristics of the melanin molecule, has a certain affinity we believe to be the process or phenomenon of *superconductivity.* However, unlike most presently known manifestations of superconductivity, this form can operate at room or physiological temperature and would be understood as a form of organic or *biological superconductivity* (Little, 1965; Langone, 1989; Cope, 1979; 1980; 1981). Melanin as mentioned above is known to be a semiconductor. The present data suggest that melanin may also be an organic superconductor under certain conditions at room temperature.

Similar phenomena have already been observed in other biological systems. Fröhlich (1983; 1970) has outlined how proteins connected in a common voltage gradient field such as within a cell membrane could oscillate *coherently* and thereby introduce long range cooperative effects by which proteins and nucleic acids could communicate in biological systems. A vibrational (phonon) or rhythmic mode of coherent excitation can be created and briefly sustained in the layers of ordered water and ions subjacent to these membranes. These biological effects of coherent excitation and long range cooperativity from Fröhlich's point of view are not temperature effects. Rather because of the coherent vibrations of these biomolecules in space and time there may be a holographic information medium in operation here. Fröhlich further suggests the real possibility of propagating waves due to the *lack of resistance* in these biomolecules and their associated layers of ordered water or what is referred to as Debye layers. In other words, a form of biological superconductivity.

For us as we discuss the possibility of life-force or living evolutionary current moving up and along the spinal line, there is a natural connection between this potential subtle current of neuromelanin biological superconductivity in the brainstem, brain, and the higher cortical processes of the neocortex. But to move from current to spreading wave-fronts, from energy to intelligence clearly requires some form of light and life-energy "transducer" or transformation. This may not be as difficult as it first appears. If we remember that *both* the spinal energy and the higher cortical processes are each an intelligent, purposeful, and working process in which light itself is being transformed ($E = mc^2$), then we need only look at parallel processes in other areas of science for heuristic analogies and homologies to help our understanding. Remember that melanin is not only an excellent photon- (electron) -phonon and electromagnetic semiconductive agent, but also transduces both acoustic and electric energy fields (Barr, 1983).

A simple light bulb has a current flowing through its special filament activating electrons so that light waves are given off or produced providing illumination to the room. A more sophisticated example is Einstein's photoelectric effect. While this theory was in support of the particle theory of light in quantum mechanics and involved a light current of photons activating energy, i.e., electrons in a metal to produce an electrical current, it still serves to suggest that light and current can be transformed one into the other. A further example in this vein is the laser and hologram interaction.

A laser or beam of coherent light, when appropriately aimed at an object and mirror, is capable of producing a unique photograph of the object. If one then took a section of this photograph away and illuminated it correctly, one could literally reconstruct the entire photograph from this fragment. All aspects of the photograph are enfolded into each aspect of the photograph. The laser can interact with the hologram in energetic ways to liberate information, energy, and other properties (Kock, 1981). What is critical here in our focus on *transformations* is that the laser light *transforms* into waves in the hologram. Also sound or acoustic and liquid surfaces acoustic holography is technically possible, as are hologram computer memories. Since melanin absorbs light, it seems that sound, possibly heat, and certainly light, are all capable of going from certain photon-phonon modes and levels to other waveforms.

Intuit for a minute a kind of neuromelanin organic or subtle biological superconducting process, or life-current, transforming or transducing itself into an innumerable network of lower and higher level cortical wavefronts in holographic or holonomic fashion in the brain with all its implications in terms of energy, intelligence, and information processing. It is known that in the brain the subiculum within the hippocampal formation is a focal area where phasic theta wave-related ratiocination/comparison occurs (Gray, 1982). The hippocampus accumulates neuromelanin formation and derivatives and the subiculum holds a significant amount of melanin with its range of electronically-coupled dendrites. This makes it an ideal location for some aspects of holographic processing (Pribram, 1980). It seems nature is more ingenious than we know and we believe has encoded this in our bio-psychological inheritance. We are left to explicate and unfold its many processes. Again all these models and facts are only that–models and facts–and someday will be supplanted by other, more inclusive ways of explaining and explicating this ancient method and intuition. They serve now to point the way into light. Indeed, all is light, light the substratum and matrix of all that exists. All that exists is a relative of light.

It is a curious fact that melatonin, a cousin of melanin but not hallucinogenic, can easily convert to the powerful hallucinogen 10-methoxyharmalan (Lansky, 1979). This may occur in a flash or slowly. It may also be stimulated by other endocrine processes associated with the brain's pineal gland, a gland long known to receive light and dark and information from the eyes and perhaps elsewhere in the biosystem or body-mind. We must keep in mind that even for our ancestral mother, the light that affected the iris in her eye also affected the neuromelanin in her central nervous system and brain. This may be partially why the mind and consciousness are so intimately associated with light.

As we mentioned earlier, the world's cultures are rich with references to "life-force" movement and a certain evolutionary impetus and trajectory up along the spine. Chinese acupuncture notes a "major extraordinary meridian" called the governor vessel meridian. It too seems to follow an almost parallel path and unfolds along the spine from the tip of the coccyx to end at the upper lip. It is said that the life or Ki energy is stored in this meridian like water in a lake. The Ki flows through the twelve ordinary meridians and is likened to rivers which distribute this luminous energy to the various organs and tissues (Motoyama, 1981).

The Indian Yogis called the energy Prana Shakti and its tube or cord the Brahman Nadi or Sushumna Nadi. The Egyptians and long dead Dravidians had even older terms. Before that were names we shall never know.

Some researchers even believe that this Ki or Ch'i energy moves in the opposite direction of the sympathetic nervous system, therein giving the overall system a dynamic balance (Motoyama, 1979; 1981). This could identify or at least correlate and parallel the evolutionary energy and flow with the parasympathetic nervous system which we now know is activated in meditation and healing of every kind.

There are numerous other references we can cite to indicate an evolutionary movement toward expansion and intelligence coursing up and parallel to the spine. It is a perceptable current of living energy the frontal self or personality and ego must adapt to and travel. The ego and personality can be understood as conduits for this localization and directionality of energy flow. They provide it some order, some individualizing process to stabilize and control.

The ego itself in this context arises as only one in the latest processes of stabilization in the psychic dimension of our consciousness. This process of stabilization of increasingly more complex and subtle processes is a reflection of the teleos or evolutionary impulse seeking wider and wider expression in the life course of our species. When the ego itself becomes the ossifying principle on stage then crisis occurs. This, we suggest, is what each personality syndrome struggles with. It must be acknowledged at every point. This is the task the next few chapters will try to unfold.

But beyond even that, our luminous inheritance can be seen to interconnect us all to each other from sources and connections reached long ago. The mitochondrial DNA of all our diverse races and bloodcells can be seen to have commonly crossed in an ancient ancestor, our She-who-has-no-name, perhaps 200,000 years ago. That ancestor in all likelihood was of African lineage and we, all her descendants, are of this common genetic stock. While she has not been definitely located in sub-Saharan Africa, the preponderance of evidence in fossil remains and morphological data and the fact that most of the humanoids, including *Australopithecus africanus* and *Homo sapiens sapiens* arose in Africa lends exceedingly strong support for this view of genetic interconnectedness. This somatic and genetic interconnectedness is paralleled by our common psychic interconnectedness as witnessed by common imagery, common experience and the binding matrix of the family and the collective unconscious. We will see later how this implicate interconnectedness intimately affects the process of healing on many levels. This will be the chapter on psychosomatic and family processes. For now we need to stress how consciousness, our very consciousness, is not a passive, isolated observer in the universe, but an active, subtle, and sometimes forceful psychic influence in the material world (Jahn and Dunne, 1987). Indeed, we are all creatures of a common light.

This excursion will proceed with these new assumptions concerning the development of the human through various stages of cognitive, affective, or emotional and psychological development. We go from the earliest stages prior to birth on through to the necessary egoic stages where contemporary psychology abandons us on to transegoic states that lead toward transcendence and translation into the Absolute. After establishing these assumptions in observations, we will begin to look at the many offspring that thrive ten thousand generations after the root-gatherer and mother of compassion first reflected on her life and family by the lake. We will look deeply at a representative relative not so far down the evolutionary tract from that ancient one.

In contemporary language we will see how her progeny deal with the forces and vectors of nature in the intimate crucible of the psyche. We will see how the borderline personality and behavior is in many ways a reflection of a frustrated and repetitive boundary breech, the failed attempt to recognize and balance the Absolute in themselves and others in addition to other psychological problems. The presentation will then progress on to the Obsessive Compulsive personality style and the ways that this Obsessive Compulsive deals with the actual tangibly experienced reality of the transcendental flow of life-force that we believe is the substratum of all intelligent energy. The next chapter will proceed to that paranoid panicky attempt at integration of true insight with its tenuous egoic attempts to master this flood of extraordinarily luminous and frightening energy into its system. Finally it will be stressed how the last one, the multiple personality, is in many ways lost in a wilderness of mirrors, a forest of splintered selves, all of them, in some ways, actually true. Theirs is truly a fragmented and failed manifestation of the search for a higher unity, not only in the waking state but in various other states of consciousness.

The so-called psychosomatic or conversion disorders require some scrutiny because they indicate a profound involvement of the physical and energy body that is currently treated in hypnosis and behavioral medicine. Attention will be drawn to the effect of the mind, mental states and egoic influences upon and within the organism. Permeating all this will be the influence of family dynamics, energy patterns, and ways in which the influence of mind and personality patterns profoundly affects the flow of energy in the human body-mind. Behind it all is the radiant life-force intuited by the Vedas, by the mystery schools scattered throughout antiquity, by all peoples and all cultures. It is seen in meditation, breaks through in art, flows through occasionally in the dream, and points to that Absolute rooted in our genes, our bodies, and our minds. It creates the trajectory of attention and intelligence back to its source in consciousness itself. This is the story of the ancient one's descendants through history and her-story. Its rhythm and thread are not anchored on some distant shore millennia ago, but registered in the blood cells, heartbeat, and mind of her progeny in this hour.

REFERENCES

Ardrey, R. *African Genesis*, Dell Publishing Co., New York, 1967.

Asante, M. K. "The African American Mode of Transcendence," *Journal of Transpersonal Psychology*, Vol. 16, No. 2, 1984.

Avalon, A. *The Serpent Power: The Secrets of Tantric and Shaktic Yoga*, Dover Publications, New York, 1974.

Barr, F. E. "Melanin: The Organizing Molecule," *Medical Hypotheses*, 11, 1-140, 1983.

Bohm, D. *Wholeness and the Implicate Order*, Routledge, Kegan Paul, London, 1980.

Capra, F. "Modern Physics and Eastern Mysticism," *Journal of Transpersonal Psychology*, No. 1, 1976, pp. 20-40.

Chan, W. T., Faruqi, I. R., Kitagawa, J. M., Raju, P.T. *The Great Asian Religions*, Macmillan Co., New York, 1969.

Cope, F. W. "Magnetic flux trapping in double diazo and other dyes as evidence for possible superconduction at room temperatures," *Physiological Chemistry and Physics* 12: 179-186, 1980.

Cope, F. W. "Remnant magnetization in biological materials and systems as evidence for possible superconduction at room temperature: a preliminary survey," *Physiological Chemistry and Physics* 11: 65-69, 1979.

Cope, F. W. "Organic superconductive phenomena at room temperature. Some magnetic properties of dyes and graphite interpreted as manifestations of viscous magnetic flux lattices and small superconductive regions," *Physiological Chemistry and Physics* 13: 99-110, 1981.

Cotzias, G. C. Melanogenesis and Extra Pyramidal Diseases, Fed. Proc. Vol. 23, 1974, p. 713.

Dillion, D. and Dillion, B. *An Explosion of Being: An American Family's Journey into the Psychic*, Parker Publ. Co., West Nyack, NY, 1984.

Diop, C. A. *Civilization or Barbarism: An Authentic Anthropology*, Lawrence Hill Books, New York, 1991.

Diop, C. A. "Africa's Contribution to World Civilization: The Exact Sciences" in *Journal of African Civilizations* (1985) 1984, Vol. 6, No. 2, pp. 69-83.

Diop, C. A. *The African Origin of Civilization*, Lawrence Hill and Co., Westport (1955) 1974.

Dobzhansky, T. *The Biology of Ultimate Concern*, Meridian Books, World Publishing, New York, 1971.

Edgerton, R. B. "A Traditional African Psychiatrist," *Journal of Anthropological Research*, Vol. 27, No. 3, 1971, 121-136.

Fairservis, W. A. *The Ancient Kingdoms of the Nile and the Doomed Monuments of Nubia*, Thomas Crowell Co., New York, 1962.

Filatous, J., McGinness, J., and Corry, P. "Thermal and electronic contributions to switching in melanins," *Biopolymers*, 15:2309-2312, 1976.

Fröhlich, H. "Evidence for coherent excitation in biological systems," *International Journal of Quantum Chemistry* 23, 1589-1595, 1983.

Fröhlich, H. "Excitation in Enzymes," *Nature*, 228, 1093, 1970.

Grant, K. "Cults of the Shadow," in *Kundalini, Evolution and Enlightenment*, Ed. by J. White, Anchor/Doubleday, 1979, pp. 395-398.

Gray, J. A. "Precis of the neuropsychology of anxiety: an enquiry into the functions of the septo-hippocampal system," *Behavioral and Brain Sciences* 5:469-534, 1982.

Griaule, M. and Dieterlen, G. *The Pale Fox*, Continuum Foundation, P. O. Box 636, Chino Valley, AZ 86323, 1986.

Hutchinson, J. A. *Paths of Faith*, McGraw-Hill, Inc., New York, 1969.

Jahn, J. *Muntu: The New African Culture*, Evergreen Books, Grove Press, New York, 1961.

Jahn, R. G. and Dunne, B. J. *The Margins of Reality: The Role of Consciousness in the Physical World*, Harcourt Brace Jovanich, New York, 1987.

Jaynes, J. *The Origin of Consciousness in the Breakdown of the Bicameral Mind*, Houghton Mifflin Co., Boston, MA, 1976.

Johanson, D. J. and Edey, M. A. *Lucy: The Beginnings of Human Evolution*, Simon and Schuster, New York, 1981.

Katz, R. *Boiling Energy: Community Healing Among the Kalahari Kung*, Harvard Univ. Press. Cambridge, 1982.

King, R. D. *African Origin of Biological Psychiatry*, Seymore-Smith, Inc., Germantown, TN, 1990.

Kock, W. E. *Lazers and Holography: An Introduction to Coherent Optics*, Dover Publications, New York, 1981.

Krishna, G. *The Biological Basis of Religion and Genius*, Harper and Row, New York, 1971.

Langone, J. *Superconductivity: The New Alchemy*, Contemporary Books, Chicago, IL, 1989.

Lansky, P. "Neurochemistry and the Awakening of Kundalini," in White, J. (Ed) *Kundalini, Evolution and Enlightenment*, Anchor Books, New York, 1979.

Leakey, R. E. and Lewin, R. *Origins: Emergence and Evolution of Our Species and its Possible Future*, E. P. Dutton, New York, 1979.

Lemonick, M. D. "Everyone's genealogical mother," *Time*, January 26, 1987, pp. 66.

Little, W. A. "Superconductivity at room temperature," *Scientific American*, 21, February 1965.

Lukoff, D. "The diagnosis of mystical experiences with psychotic features," *Journal of Transpersonal Psychology*, Vol. 17, #2, 1985, pp. 123-154.

Lumpkin, B. "Mathematics and Engineering in the Nile Valley," *Journal of African Civilizations*, (1985) 1984, ibid.

MacLean, P. D. *The Triune Brain, Emotion and Scientific Basis in the Neurosciences*, F. P. Schmitt, Ed. The Rockefeller Univ. Press, New York, 1970.

Marsden, C. D. "Pigmentation in the Nucleum Substantiae Nigrae of Mammales." *Journal of Anatomy*, V. 95, 1961, p. 162-256.

Mookerjee, A. *Kundalini: The Arousal of the Inner Energy*, Destiny Books, New York, 1982.

Motoyama, H. "A Biological Elucidation of the Meridian and Ki-energy," *Journal of Research for Religion and Parapsychology*, August 1981.

Motoyama, H. "PK influence on the Meridian and Psi-energy," ibid, 1979.

Motoyama, H. *Theories of The Chakras: Bridge to Higher Consciousness*, Quest Books, Wheaton, IL, 1981.

Newsweek, March 10, 1984, "Raising Children Who Care," p. 76.

Pappademos, J. "The Newtonian Synthesis in Physical Science and Its Roots in the Nile Valley," *Journal of African Civilizations*, (1985) 1984, ibid.

Pribram, K. *Brain and Perception*, Lawrence Erlbaum Associates, NJ, 1991.

Pribram, K. *Languages of the Brain*, Brandon House, New York, 1971 (1981).

Pribram, K. H. "Mind, brain and consciousness: the organization of competence and conduct," *The Psychobiology of Consciousness* by J. M. Davidson and R. J. Davidson, eds., Plenum Press, New York, 47-63, 1980.

Sannella, L. *The Kundalini Experience: Psychosis or Transcendence* Integral Publishing, (1976) 1987.

Satprem, *Sri Aurobindo or The Adventure of Consciousness*, Harper and Row, New York, 1968.

Scherer, H. J. "Melanin Pigmentation of the Substantia Nigra in Primates," *Journal of Comparative Anatomy*, V. 71, 1939, p. 91-95.

Schmeck, H. M. "Modern man's origin linked to a single female ancestor,"*The New York Times*, March 26, 1986, pp. 24.

Schuon, F. *The Transcendent Unity of Religions*, Quest Books, Wheaton, IL, 1984.

Schwarz, B. E. *Psychic-Nexus*, Van Nostrand Reinhold Co., New York, 1980.

Stone, M. *When God Was A Woman*, Harcourt Brace Jovanovich, New York, 1976.

Taub-Bynum, E. B. *The Family Unconscious: An Invisible Bond*, Theosophical Publishing House, Wheaton, IL, 1984.

Thakkur, C. G. *Yoga: Yoga Therapy, Yogic Postures*, Yoga Research Center, Ancient Wisdom Publications. Bombay, India 1977.

Watson, L. *Lifetide: The Biology of Consciousness*, Simon & Schuster, New York, 1980.

White, J. and Krippner, S. (Eds.) *Future Science: Life Energies and the Physics of the Paranormal*, Garden City, New York: Anchor Books, 1977, 550-555.

Wright, L. and Tierney, J. "The search for Adam and Eve," *Newsweek*, January 11, 1988, pp. 46-52.

Chapter 2

Development: The Roots of Transcendence

THE TRIPLE ASCENT

> Development is evolution; evolution is transcendence.
>
> –Wilber
> *The Atman Project*

> If a spiritual unfolding on earth is the hidden truth of our birth into matter, if it is fundamentally an evolution of consciousness that has been taking place in Nature, then man as he is cannot be the last term of that evolution: he is too imperfect an expression of the spirit, mind itself, a too limited form and instrumentation; mind is only a middle term of consciousness, the mental being can only be a transitional being . . . if his mind is capable of opening to what exceeds it, then there is no reason why man himself should not arrive at supermind . . . or at least lend his mentality, life and body to an evolution of that greater term of the Spirit manifesting in Nature.
>
> –Aurobindo
> *The Life Divine*

She-who-has-no-name passed her life amid the clutter of deaths, upheavals, and periods of long, stable rest. Her grey-marbled hair and age where the vast course of life flowed through her were testimony to her strength, her power, her great value to her clan. Herds of unnameable beasts roamed near her but always retreated when she yelled or approached them. Sometimes they provided a meal; sometimes a dream animal painted on rock-wall relief. Beside the bird-lined shore and shell heaps of the great lake a quiet pool or inlet would create the perfectly still water where she reflected and discovered her own face.

Peering into the place of fish and her sunken feet she braided her hair, washed her face. The fingers folded ropes of hair into patterns unique to tribe. Even family linkages in amulets were tied into styles woven by her skill. A hunter's hair was knotted differently than a child's or a healer's or even the small contingent that usually guarded while the others would sleep. She fleetingly reflected in the mirror of waters, quietly braided her thoughts into early magic and technology for herself and future generations. Her own ancestor "Lucy" had been sleeping nearby, braided into the soil for at least 2 million years. We pick up and braid a few strands of this perennial, multisectored spiral of her progeny's human development.

Given that there are so many diverse aspects to this unfolding process it will be useful to look at it from several angles. This will allow the cross-currents to be seen and also the divergences to be taken into account. To keep track, a simple device will be used. Sections will be presented to show the contribution to the shared fabric and also to break up long discussions into digestible amounts. Human development in each person's life embraces an epochal span between the time prior to birth to, at least from the evidence we have from near death experiences (NDE), some brief "psychological" time after clinical death. It is obviously not easily reducible to a brief excursion into developmental psychology. The major schools of human development will be introduced, their organizing principles elaborated, and then the primary exponents and theoretical champions of these schools will be explored. We will begin before birth and hopefully provide enough observational and research material to fill out the cloth of the story. Eventually, the specific findings of each school of methodology will be integrated into the arch that is human development. Several charts with these specific developmental markers will be provided in the text to make a quick reference to. We will look at emotional, psychophysical, cognitive, and noetic development. Clearly, not all can be said and not every theorist given full due. However, hopefully, at least we can attain to the essential between our first emergent self-consciousness in She-who-has-no-name and our progeny's trajectory into the stars.

Many different theories of individual human development scatter the evolutionary light into diverse areas, all these necessary, all these perceptions true to some degree. Yet underneath all these multiple theories there is a central guiding vision. All of these theories begin with an undifferentiated unity, proceed to differentiation in various ways, and return again to a sense of greater integrity or unity. They may speak of this in terms of seeking a "balance" between assimilation and accommodation, a "balance" between the ego, id, and superego, etc., or between anima and animus, etc. They may even speak of a sense of balance in cognitive structures in a very subtle, but specific, process. These are all true and these are all multiplicative ways of perceiving the One. It is assumed that all these major theories and perceptions are in various degrees true and, therein, we feel free to draw from these where it seems appropriate in order to flesh out the different limbs of the developmental structure that will be presented. The fabric woven of these different theories hopefully will grace, yet will never completely cover, the whole body of this subject. Attention will be called to focus whenever one area is braided into another. After exploring these in some minor detail it will be easier to draw clearer references and perspectives concerning the primal rootedness of the Absolute and of the seed of transcendence unfolding in our nature. Body, mind, and the noetic, or spirit, are the three pillars of this great ascent.

Three Theories

The major psychological schools of human development may be organized as follows in three groups. The first group is the organismic vision of which the "organic lamp" theory of Heinz Werner is a principle landmark. Here the *autogenetic* thesis is found, which emphasizes that man develops into what he or she makes themselves by their own actions and unfoldment in the world. Creativity itself is seen as basic to development here, particularly, as we shall see in cognitive development. It has given birth to many similar theories. Both Kant and Coleridge had contributed to the notion of self-organizing or self-generating processes in development. This idea of self-organization is extremely helpful in our own consideration of development. Some allied theories, such as that of Piaget, which will be discussed in depth, accept the idea of self-organizing processes, but for Piaget, emphasis is placed on other dynamics within the developmental process, namely on the equilibration, or seeking of a balance, in functions. These occur in definite stages at certain ages and, we believe, have specific neural substrates of growth which we will mention.

The second great vision of human development is the *psychoanalytic* vision, or position, that takes a different view of the internal and external forces acting on the developing being. It stresses conflict and attempted mastery, repression and resolution. This great vision has spawned many others, such as Mahler, and Loevinger, in addition to some that parallel it in many ways. These too will be braided into a useful, but limited, cord of development. Also Sullivan and Kohut must be threaded into the story. These two are really the basic psychological theories of development in which "something" emerges and changes in the organism because of its innate processes.

The third approach comprises the *behavioral* theories of development, which simply reduce the organism to a contingently complicated, or embarrassingly simple and totally reactive plaything of the external environment. These latter theories cannot adequately account for creativity or the quantum leap in intelligence afforded by the generation of language in humans (Chomsky, 1965), much less the place of intuition or higher unfoldment in the individual. For that reason, we will not seriously explore them as theories of development. They shed light on reactive behavior in the early stages, yes, but not on creative development.

This is not to say that the integration of reactive behavior into the organism's system is not important, for indeed it is. While the behavioral models cannot account for generativity and creativity, nor do they posit any inherent directionality (teleology) or purpose beyond fortuitous occurrences in nature and environmental contingencies, they do serve a valuable part. These approaches account for certain external and physicalistic necessities which are an essential aspect of the overall process. They appear most early in the life course and focus on the ways of controlling the body, comfort, and staying alive. They account for the outer sheath or dimension of our lives. The only implicit sense of creativity is found in the notion of generalization of behavior to novel situations. This actually is an organismic notion embedded in a mechanistic system. The ground or fundamental assumption of all behavioral theories of human development appears to be that mankind grows to be what he becomes by way of his environmental exigencies only. Even when the environment itself changes and requires a creative solution on the part of the organism in order to survive and flourish, it is really an implicit potentiality of the organism involved, not the external environment. Just because an organism seeks to sustain itself is not a clear indication of "telos," rather only a memory, or history of adaptation to the world. No, telos or teleology is implicated in the evolutionary novelty of self-consciousness itself.

The Mental and Affective

The psychoanalytic vision tends to focus its lens primarily on the affective-emotional dimension of development. This is deeply embedded in the emotional and energetic level or sheath of our existence. A process called "sublimation" is recognized here, where raw energy is made more subtle and finds expression in more sophisticated forms of behavior and cognition. This level is amply covered by Freud, Sullivan, Mahler, and others. The notion of sublimation feels like an implicitly teleological or purposeful notion at the very heart of psychoanalysis. It is the process of leading or drawing the psychic energy to "higher" levels for various purposes. It is the proverbial Trojan horse in the mechanistic city.

In a very real sense, Werner, Piaget, and others of the organismic approach focus primarily on the classically "mental" theater of our evolutionary drama. That sheath or level is most concerned with cognitive impetus and unfoldment. Beyond that mental level we might posit a level of pure discrimination and body-alive sense, which many refer to as the bliss sheath. We will say more of that eventually. Suffice it to say here that they all interpenetrate each other and perhaps even unfold out of each other, with the subtle discriminative or blissful level being the innermost level. Each has a particular and necessary thread to bring into the emerging fabric. They must all braid together at a certain stage in order to quiet the ego enough to be translucent to its cognitive and affective turbulence. This is facilitated by the highest levels of post-formal cognitive operations. But slow down, we are getting ahead of ourselves.

These sturdy theoretical structures account for a great deal of human development up to and including ego development. They each view the process from a different, useful perspective. For some reason they all assume that evolution stops there and that there is nothing beyond, thus perceiving any behavior or action/insight that might not fit into these patterns as regressions to lower structures. This is the reductionist bias so often seen in contemporary science. This study, however, will present and explore those cognitive and developmental levels and structures that emerge in states and conditions beyond the conventional limitations of ego development. Hopefully, out of this will emerge a new witnessing of teleological forces and a new perspective on symptoms and symptom formation. Now let us look at, and attempt to braid more detail into these structures and theories of human development. It is a long, detailed story, full of odd corners and surprising turns. Only its general outline can be found in less than a thousand pages. Bear with me as we braid together these threads and motifs, focusing at times, here, with this theorist, and then focusing at times, there, with that data. It is necessary to criss-cross, to cross-fertilize. However, the fabric will always turn back upon the living weave of evolution itself.

Let us begin. And where else to begin, but at the very beginning, before birth and breath itself.

Prior to Birth

The seamless peace is disturbed. After a timeless duration in the sea of the mother's womb the world begins to tighten, constrict, and move with an unpleasant sense. Soon the universe itself is caught in a cataclysmic struggle; terror and nameless panic rifle its existence. Then the sea bursts open into blood, urine, feces, and light. Birth trauma and the first crisis of breath has dawned.

These, of course, are the stages of birth prior to face-to-face contact between infant and family. Grof (1985) has delineated at least four stages prior to birth through which we pass and have our formation. These "perinatal matrices" are profound and have their impact on subsequent behavior beyond the womb. The first one is that realm of the undisturbed intrauterine state of no boundary and seamless bliss. It is the ocean prior to differentiation. It is the real source of "thalassal regression" but not at all identical to what some would call the mystical state! A child's unborn eyes here will turn toward light. It will react to pain, to music, to stimulation from the outside. The extensive research of the Pre- and Peri-Natal Psychology Association of North America presents every year now medical and scientific support for the active existence of human consciousness prior even to birth (PPPANA).

The second great matrix arises at the onset of biological delivery. It announces a certain disquiet in the world and ushers in constraint, tension. The passive, formally blissful, fetal life is inundated with pain but has no way to escape its tight world.

The third perinatal matrix is robust in its struggle of great forces in the womb and birth canal. All the primal emotions and conflicts take center stage. The world of the fetus propelled through the pressurized cavern of birth is fraught with pain, powerful energies, and new demands on the organism. All manner of intense life energies are stimulated, e.g., self-destructive, intense erotic arousal, aggression, and physical pain.

Finally, the fourth perinatal matrix unfolds. After a *sense* of near total annihilation comes the rush of birth. Energy, light, sound, and texture are all enormously expanded. Death and re-birth have occurred before the first vocal discharge is uttered aloud.

This sequence is the one we generally take en route to this life. Grof has opened it up fully for our inspection. He has built on the earlier work of Otto Rank (1929), Nandor Fodor (1949), Lietaert Peerbolte (1975), and others. The influence of these stages on later cognitive development, let alone its influence on affective and symbolic expressions is beyond dispute. Yet it may not always reach the surface and certainly is assimilated differently than is an "experience" conditioned by attention and consciousness.

Grof's birth trauma provides much of the *intense* memory of somatic, physical, and other cataclysmic processes that occur in traditional delivery events. It is questionable whether the fetal being has an image or idea that it is an organism under attack. It has a *sense* of self and is infused with raw affective energy that needs to be forgotten or repressed because of its pain and organismically perceived potential for dissolution of the organism. There is awareness, but not in the "I" sense of the born psyche. Thus there is no "experience" as we conceptualize experience. There is intelligence, but no arena of words, images, cognitions, or symbol/signs as we know it. The "memory" of events is embedded in the neuronal structures and muscles and is elicited or emerges through development under certain circumstances. We point this out here because there is a subtle tendency to reduce or trace things back to the womb in a vaguely reductionist manner. The saline sac is where we start but it does not contain our psychospiritual destination on the evolutionary arch.

So what does the infant come to us with by the hour of birth? It has lived a saline history in which it has partially recapitulated the organic development of its racial lineage or phylogeny in its own psychophysical or ontogenetic development and yet has still managed to go further and bring more novelty into the world. In its embryonic unfoldment from neural tube to spinal cord, the cells along its length have evolved into melanocytes and all the endocrine glands, from pineal to pituitary to thyroid and others. Melanin and melanocytes are intimately involved in biochemical and hormonal interaction with light.

It has brought a recent history of the brain. At its core is the reptilian anlage from the lizard and dinosaur. Then the mammalian upsurge is seen in the limbic system and its associated structures that integrate affect, emotion, and the precursor of thought. Finally, the neocortex spreads over the surface and provides the pathway for primates, *Homo sapiens* and who knows what else. This, of course, is the evolution of the triune brain (MacLean, 1970) well researched in the neurosciences. Yet note the evolutionary trajectory of the life-force, from primitive to more complex interactions with the environment and light, manifested from coccyx to crown. It is the luminous chord in potentia.

Then there are the blood and saline dynamics of birth. The perinatal matrices galvanize the fetal aquanaut, infusing and embedding in its muscles soma and neural processes, powerful affective tendencies, and precursors. Much of this psychic energy informs (in-form-mation) the real life river of imagery, affect, and states of attention that suffuse the process of our later psychological life.

However it has no "I" or boundary and as such, paradoxically, has nothing that would appear to us as "experience." That last statement will become clear, hopefully, in the later section on post-formal cognitive operations.

These are the embryonic tributaries that flow prior to actual birth and then wash into the vast, bright, bewildering ocean of life with others. We each come to it with different tendencies and potentials embedded in our genetic, neural, and still unknown make-up. It unfolds from birth onward, nursed or punished by the shifting environment, yet pulled beyond all this by the evolutionary force. In all this the psychological or cognitive structures must stabilize the mind, must localize the flow of intelligence and light.

So the child is here. In the early minutes after delivery the first reflexes are seen outside the womb. He or she may have sucked a thumb in the mother's recesses but to see the infant sucking the nipple untaught by you or me is a whole new occasion. The average skeptic is moved by this. Something, for a brief moment, stops the concertizing and localizing, opening a quick door in the heart for the prophet Elijah to pass through our lives.

Consciousness at Birth

But what about intentions, desires, will, and "expression?" Does the newborn or neonate have conscious processes in any way similar to our own? In other words, while there are certainly events and interactions right after birth, is there in any sense *consciousness* at birth in the sense that we mean it as adults?

Recent experimental and observational studies tend strongly to show that there is indeed conscious activity and process at and right after birth. "Starting from birth infants regularly occupy a state called 'alert inactivity,' when they are physically quiet and alert and apparently are taking in external events" (Wolff, 1966). The infant is not only sleeping, eating, crying, and moving during these earliest hours and days. This state of alert inactivity can extend up to several minutes from birth on.

Other observational and experimental studies point to the gentle fact that infants can turn their heads to *selectively* choose their mother's milk over others (MacFarlane, 1975). They can increase or decrease their rate of sucking (Friedlander, 1970); they can visually move toward human faces versus other such images (Fantz, 1963); they can reflect other subtle signs of choice, intentionality and will. All their primary sensory modalities orient as gracefully toward the mothering one as melanin orients toward light. It is no coincidence that melanin is highly localized in the eyes, ears, GI tract and heart. It efficiently transduces visual, auditory, and thermal energy.

Interestingly, infants seem to come equipped innately with what is called amodal perception. This is the capacity to take information from one sensory modality and translate it into another sensory modality (Stern, 1985). As Stern points out, this is "probably not experienced as belonging to any one particular sensory mode. More likely it transcends mode or channel and exists in some unknown supra-modal form." This of course involves or implicates "some form of encoding processes." Also important for our later exploration in this present study is the related notion, put forth by Stern and others, that, in reference to intelligence itself, the infant seems to be able to experience the process of emerging organization as well as the results or consequences of this increasing organizational complexity.

From our point of view here, the "experience" that the neonate/infant passes through is radically different from the boundary-informed egoic experience of childhood and adult life. Yet clearly intelligence and consciousness are involved. This particular problem, this specific disjunctive, will be taken up again and again in the later unfolding developmental arch. With thought and language we will see it emerge and separate, in the stage of post-formal operations, we will see it repeat this process.

Yes, it seems that even at birth itself, some form of consciousness has beached itself successfully outside the womb. The various developmental tapestries and theories that we will now present are all attempts to describe and make explainable what occurs with these birth-given tendencies as they unfold along the path. Each one, from Werner to Piaget to Vygotsky and others, seem to do best in the regions of early cognition and neuropsychology. Mahler, Freud, Sullivan, and others describe best that dimension of ego, emotion, object anxiety, and interpersonal arrest. Still others, Riegel, Koplowitz, and unmentioned others paint clearest those stages of the intellect and cognition we unfold long, long after birth. Finally, Wilbur and Kohlberg weave the moral and spiritual trajectory at its best. Each one we will cover and draw from. Again I apologize for the shortcomings that this attempt will no doubt reflect. While inadequate in many ways and certainly incomplete, it will hopefully still fulfill the need to catch a glimpse of consciousness and a full cycle of human life in its triple ascent.

The Western Map

All approaches to the maturation or unfolding of human potential begin in the ground state where those material and organic forces are dominant and still consciousness has reached out to this shore. I ask you at this moment to remember this as we move toward a closer look at how the psychological structures and functions seem to arise from a Western psychological perspective. I also ask you even more importantly to remember that the material world or matter itself is the translation or reflection of energy or light. $E = mc^2$ is *really true*. This root premise will re-emerge in the final section of this chapter in a most natural and culminating way.

Heinz Werner

As mentioned earlier, Heinz Werner (1948), in the autogenetic tradition, elaborated what he called the orthogenetic process in human development. The central idea in the orthogenetic process is that the initial stage of the child's mental organization is global. That is to say, it is composed of functional structures that are structurally undifferentiated and functionally unrelated. The orthogenetic process is directed (teleology) towards increasing differentiation, centralization, and hierarchical integration in the child's mental processes. Here the process of development is seen as active and self-regulating while hierarchical in description. We might add that it also seems to unfold from a generally enfolded process. In Werner's words development proceeds toward:

a. increasing differentiation and specification of primitive action systems that are initially fused with each other in one global organization, causing

b. the emergence of novel and increasingly discrete action systems that are also increasingly integrated within themselves, such that

c. the most advanced (differentiated, specialized, and internally integrated) systems hierarchically integrate (functionally subordinate and regulate) less developed systems.

This model does appear to fit the observed description of the development of specific behaviors except that it perhaps may not be confined to a "hierarchical" process exclusively. It is quite possible to see these processes "unfolded." Truly, as developing functions progressively differentiate into increasingly discrete yet internally balanced systems of actions, their structures have indefinite boundaries at first, then more integrated networks, and finally, well articulated functions. The fact that they are locally discrete yet also non-locally integrated and directed from the very beginning implies to us a deeper order or teleos that is not initially seen by the exclusively analytic lens. This deeper order is felt, however, by intuition and born out by subsequent development. It would appear that processes do hierarchically integrate, but that they also unfold from a higher enfolded unity. This implicit integration of both hierarchical and enfolded processes is a more balanced representation of these creative processes than the primarily "masculine" imagery of the raised hierarchy. The creative organs from the very beginning are both male and female. More variation, creativity, and spontaneous play is possible in this way.

Given the sometimes abstract notions that appear to underlie or give rise to these behaviors and structures, it would be helpful to be specific at times as to the exact behaviors, etc., that we are talking about. Otherwise things could seem adrift in a sea of loose abstractions. A table is provided that gives a general sequence of the actions and behaviors at hand. It is not absolute because we all have our own developmental curves and Oxbow Lakes. It is, however, a map of the general course and current of the river. Let us look very closely at the first year. Please note Chart 2.1.

CHART 2.1. Developmental Milestone

	0-2 months	3-5 months	6-8 months	9-11 months
Perceptual	Follows moving object past midline. Stares at object, does not reach the object. Stares at surroundings.	Reaches for dangling object. Integration of grasp reflex. Moves head to track moving objects.	Retains 2 objects when 3rd is offered. Scoops up food and attains it. Uses thumb opposition.	Pokes with isolated finger. Uses pincer grasp with objects. Attempts to scribble with crayon on paper.
Cognitive	Coordinate eye movement. Visually prefers people to objects.	Repeats random moves (primary circular reaction). Watches place where moving object disappeared. Coordinates two actions in play.	Attains partially hidden object. Imitates sounds and hand movements already known. Likes to look at objects upside down and create changes in perspective.	Shows knowledge of toy behind a screen. Imperfectly imitates sounds and movements not performed before.
Social and Emotional	Quiets to holding, voice, or face. Body tone improves. Smiles or vocalizes to talk and touch.	Laughs. Awareness of strange environments. Smiles at image in mirror. Reaches to familiar people.	Withdraws or cries when stranger approaches. Shows dislike when familiar toy is removed.	Shows displeasure when separated from mother in new place. Repeats vocalizations or activity when laughed at. Participates in pat-a-cake and such games.
Gross Motor	Virtually all arm, leg, and hand movements are still reflective. Startles spontaneously (more reflex). Grasps becoming involuntary	Plays with toys in hand. Fingers own hand in play at body midline. Prone: rolls to supine. Integration of more reflex.	Rotates wrist, manipulates objects. May begin to crawl. Reaches for objects with fingers overextended.	May build tower of 2 blocks. Stands alone. May use hands in sequence, e.g., feeding. May pull off socks, untie shoes.

CHART 2.1. (continued)

	12-15 months	16-19 months	20-23 months
Perceptual	Turns page of cardboard book. Removes cover from small boxes.	Places round form in formboard when 3 forms are presented. Imitates crayon stroke (crayon held with butt end tightly).	Makes vertical and circular scribble after demonstration. Folds paper imitatively. Can place 6 or more pegs in pegboard in half minutes.
Cognitive	Repeatedly finds toy when hidden under one of several covers. Balances many cubes or blocks on top of each other.	Uses a stick to try to attain object out of reach. Uses trial and error to exactly imitate new sounds, words and movements.	Imitates sounds, words, body movements, immediately and exactly without practice. Deduces location of object from indirect visual cues.
Social and Emotional	Initiates ball play or social games. Offers and releases toys to adults.	Uses mother as secure base, checking back with her frequently (refueling).	Often clings to or pushes away adult. Picks up and puts away toys on request. Plays near other children.
Gross Motor	Can place 1 or 2 pegs in game board. Scribbles spontaneously; walks alone; walks backward.	Can place 6 or 8 pegs in game board without help; "Runs" stiffly. Builds 3 or more block towers. Creeps backward down stairs.	Walks down stairs with one hand held. Jumps in place. Squats in play; then resumes standing.

That First Year

By the end of the first month after birth you will notice that virtually all the child's arm, leg, and hand movements are still reflexive. The unsupported head sags, flops forward and backward, creating a good deal of anxiety in the parent who feels that the kid is very fragile. They have often begun to stare at "objects" but do not yet reach for them. Significantly enough in this early period of perception these object patterns are most noticed when they are large and bright or of vivid color. Patterns as energetic sensory fields are perceived on all levels of feeling, auditory, visual, etc., in a buzzing, highly undifferentiated way. The gradual emergence of "form" and localization of function, feeling, etc., reflects the emergent connections between the brain and CNS and its bodily sensors. In-form-mation of this highly unstable but teleologically emergent kind seems to influence what appears to be enfolded or encoded in the greater energy field of the growing brain. This is why we believe that consciousness not only arises but also descends into human development. Localization and perception of external objects in the world occurs as the representations and patterns of the object are localized and encoded in the brain. When localization is stabilized in the brain's neural processes an "object" is perceived. The object unfolds from the prior implicate field of energy.* The holographic analogy to this neurological process is exceedingly useful in grasping this sequence of events and has acquired an enormous degree of experimental support in recent years (Pribram, 1971; 1981).

Socially, by now, he or she cries deliberately and the child's eyes will fix on the mother's face in response to her smile. The little bodies are experimenting with muscle actions and they will adjust their posture to the person who is holding them. This is an intimate communication, just as is their capacity to recognize the parent's voice. In the midst of all these warm, vulnerable, and gentle feelings between parent and child, the parents generally fail to notice that most of the time the little one's facial expression is vague and impassive! A deeper communication has already taken root.

---

*The observer seeks a stable or invariant image amid the blurred phenomena and information. In a sense, it seeks to explicate out of an implicate or enfolded meaningful order.

By two months or so, they will startle spontaneously. This is just the Moro reflex. The little hands are grasping voluntarily and may even swipe at objects sometimes. Many infants by late two months are coordinating eye movements in a circle in regarding objects and light. Many can follow them from the outer corner of the eye past the middle of the body, in some cases. In fact, the moving or contoured objects seem to keep their attention longer. Interpersonally and emotionally it is a good time for the parents because their loved one has started to visually prefer people to objects. They will stare, seemingly deeply, into the parents' faces. The whole body has improved by this time.

By three months, you will sense a real person there. Saliva, saliva everywhere! They have begun to sense that their hands and feet are extensions of themselves; they respond with the whole body to recognized faces, and, in some instances, they have even begun to vocalize when spoken to. Mind has begun to reach out physically to the world. Swiping with closed fists is common or reaching with both hands. They can retain objects in the hand intentionally now and have a pretty good grip. The hands are everywhere, in the mouth, the eyes, the face. Waiting for an expected feeding betrays the dawn of memory. The body's arms and legs can be better coordinated in side movements and the head bobs back and forth less like a baby bird now because the back and neck muscles have become more sturdy. Smiles come immediately and spontaneously. They even seem to sometimes become bored with repeated sounds and images. In essence, they seem to be aware of themselves.

Generally, near the end of four months, there is obviously a real and distinct psyche inhabiting their body! While swiping at objects may still be inaccurate, the hands may be able to take and hold small objects between the index and second figures. Memory span may be as long as seven seconds. They have already begun to adjust their responses to people and to notice the distinctness of their actions from the external result. In other words, they have come to notice themselves as distinct from the outer world and other objects. The moods are vocalized with laughter at times, and wailing with loss at others. Some become interested in their image in a mirror and all show interest in playthings, even a special toy. The really nice thing is that they can *imitate* at least several different tones!

By five months or so, there is a literal explosion in social, cognitive, motor and other behavior. When lying on their stomach, now, they can push on their hands and draw up the knees. If bottlefed, many can hold the bottle by themselves. Objects of interest are exchanged between hands. Sensorimotor coordination has enormously improved. When out shopping, or at another home, they will turn their head deliberately to a sound or to follow a disappearing object. Indeed, the world is now full of reachable objects. They will raise their hand quite deliberately in the area of an object and alternately glance between their hand and the object. Visually, they will search for fast moving objects and look for fallen objects. In the family matrix they have come to differentiate parents and any siblings from others. Mother and self are recognized in a mirror. Fear of strangers arises. They understand the names of people in many instances.

Sometime near the end of the first half year, the whole family has had to adjust. There is a great deal of communication with and through the child who now has become a knowing person. Most smile at their mirror image and try to imitate facial expressions. They prefer to play with people, especially cooperative games. Babbling is constant. There are rivers of saliva. The objects they like are held upside down to create different perspectives. They are also held out at length. Many children have come to play by holding one block, reaching for a second, and then noticing the third almost immediately! They can rotate their wrists and turn the head freely.

Vowels have generally begun to be interspersed with more consonants (generally the f, v, th, s, sh, z, sz, m, and n) and there is great variability in volume, pitch, and rate of utterance. These babbles become even more active during exciting sounds. These are the roots of real language.

Near the end of seven months, for the average child, vowels and consonants occur at random and they may try to imitate sounds or sound sequences. To the overawed parent they may even say "dada" or "mama." They have usually come to distinguish near and far objects and space. They can compare and be aware of size differences of similar objects like blocks and balls. With the head now well balanced they can hold two objects, one in each hand simultaneously, and bang them together. This adds to the noise level in the house.

By the passing of eight months he or she will push away these objects when they are not wanted anymore. They may have a hard time with confinement, which can harry a busy parent. Shouting for attention itself is frequent. The fear of strangers continues as the child becomes intensely attached to the mother. The fear of separation is usually very strong, making this a difficult period interpersonally for both. When we talk of Mahler's work on individuation and borderline behavior we will return to this.

The child can, however, often use two-syllable utterances. "Dada" and "Mama" have become specific names. She or he will listen selectively to familiar words and would seem to recognize some of them. This appears to occur as the child is able to recall past events and past actions of its own. They can anticipate events independent of their own behavior. In most instances, they are crawling by now, have a good pincer hand grasp, and combine known bits of behavior into new actions. These are the advanced sensorimotor schemes outlined by Piaget.

Nine months brings the social theater. The child, by this stage, will perform for a home audience, repeating little acts and behavior if it is applauded. Simple words are understood in the notion of possession or "my toy."

In terms of objects, they generally recognize dimensions of objects by approaching small objects with, say, a finger and thumb, but approach a large object with both hands. Building things with blocks is intrinsically interesting and in some cases helps keep a series of ideas in mind. The tenth month continues in this vein. This time sequence, again, is variable even though the sequence itself tends to be the same.

During the eleventh month parents notice that their child now actively seeks approval and tries to avoid disapproval. Guilt arises. Speech is partially gibberish with an increasing number of intelligible sounds. Anywhere from 3 to 15 words may be known. The words are recognized as symbols for objects such as toy, food, dog. They can often easily place and remove objects in boxes and appear to be aware of their own actions and their implications. They can associate properties with things like barks for dogs and pointing upward when a bird is sighted. For some annoying periods of time they may repeatedly remove their shoes, socks, and clothes, and find this funny. It is almost that funny to the parent. Many, many other such social and cognitive behaviors unfold.

Eventually by the end of this first year, for the normative child, many emotions are expressed and recognized in others. The bodily self is clearly distinguished from others. Their need and ability to undress themselves has increased as has their interest in unwrapping objects, toys, and other things. Objects are perceived as detached and separate and they can search for them if lost. Memory has greatly increased in these cases. However, negativism has also increased and they may refuse a meal, or even throw a tantrum. The parent hopefully learns to develop even more humor and patience. Brief "sentences" may appear.

All of the above is the general content and sequence of unfolding behaviors that first year. Obviously some children acquire certain behaviors sooner or later than others. The process is by no means absolute as to the dawn of specific behavior. However, the general process and sequence describes this unfolding for the average or normative child. Please refer to Chart 2.1 for this sequence and also for behavior and cognitive/social/motor unfolding beyond the first year. To describe each year would take too much time and space in this long chapter. A similar suggestion is made for Chart 2.2. Let us leave observations and return now to the more theoretical side of this study.

Variation is allowed and, indeed, the place of consciousness is implicit as these action and cognitive systems become more integrated and complex. Each level allows higher structures to emerge but, also, one can revert or regress to a lower, more primitive, and earlier structure. If you have a second child within several years of the first, you can readily see the regression in the behavior of the first child for awhile. It is easy to see how this theory and brief outline of early development lends itself well to other areas of interpretation, especially in psychopathology and comparative anthropology. Many useful but limited parallels can be drawn between the reasoning structures of the child and the reasoning structures of the "primitive mentality." Take, for example, our early mother of the lakes. Many of her primitive or archaic reasoning processes can be vividly experienced, of course, in the actual experience of schizophrenia or psychosis that is devoid of noetic urgency. Many of these same processes can also be seen in the experiences of those who are transcending those very structures of the ego-mind that give rise to those particular structures and defensive patterns in the first place. The former is illness, the latter is what is termed a "spiritual emergency." Werner's work is compelling and powerful in its scope not only because it fits the mold of the vital and human mental world so well, but it has the intuitive pull of a great and vastly intricate, yet unfinished, poem.

Jean Piaget

Piaget's (1952) great humanizing work also parallels the self-regulating processes of maturation, particularly physiological maturation as outlined by Gesell (1946). Piaget saw human development as a continual process seeking higher and higher equilibration or balance. For him, development proceeds from relative disequilibrium to increasing equilibrium. The child's innate biological needs to feed and survive, and unfold, pull like the arch of evolution upward to lead the system to take in or incorporate material and data from the external environment. This is called assimilation. The child must then subtly and intelligently alter the system itself in order to deal with the assimilated world. This latter process is simply termed accommodation. Thus, assimilation and accommodation work together for the transformation of the system. This transformation process is then referred to as adaptation. This dynamic process occurs continually. When the child is in disequilibrium, from an internal need or imbalance, the child or organism will operate to establish a greater sense of equilibrium. Thus the child changes him/herself and develops while learning to deal with both the changing internal and external environment. This sense of body-mind disequilibrium is helpful in moving from one transitional phase to another in development. The new behavior is fragile, the new capacity to cognitively manipulate is weak and may sometimes miss the mark, but grows with repetition and insight. These include cognitive structures up to and potentially beyond those outlined by Piaget. Here again a sense of teleology arises.

Yet is not a similar process seen in all self-organizing structures, including those of the material world? Ilya Prigogine (Jantsch, 1980), a chemist, won the Nobel prize for outlining exactly how this process of self-organization occurs in chemical processes. A new ordering principle emerges in certain so-called "dissipative structures" in chemical processes. A certain "order through fluctuation" occurs that is seemingly beyond the heat-death epitaph of the second law of thermodynamics. This apparently occurs in novelty, in open systems functioning far from normal equilibrium. This is not to reduce what the human does to the material plane but rather to show that in all the planes of organization, from the organic, which is clearly self-organized, to the material, which may not apparently seem self-organized, that the process of self-organization is alive there also. This theory and approach of self-organization can even be seen in the "new physics" in the bootstrap hypothesis of Jeffrey Chu and Frijof Capra, where nature is not so much a court of inflexible natural laws, but rather a dynamic theater of interconnected relations and events manifesting a certain self-consistency in operation (Capra, 1975).

Piaget extended this idea, of self-organization and balance of various needs and structures to attain a higher equilibrium, into the finer structures of cognitive intelligence. Piaget outlined specific and sequential stages in the development of cognitive structures. Each stage seeks equilibration or balance. These stages begin with the rudimentary sensorimotor stages, where actions predominate, and where the first notions of "objects"–coordination of objects, space, time and causality considerations and categories, originate. This stage itself has six substages of sensorimotor activity, all in sequential order. We will not elaborate each one here but, rather like with the earlier chart on developmental milestones, will summarize the highlights. In a brief section near the end of this chapter, we will outline what are seen to be the neurophysiological correlates and substrate of these cognitive growth periods. It needs to be remembered, however, that the time period of these milestones is not rigid for their appearance. Rather, their invariant sequence of emergence is the point. The patterns are purely practical or action categories, not as yet ideas or thinking. Please notice Chart 2.2 for the stages of purely cognitive development up to and beyond those outlined by

CHART 2.2. Stages of Cognitive Development.

Stage	Dynamic Processes and Transformations
Sensori-Motor sub-stage #1 Radical Egocentrism Age 1-1 1/2 months	Spatial – A constantly shifting theater. Reflexive neuromuscular coordination provides only a sense of displacement between "here" and "there." The intuition built on here vs. there vs. here again is later concept of reversibility. Temporal – Simple duration immanent in a practical series of the child's acts. Objects – As yet they have no permanent status or substantial form. Causality – Merely "a sort of feeling of efficiency or of efficacy linked with acts." Simple desire/feeling extended in the world. Summary – Global, undifferentiated feelings and needs. Reactive gestures and neuromuscular actions exercised. No ideas of inner and outer, you or me.
Sensori-Motor sub-stage #2 Anticipating and Generalizing Age 1-4 months	Spatial – Limited to consolidating, extending and coordination of previous stage actions. Temporal – Limited to consolidating, extending and coordination of previous stage actions. Causality – Limited to consolidating, extending coordination of previous stage actions. Objects – Visually follows a moving object. Then extends these movements to the body. No search yet for objects out of the visual field. Objects exist only as "things-of-action/posture-in-progress." Summary – Child begins constructing anticipatory signs e.g., crying, which gets needs satisfied. Thus arises initial transitional representation forms between signs of previous stage and signals of the next stage.

Piaget. This chart will be referred to several times throughout this chapter. It is the distillation of the scheme or unfoldment of cognitive development from the earliest sensorimotor period, when the infant is totally embedded in matter and the world, to the post-formal era where the adult, through the refinement of consciousness, becomes tangibly aware of the literal light itself that is the substra-

Stage	Dynamic Processes and Transformations
Sensori-Motor sub-stage #3 Static Coordinating Age 5-8 months	Spatial – Hand and eye coordination lead to first cognitive system of actions in space. A tactile-kinesthetic sense of space evolves. Child begins to observe itself and its actions. Temporal – Sense of before and after in experience emerges. A sense of temporal series and memory arises through actions bearing on several objects months at once. Causality – Differentiation between desire, action and result. Objects – Memory of immediately past things-of-action. Begins to look for objects out of the visual field. No real sense of permanence however. Summary – A functional coordination between various schemes of action appears. Intentional grasping occurs, thus indicating the primitive arrival of analysis and generalization. No imitation yet of actions suggested by others, yet able to reproduce already learned actions. Thus the first communication and signal-to-action scheme arise.
Sensori-Motor sub-stage #4 Mobile Coordinating and Signaling Age 8-10 months	Spatial – Child sees things as existing in space beyond the immediate visual field. Differentiation between changes of position and state. No reversibility yet. Temporal – Series begins to become objective. Coordination of actions and goals spells simple reversibility of time sequences, although only primitive. Causality – Transitional phase because "causality becomes detached from the child's action without, however, being attributed once and for all to objects independent of the self." Yet the child also realizes that it is not the sole source of causality or action. Objects – Objects become permanent in the past and the present as things-of-action. The child looks for hidden things. Summary – Child develops signal activity and sets the stage for later truly symbolic activity. Signals are expressed in posture and sound that mimic the desired situation. This however is not yet make-believe play.

CHART 2.2. (continued)

Stage	Dynamic Processes and Transformations
Sensori-Motor sub-stage #5 Experimentation Age 12-15 months	Spatial – Because the search for objects beyond the immediate visual field occurs, there occurs the elaboration of the relationships of movements within space. The child can account for displacements yes, but can as yet only perceive space, not imagine it. Temporal – For short periods the child has accurate memory of the above spatial and object displacements. Causality – The child sees himself no longer as the center of actions and begins to conceptualize a dependency between its actions and separate objects in space. Objects – Things are permanent as long as the changes in position occur within the same visual field. Summary – Intentional actions now lead to active experimentation with creative, new actions to meet needs. It goes beyond the immediate body to gestural representation of other things in the environment. Soon unrelated gestures are coordinated. Pointing is a good example.
Sensori-Motor sub-stage #6 Symbolizing Age 15-21 months	Spatial – "The child is now able to locate a hidden object even when he has not perceived its displacement because he can now represent the displacement to himself." The notions of behind, inside and upon have arrived. Temporal – The child constructs an extended past. Causality – Causes can now be constructed in the presence of their effect without perceiving the exact action of the cause. Representation of causality occurs. Objects – "Representation permits the child to conceive of objects that are not spatio-temporally present and leads to his internal expectation that when an object disappears it does not dissolve." Summary – This last sensori-motor era sees the rise of true mental operations which are interiorized schemes of action. The child reflects and represents primarily non-verbally yet symbolization begins to unite with verbal actions. Pretending occurs.

Stage	Dynamic Processes and Transformations
Symbolic-Operations	Spatial – Spatial understanding is based on movement in the environment and limited memory capacity. Space is personal action-space.
sub-stage #1	Temporal – A future perspective emerges. Primitive symbols are used to evoke and reconstruct absent events in the child's memory.
Pre-conceptual: Gestural-Verbal Acts Age 1 1/2-4 years	Causality – Reasoning gradually becomes more independent of immediate events and is so organized. Space and time are not seen as independent, but rather to participate in each other. Physical causality is still fused with social necessity and personal desire. "The child thinks in a magico-phenomenalistic fashion such that desires for physical proximity influence objects, which are obedient."
	Objects – Object permanence remains as in earlier stages but lose their identity in different spatial locations.
	Summary – Human activity is the metaphor for all action. The Life-Force is seen to animate everything e.g., stones, trees, dogs, etc., as long as these objects are in motion. Words are primarily global in their reference to things and events. When specific words are employed better, the symbol refers to ideas mid-way between particular referents constructed by earlier sensori-motor actions and true symbols created by later mental operations. "Individual identity and . . . general class" are still confused.

tum of and which expresses and enfolds that original matter that the organism found itself embedded in. This chart draws freely from the work of Piaget (1954; 1968), Inhelder (1964), Werner and Kaplan (1963), Koplowitz (1984), Riegel (1973), Langer (1969) and their numerous co-workers.

Language

From roughly the age of 15 to 21 months, symbolizing ability usually dawns and marks the end of the exclusively sensorimotor stage of actions. We believe this period has neurological correspondences in brain growth. A later observational theorist, Margaret

CHART 2.2. (continued)

Stage	Dynamic Processes and Transformations
Symbolic-Operations sub-stage #2 Intuitive-Verbal Acts Age 4-7 years	Spatial – While developing a grasp of distance, the child still cannot conceive of pure "empty space which has invariant geometric properties that are conserved and that are partially independent of the objects in the space." Temporal – "the intuition of time is bound to the phenomenal quality of the objects he is observing and the type of movement they are engaged in." Time is highly personalized. Causality – The first pure physical explanation of causality emerges. Continuity and physical contact between objects, not personal needs, are the new basis of causality. Objects – The child now acts upon objects as though their identity remained stable regardless of location. However, the child does not understand the conservation of objects. Summary – While mental operations are still highly associated to immediate, phenomenal relations, the child begins to differentiate between "all" and "some" and create a system of wholes and parts, of classes and sub-classes. The concept of number takes root in the notion of "more" or less in a certain class or configuration.

Mahler, made much use of this newly emerged capacity for symbol activity. We will come back to this later in the discussion of the separation-individuation process. The next stage for Piaget is the *symbolic operational stage*. The slow sequencing of the child's behavior ends and more rapid cognitive styles enter. This is quickened with the dawn of language around 24 months or so. This period of cognitive development unfolds and lasts until approximately seven years of age when by the impetus of evolutionary forces a radically new series of structures emerges. At this later stage, the child can *imagine* and *consciously reflect* on the world. No doubt the mature adult's creativity in a whole host of areas has

Stage	Dynamic Processes and Transformations
Symbolic-Operations sub-stage #3 Concrete–Verbal Acts Age 7-10 years	Spatial – "The child develops a limited, objective group coordination of parts in total space . . . He begins to understand that space (the container) has invariant properties that are independent of the objects in it . . . he is now able to coordinate two reference systems." Temporal – Coordination of succession (first, second, etc.) with duration in a coherent system. The concept of velocity is possible. Causality – The discovery of other possible viewpoints in addition to one's own as constituting reality. Thus new priority and emphasis given to spatio-temporal and mechanistic aspects of relations and events. Movement and force account for change. This is based however on perceived facts, not deductive reasoning yet. Object – "The child can now related successive appearances as reversible transformations. Objects that have changed not only maintain their permanence and identity but are conserved." Number – "The child differentiates the number of objects being counted (quantity) from the actions he performs upon the objects and the configuration in which the objects are perceived (quality)." Summary – True mental differentiation has emerged. The child has a conceptualization of classification systems and has evolved an essentially physical or perceived, not yet logical, conception of space, time, objects, number and causality. This is the so-called "thawing out of intuitive structures." The new mental suppleness is reflected in the fact that: 1. "Thought is no longer bound to the particular phenomenal state of events but begins to take into account successive transformations ('detours and reversals')." 2. Thought evolves from egocentric to many perspectives. The possibility of multiplication occurs from the coordination of several viewpoints into a system and 'logical group of objective reciprocities.' 3. The child is able to isolate specific variables in a situation and apply initial reversible operations on them. This allows for the development of conservation." The logic of the cognitive activity . . . is the product of the child's differentiation of two reversible operations, inversion and reciprocity."

CHART 2.2. (continued)

Stage	Dynamic Processes and Transformations
Formal Operations Age 10-15 years	Spatial & Temporal & Object & Number Causality: After concrete operations in these areas the child constructs a formal 'logical theory of events' that is both independent of any specific episode and also open to events that as yet exist only in abstract possibility. "Formal thinking is both thinking about thought (propositional logic is a second-order operational system which operates on propositions whose truth, in turn, depends on class, relational and numerical operations) and a reversal of relations between what is real and what is possible (the empirically given comes to be inserted as a particular sector of the total set of possible conbinations)." This of course is dependent on greater mental suppleness and virtuosity, and also the "conscious discovery of perturbations" in the fabric of reality. The final mental capacity here is "the integration and simultaneous usage of the two reversible operations, reciprocity and inversion, such that they become functionally equivalent. This development leads to the structuring of a combinatorial system . . . that can be formulated by means of implications, equivalences, disjunctions, conjunctions, exclusions . . . etc., depending on the case. . . This combinatorial system consists of the grouping of four cognitive operations or mental means of transformation: direct, inverse, reciprocal and inverse of the reciprocal transformations . . . It is the integrated structure of mental operations that henceforth underlies the invariant theoretical cognition of the physical concepts of objects, number, space, time and causality."

roots in this new symbolic period. There is a greater capacity to develop other perspectives. This means some loss of grandiosity and naive egocentricity. The transient cognitive structures that had emerged and allowed for more actions in the environment and the development of egocentricity, so that the psychic apparatus could influence the environment, must now change or slowly dissipate as

Stage	Dynamic Processes and Transformations
Post-Formal Operations Age 15-?	Interdependence of Space, Time, Object, Boundary and Causality: Causality – Post formal operations construct linear causal chains. These linear chains are abstractions of larger, cyclical and multileveled chains which can always be broken down into more discrete linear chains. The reverse is not true. Causality is specific to an empirical, local event in formal operations. Causality is interconnected and nonlocal or all pervasive in post formal operations. Objects, space and time, and all boundary notions are enfolded in a higher order, all pervasive causal nexus.
Post-Formal Operations	Spatial – In formal operations space is both independent of the observer and independent of time. In post-formal operations space is recognized as a construct (as the sensori-motor period shows) that is useful. Also space is seen embedded in time as in relativity theory.Thus matter in objective space becomes an abstraction from energy pervasive in space-time. Time – Time, like space, is independent of the observer in formal operations, but is implicated in space itself by post-formal operations. It becomes a construct (again!) that can be used as a specific or as all pervasive. Objects – Objects are permanent in formal operations, their identity stable through transformations. They are independent or separate in the causal chain and exist separately from the knower. By post-formal operations, given space-time as an all pervasive continuum, objects are not solid or permanent by share identity. The knower gives meaning to the known and thus structures its discrete perception. Boundary – Thus boundary is no longer separate, closed or independent. Variables are interdependent in the post-formal mode. Discrete causes and objective boundaries are abstractions from an all pervasive, undivided whole. There are no "fundamental building blocks." The formal operation of boundary and variable isolation with "all things being equal" is no longer absolute. Interpenetration and shared valence emerges. Boundaries are functional, not absolute, and help make sense of the experience.

structures, such that more inclusive cognitive structures and information can arise. This entails some fluctuation, so there is an internal and external sense of disequilibration.

There are at least three powerful consequences that arise with this earlier stage of development of language. The first is the possibility of verbal exchange with others, which is an overture to the higher and later socialization of action. Secondly, with language comes the *internalization* of words and images. Thus, thought itself has arisen, which is nourished by internal signs, symbols and systems. Finally, with this new genie out of the bottle arises the internalization of action such that rather than only a perceptual and motor-formed reality, the child can actually *represent* reality intuitively with these internal images. Mental experiments can now be executed on reality. This is the upbeat part of the saga. On the other side of the mountain the child "discovers" that he or she is also only one element or entity amid a sea of others. These others will be experienced as external and separate from the perceiver, even though the images of these others remain "within" the child. This is an aspect of the rise of the ego. It is still pre-personal, but the long march has begun. It is the Copernican revolution we all discover and most of us pass through. At this point in development, the world is infused with the life-force and everything is endowed with life and intentionality. It is intelligent but naturally pre-logical. Yet intelligence had already entered the scene before language arrived! In a sense, pure, but certainly only practical, action-bound intelligence was in operation in the early coordination of sensorimotor patterns or schemas for handling the environment, as we saw in our description of the first year. The point, however, is that some form of real intelligence was actively existent *prior* to language. Let us go on in this slow braiding of the roots of growth.

Vygotsky

Vygotsky (1962), taking a different perspective on this momentous advent of language, tacitly supports the notion of intelligence prior to language. Vygotsky demonstrated that thought itself as well as speech had different genetic roots. This could even be seen in other, highly socialized primates. In humans the functions of thought and speech do not integrate until language dawns. "When speech begins to serve intellect and thoughts begin to be spoken" the child's world consciously transforms itself. Everything has a name! Previous to this, for Vygotsky, speech was socially echoed babble and thought was in a prelinguistic stage of image and actions. Despite this great marriage at two years old, some aspects of thought never reach speech, and implicitly, *some aspects of intelligence never fuse with thought!* This notion of an intelligence prior to thought and mental forms is crucial to our own emerging perspective on human development.

Concrete Operations

Next are observed massive changes that ensue through the following five years in four sequential stages, resulting in the ability to go beyond strictly phenomenal data, to work with "pure" concepts such as numbers. It is the dawn of true reason. Moral reasoning is clearer and less egocentric and he or she can actually accept the position of the "other." This, at about seven to ten years of age, sets the stage for what are called "concrete operations." This stage, as we shall see in the later brief section on neural correlates of cognitive development, is accompanied by surges in brain growth in specific areas. For now it is good to know that these concrete operations are "formed by a kind of thawing out of intuitive structures, by the sudden mobility which animates and coordinates the configurations that were hitherto more or less rigid despite their progressive articulation" (Langer, 1969). The result of this greater field of cognitive operation at the stage of concrete operations is that:

1. Thought is no longer bound to any particular state of events, but begins to take into account successive transformations ("detours and reversals").

2. Your child's thought can and does change from egocentrism to perspectivism, and it becomes possible for him or her to perform multiplicative operations. The child begins to coordinate different points of view into a system or logical group of objective reciprocities. He or she begins to realize that the nature of things is not rigidly absolute but relative to the viewpoint from which it is coincident. For example, when your child views liquid being poured from one container into another, he or she no longer sees only the

change in height or in width but both. Simultaneous recognition that from one viewpoint the amount has increased, while from another viewpoint it has decreased, is necessary for the multiplicative coordination of these two variables.

3. The child begins to be capable of mentally performing transformational operations upon phenomenal configurations. This means that he or she can mentally isolate the relevant variables of a display and can apply reversible operations upon these variables. This ability is the mental source of the ability to form such concepts as conservation. Thus the logic of the cognitive activity that develops through this whole stage of concrete operations is the product of the child's differentiation of two reversible operations, inversion (the operation of negation) and reciprocity (the operation of compensation for a difference such that the product is an equivalence operation or relational structure). It should be noticed, however, that reciprocity and inversion are not really coordinated until Piaget's final stage of formal operations.

The Rise of Formal Operations

The final stage in Piaget's system includes formal logic, the easy reversal of relations between the real and the possible and the general ability to be independently reflective on thought. Many other structures come into play that allow for the numerous adult cognitive abilities, including a *linear* conception of causality, boundary formation, and purely creative conceptualization. This stage is the stage in which most good technical and other thinking occurs, but we suggest here that there are stages even beyond these of formal operations which generally begin around the age of 12 to 15 or so. This stage, too, has a neurological substrate.

This stage of formal operations appears to engender a "logic of propositions" in marked contrast to the logic of relations, classes and numbers engendered by what are termed the earlier concrete operations. This system of implications that orders these propositions is an abstract translation of the system of "inference" that governs the concrete operations. These formal operations which are the groundwork of adolescent cognition introduce a radically new ability which helps detach and *liberate cognition* from concrete reality, thus allowing and even facilitating more self-reflection and theory construction.

It is extremely interesting to observe the revolution of thought at this period. Adolescent egocentricity takes the peculiar form of belief in the omnipotence of reflection. Idealism is the lifeblood of adolescent conception. The adolescent often has his or her first serious encounter with philosophical and metaphysical insight. Religion as theology becomes important, not merely as faith! The adolescent constructs world systems, usually idealistic and altruistic with a good dose of grandiose design that may touch upon megalomania. Devotional feelings arise along with a greater sensitivity to his or her social perception by others. However, the adolescent, given this first true flush of the adult world, will generally not test out their great propositions with others. An interest in politics or religion may arise in this period of hypothetical-deductive reasoning. This is a great and marvelous stage of unfoldment to the deeper mysteries and intelligences of life. It is also deeply enmeshed in egocentric idealism. At best, the adolescent touches deep, archetypal images and reservoirs of knowledge and intelligence. At worst he or she becomes withdrawn, misunderstood, schizoid, and depressed. We will return to this stage in the subsequent chapter on the fall into paranoid thinking. Let us go on to those stages which are presently unfolding that were not touched by Piaget.

The stage of formal operations pulls for linear causality, boundary formation, and is imbued with a sense of being separate or alienated from the object of study. It does not allow for the dialectical or reversible in causality which appears in the new contemporary systems thinking in science. It does not account for creativity beyond linear relationships. Circular thinking, spontaneous symmetry breaking, and inherently changing boundaries are not adequately accounted for. Yet these forms of thinking abound in modern science. Thus beyond this stage of formal operations one observes a post-formal stage of cognitive operations (see Chart 2.1). It has been termed the stage of dialective operations (Riegel, 1973) where apparently contradictory thinking is valid. Others see this stage as more fitting for general systems and open boundary processes (Koplowitz, 1984). Here the principle of undivided wholeness of processes is seen. It is a level or perspective that is much in keeping with the yogic perspective of unitary thinking in which, as Bateson pointed out, ontology and epistemology become fused because the subject, in the process of knowing, becomes identified and fused with the object of knowing in a common ground. This wellspring of insight and intuition will come up again later. Right now it is mentioned in order to round out the schema of cognitive development.

The First Sense of Ego

The ego develops in this overall system from a state of dominant naive biological drives and associated psychophysiological tension states and other rudimentary associations, to a prolonged period of egocentricity in which the environment is progressively mastered to the awareness of conscious intelligent functional others in the world. In each stage and series of substages, the ego, which experiences the "I" sense, must identify with and use the cognitive structures it acquires and develops. This process itself reaches a crisis when later that "I" or ego must itself become a stage or tool for the higher cognitive functions to evolve! The subsequent identification and consequent disidentification of the ego or "I" sense with these emergent structures is a less well-understood process. Suffice it to say here that the root of the ego-sense arises initially from states of "tension" arising from psychophysical zones of interaction (Sullivan, 1953) and as such it is asserted that all egoic development, regardless of how mental and sophisticated, arises from these earlier sensorimotor actions in the organism and reflects this at some level, and at some level, always remains concerned with the *perpetuation* of this sense. This ego-tension is a balance between absolute terror and euphoria. This tension is initially an experience of the body and therein it is necessary to braid this part of the story together in order to make a point. This means, to some extent, to touch the ground floor of development again. For that, we focus our lens on that other pillar of ascent in the saga of human development, the ground state and trajectory of the ego.

BODY TENSION AND THE RISE OF EGO

While relaxed at some time, have you ever noticed that when there is very little "tension" in any part of your body that there is also no discrete sensory data? All feels diffuse, unbounded. Very low levels of tension are experienced as profound relaxation. Beyond this, in situations of almost no body tension at all, the human reactions can range from extreme fear of loss of control (ego-death) to rejuvenation and mystical elevation (re-birth). At this point, a person mentally projects wildly as in sensory deprivation experiments, or even allows OBE (Out-of-Body Experiences) to occur. In Yoga, when this is learned in a controlled manner, it is called pratayahara, or conscious sensory withdrawal.

As the mind and cognitive structures become capable of abstract conceptualization and freedom from all psychophysical references, the more difficulty the ego has in directing or owning the whole process. The roots of the ego arise initially to help govern a physical and subjective environment that requires action upon it in order to survive, compete/cooperate, and exercise power of many kinds. It has survival capacities. Like any system, biological, social or religious, it seeks to stabilize and perpetuate itself. The ego, as a function, generally does well in the management and balance of tensions and needs.

It seems that the increasingly complex action systems of the organism that begin to co-ordinate the needs and satisfactions of the child's world become more stabilized with use and success. The sensorimotor schemas that have been spoken about are held to reflect, biologically, the operations of the physical world and as such have intelligence *imminent* and *implicit* in them in the form of potential actions of increasing complexity. The tensions naturally arise from biological needs and drives that must be reduced or satisfied in an organized way if the child is to survive. Piaget referred to these tensions as periods of internal and external disequilibrium which demand change and adjustment. With the success of these operations or actions in the world, patterns of satisfactions and nourishment become stabilized. Awareness localizes around these episodes and zones of interaction in the body, e.g., mouth, hands, anus, etc. With the increasing stabilization of tension-satisfaction interactions, a primitive sense of organization imbues awareness. Out of this fleeting process arises the earliest eyes of the ego.

The ego then is not an entity, it is a process. The ego is not consciousness itself, but rather participates in consciousness. The ego is only awake! When we dream, there is sometimes an observer of the dream process itself, usually there is only the dream process occurring in the unconscious terrain. When the conscious dreamer in the dreams turns attention back on the observer itself, all observing ego dissolves in a sea of light and yet consciousness remains.

This emergent ego plays well as long as the cognitive structures are compatible with duality. The ego appears rooted in duality. However, as the cognitive structures continue to evolve, as elaborated in the last section, a greater schema of structures reflecting unitary conceptualization in a more sophisticated way emerges in the human cognitive system. These stages are post-formal operations, mentioned earlier, that emerge after Piaget's structures. These latter systems are as radical an improvement over egoic and dualistic cognition as the dualistic cognition was originally a great leap beyond primitive concepts of the One. We here are distinguishing between *primitive mental concepts* of the One and the primordial intuition of the One. To be sure, the ego can regress, as Werner and others point out, to more primitive modes of cognition in states of illness, but these all involve fear and the threat of ego-death and psychophysical extinction. In yogic terminology these are referred to as root chakra preoccupations. In other cases, however, where there is conscious movement to other levels that necessitate the diminution of the ego, there is profound peace and the intuition or recognition of luminosity. This is the transcendental framework. The latter appears to be more compatible with these later cognitive developments than the former. Let us now move away from primarily cognitive development and look at how this emergent process called the ego deals with the powerful *affective* currents of early development, how it creates structures that are useful and necessary, but which also hinder development at a certain point. When the ego is healthy, its structures are functional and manage information and then *dissipate* when no longer functional. When unhealthy, these structures seize and constrict in the face of internal or external crisis.

THE PSYCHOANALYTIC VISION

The psychoanalytic theory, that brilliant synthesizing vision that emerged from the genius of Freud in the last century, does not see the child's behavior as those two theories of Werner and Piaget outlined above. Piaget and Werner present very *rational* systems of cognitive, and to some extent affective or emotional, development. Rather the psychoanalytic theory does not see man as primarily rational at all. Man is perceived as basically affective and *irrational.* This is a profound difference that eventually leads to very unsubtle differences in world view.

The child in psychoanalytic mythology is seen as reluctantly learning control over his or her behavior, impulses and passions which, of course, always means coming to terms with frustration and conflict. Thus, at the very basis of this psychoanalytic view, the child is seen as a being who is in conflict with society and is driven to action and growth by passions or instincts and external forces adjusting to internal needs and demands. It all feels like a great J. M. W. Turner painting of the Hudson Valley School, where the small conscious and reasonable lives of humans are acted out against the backdrop of immense primordial pressure and elemental contacts.

There are more mellow and gracious expositions of this very heroic and Romanticist view. Erik Erikson might be called a Freudian revisionist since so much of his work is permeated with a nurturant insight and upbeat genesis that it gives light to the sometimes pathology saturated lowlands of psychoanalytic exploration. He pointed out that at different stages of development in this process, a process which Erikson (1963) calls epigenetic stages in human development, different needs and dynamics unfold and come into play. At each stage in this epigenetic process, the affective instinctual energy which the child is born with is invested in different parts of the body in a proscribed sequence at determinate times in the life cycle. That specific function, such as oral sucking, etc., becomes the child's predominant mode of action, etc., at that particular period. It characterizes a stage of child psychosexual development which has profound implications for his or her later involvement in the interpersonal and intrapsychic world. Here we can see that a pattern of recurrent transactional patterns emerges at specific stages and develops deeply structured ways of handling emotional or affective energy. Because imagery is primitive and affective charges are *largely* based on family/intimate patterns, and also because much of this occurs before the stable, intact, separate "ego" is a daily reality, one sees the profound development and influence of the family's unconscious modes of learning.

There are implications for the family matrix into which the child is born. The family matrix influences the currents of development within each psychosexual stage to a profound degree. The work of Harry Stack Sullivan (1953) and Margaret S. Mahler et al. (1975) offers insights that are to some extent allied with the psychodynamic vision. Mahler, clearly, is firmly established in the Freudian psychoanalytic object-relations tradition, whereas the tradition of Harry Stack Sullivan involves different assumptions that in many ways include psychodynamic similarities. All other theories of development from this point of view are actually variations from the basic ones previously outlined.

There is a general consensus that these intrapsychic structures consolidate somewhere between the rise of the ego and language at around two years old, *and* the end (in the West) of the Oedipal period. Repression as a function of psychic energy is then a stable process. What is not an acceptable aspect of the system is considered "not-me" or ego dystonic and repressed. The borderline and psychotic tendencies are seen rooted in processes established before this secure stabilization of repressive capacities. The psychoenergetic process of repression moves like a wave-form to suppress unwanted and disorganizing images and impulses and thereby gives rise to the psychoneurotic tendencies, e.g., obsessive-compulsive and paranoid. We will return to this in subsequent chapters.

It is stressed here that in addition to the intimate family and intrapsychic dramas above that there is also the need to recognize the biologically rooted process of the human being that arches toward the Absolute in his or her experience. In the light of recognizing the Absolute as rooted in the very nature of the human aspiration, it is helpful to look very closely at the marvelous work of Ken Wilber (1981) and his perceived two forms of ontogenetic development. His work is especially noteworthy because in many ways he comes closest to integrating the powerful insights of the Western model for structures of conscious and cognitive development and integrating those perennial structures and stages of consciousness that have been studied in the Eastern introspective traditions.

The reader of Wilber's work is asked to note the difference between transitional psychological structures, which the child uses for a while then discards in the path of development, and perennial structures, which are formed around basic needs and states of consciousness. Wilbur has outlined them very well, and they are touched on elsewhere in this work. These two patterns of development, including transitional structures and more perennial structures criss-cross and interconnect with each other constantly. In all these theories of development, however, one goes through a pre-ego state to various levels of ego identification and involvement with psychological structures where the approach of the psychoanalytic, the orthogenetic, and the Piagetian approach end. There are stages beyond intact ego which Wilbur has outlined as transegoic states. These include states of consciousness that have been explored in depth in the traditional introspective scientific traditions of the Eastern meditative practices. In the latter part of this chapter, cognitive structures that are most highly developed and are conducive to these transegoic states are briefly identified .

All of the structures discussed here, from those of the psychoanalytic theorists to the work of Mahler and other people, are seen to be embedded in the unconscious in potentia. That is to say, the states of consciousness that are explored in yogic terms, as well as Piaget's and Werner's, all exist in the great unconscious of the infant at birth. Thus the notion of the unconscious must be *expanded* so that all these potential levels, including the potential transpersonal levels, are seen to exist in potentia at the outset. In addition to the intrapsychic unconscious, and the collective unconscious, but there is also the family unconscious that enfolds affectively and unfolds through development.The individual's consciousness is seen to be embedded in this expanded unconscious and through development, more articulated and hierarchical structures unfold from more subtle and inclusive orders. In this way, the transegoic structures can emerge in development. These include the subtle, causal and ultimate levels of consciousness. It includes the family unconscious also, which is a more "embedded" unconscious from which the person never completely emerges; nor is it necessary that the person emerge from totally in order to achieve a healthy differentiation. Each level unfolds through development and each has levels and patterns unique to it. One cannot be reduced to the other. At each level, the child seeks balance and unity as part of its very nature. This process is carried through to the highest stages of human evolution, in which one witnesses that flow of energy that is prior to cognition, radiant by nature, and intuitively known as the Absolute.

PRIMEVAL SYMBIOSIS AND THE LOSS OF THE ABSOLUTE

Narcissism

Mahler (1975) braids together these early years of the child with a perceptive and scholarly eye. She points out that "the biological birth of a human infant and the psychological birth of the individual are not coincident in time. The former is a dramatic, observable, and well-circumscribed event; the latter a slowly unfolding intrapsychic process."* The separation-individuation period of the child is a long march to autonomy. There is initially a predominance of inner or intrapsychic phenomena while external, or what are called interpersonal object relations, generally occur later between approximately the fourth month and develop on through the thirty-sixth month (three years). As alluded to earlier, Sullivan (1953), saw the rise and fall of physical and biochemical organization creating tension zones that lead to the first fragmentary moments of awareness. The child's needs get satisfied and early self-object relations (Mahler) are established. According to Sullivan, tension in the child leads to tension in the mothering one, which evokes a sense of tenderness in the parent. This is seen as the dawn of relational empathy. It is Sullivan's theory of "reciprocal emotion." Both Mahler and Sullivan have recently become experimentally supported by the work on

*We would also point out that the same is apparently true for death. That is to say that NDE, or near-death experience research, strongly suggests that for many, *clinical* death has not been identical to psychological death since some form of psychological or "personal" experience or awareness and intelligence continues, at least for a brief duration. We will not expand on this here; however, this notion is implicit throughout and rounds out a full human cycle of embodiment (see Moody 1988, 1975; and Sabom, 1982). We will look at it more closely in this chapter in the section on consciousness at death.

early child development and empathy. This seems to indicate that at least possibly the experience of tenderness and compassion is rooted in these first moments of awareness of the child and seems to be embedded in the root of the child's experience.

As stated earlier, it appears that the organism of the child seeks unity and self-organization as do all other natural phenomena in the very early stages of development. During this period one can often notice the primitive experiences of psi or ESP as exemplified in the explorations of mother-child symbiosis by Ehrenwald (1971). Here the emotional or affective field of mother and child is shared openly. There is a *shared* boundary, a *common ground* of affect and psychic causality.

Recent studies by the National Institute of Mental Health show that empathy can be seen to naturally flourish at an early age and may very well be biological or innate (*Newsweek* March 12, 1984, p. 76; Adler, 1990; Brothers, 1989). It appears that from the dawn of actual rudimentary awareness the child intuits or senses that there is an undivided whole or is undifferentiated from this undivided whole by the sense of empathic linkage to others in innumerable ways. It is the root of the child's unfolding spiritual sense. This empathic linkage has no boundary, yet emerges through its development. This bares a striking parallel to the Buddhist notion of the world pervaded by compassion. Remember that in the earliest stages of mentation for the child the world is indeed undifferentiated. The child experiences, especially in some stages of real cognitive development, that the whole world is literally "alive." In other words, a child thinks, perceives, and experiences every aspect of the world–chairs, animals, visions on TV, etc.–as actually alive and permeated by a current of living energy. Naturally, however, with progressive ego tensions and boundary formation, the body-mind becomes the object of experimentation by the newly awakened consciousness. Thus a sense of the potential loss of this body-mind island of sensation and security, with the subsequent fall back into undifferentiated wholeness, emerges in ego consciousness.

At this juncture there is *both* the experience of a "primary narcissism," and a primitive, transcendent, undivided wholeness of self and universe. One does not exclude the other. They both exist in potentia at this point. The sense of basic aliveness becomes intensely *localized* in the physical body by the developing ego. The psychic process uses the body to stabilize itself but later becomes completely identified with this body and its relations. It is much like how the force of gravity, which is invisible and boundaryless in the universe, works on matter to condense it into a solid, rigid form. Its ultimate expression is a black hole that allows no escape from its narcissistic relations.

The Emergence of "Objects"

This localization of body tension zones with the early "I" sense implies a rather subtle process of affect, perception, and bodily intelligence. Remember the earlier discussion of the young infant's behavior, especially the beginning of staring at parents or objects, etc. It appeared as the earliest attempts by the organism to cognitively focus attention on something. That stare, which the parent so warmly recognizes as real communication, also reflects the organism's attempt to focus the sense of "objectness" in its rudimentary cognitive framework. The stare helps the mind to recognize what was initially merely a "pattern" fleeting through the boundaryless, buzzing abyss. As the sense of object takes root in the perceptual field, the notion of object is localized in the brain out of more nonlocal, active fields of patterns and relations. Energy and pattern are primary; objects localize and unfold out of them. Therein arises the universe of objects. The funny part of this is that much later in life, in adult meditation, one finds that if one focuses direct attention on any specific thing exclusively, it tends to perceptually deconstruct or disappear into pattern and energy again, dissolving the mirage of discrete object!

This seemingly nonlocal psychoenergetic field that localizes body tension zones with the roots of the "I" process has another side. With this arising synthesis and *functional* sense of boundary comes the capacity for repression and differentiation. They occur together, at least initially. The more stable the emergent "I," the better repression is as a *permeable* boundary. What is repressed, in order for the infant organism to survive, are perinatal proto-experiences: amniotic fusion, sudden organism danger, cataclysmic struggles in blood, pain, and water, and the birth of unbounded light.

Psychoanalysis sees only a potentially regressive trend or, at best, an "Oceanic feeling" in this process. The subject feels omnipotent and supposedly omniscient. This oceanic feeling is, in principle, an unattainable ideal because the later ego has boundary functions and limits.

> When we are proved otherwise than omnipotent and omniscient, there is resentment, followed by an effort . . . to repair the gaps and lesions in this primal feeling . . . Many have sought and still seek in learning and in scientific work the restoration of an infantile confidence and sense of perfection. (Lewin, 1958; *J. of the American Psychoanalytic Assoc.*)

But this is to limit highly conscious intelligence to the ego alone; it is to collapse or constrict intelligence to form and content and actively repress boundaryless process and flow of life-current. Objects per se arise in the life-current or process and their actions and dynamics are then internalized by the organism.

Later at around four to six months of age the child develops the sense of object constancy. He or she begins to fear the loss and separation of others, other objects, etc. It is a complicated time. The rudimentary reflections of the child are seen in the patterns and objects of its environment–physical, emotional, and perceptual. When these dissolve or disappear the emergent mind is reminded of its own potential dissolution.

In the period of objects arising comes the fear of strangers. By now "other" has clearly arisen and to often "where there is other, there is fear." Scratch a little deeper than this and one finds the earliest intuition of death.

This whole era in the arising and stabilization of early awareness in the fluctuating sea of objects, events, and relations is fraught with potential dissolution. This early clinging to objects and forms creates a certain kind of suffering. It is a subtle pain similar to the Buddhist notion of Dukkha-viparinama or "suffering caused by change" and the fear of change. It is apparent prior to age two and evolves beyond.

Abhidhamma or Abhidharma (Hall and Lindzey, 1978) is the Eastern introspective traditional name for the psychological system that addresses this process of conflict with "objects" of various kinds. First there is what is termed Dukkhadukka, which is ordinary psychoneurotic object conflicts with others, one's own impulses, etc. Then there is the above-mentioned Dukkha-viparinama, which is a very primitive fear of any change in object status. It is less a root of psychoneurotic conflict than even more primitive borderline and psychotic processes. Here the intimate fear of the actual dissolution of the self-sense can occur with enough anxiety and boundary disturbance. There is also Samkhara-dukkha: the delusion of objects and object seeking. It is a perspective more rooted in the realm of energetic and field perception in which objects are seen to emerge or localize or unfold out of undivided and interconnected whole. Each "dukkha," so to speak, addresses a certain level of object-seeking pathology.

I do not wish to create the impression that everybody experiences objects the same way, or even develops object relations in the same exact manner. There are probably some sexual and cultural variations in human development around this emergence that can be more readily seen in related behavior. Gilligan (1982) points out that in crucial ways the scheme in cognitive moral development is somewhat different in males and females. This difference leads to different values and behaviors. This raises the question of other deeper differences in cognitive developmental processes that are reflected in our relationships with others, and in certain concepts that are held to arise from early object dynamics and object relations, e.g., reciprocity, rule flexibility and rigidity, role taking, empathy, and responsibility. This is echoed by Chodorow (1978) in her view of the family matrix:

> A girl's family setting creates a different endopsychic situation for her than for a boy. This second major difference between feminine and masculine Oedipal experiences both results from and gives further meaning to the first, to the greater length and intensity of the pre-oedipal mother-daughter relationship, and it contributes to further differentiation in relational capacities and needs.

Note how embedded here is the notion of very early "object-splitting" of internalized maternal images, etc.

This is all grist for the mill, this arising of objects in the initial and primal sea of non-localized affect, energy, and patterns in relation. It occurs as the new "I" sense arches up toward stabilization in the process called the ego.

Epistemology

It can be seen now that in the process of cognitive and ontological development, the child goes from this prior undifferentiated dim experience of unity to frustration-created isolation. The ego develops eventually on toward a sense of epistomological loneliness of the self, in which the child begins to experience a greater sense of isolation and alienation, a sense of being an island or planet of consciousness separated in a sea of ignorance with only other isolated islands of consciousness called other people to be around. The child begins to withdraw the consciousness principle from the numerous formerly "alive" things in the world. It is also held, however, that through the higher stages of development, particularly the transeogic states, the consciousness again reawakens to its prior experience of a radiant transcendent living energy pervading all the planes of consciousness and also the material-energy world. For when the more inclusive cognitive structures emerge, the schemas of greater wholes or unities appear. This allows the witness state to *expand* the prior and dim intuition of omnipotence and life-current rooted in the earliest cognitive perceptions and gradually loosen the functional hold of the dualistic ego condition on the psyche so that a more luminous and integrated sense of unity can emerge. This is the trajectory of our evolution. It is the realization of the early seers of Kemetic Egypt, the Vedic Rishis and also the testimony of mystics of every age, including our own. This realization is periodically seen in the insights of poets, occasionally in dreams, obviously in mystical states and occasionally, in an injured way, in psychosis. Again the failure to integrate and transcend into this next level of necessary human development is the fall into neurosis and psychosis.

In the pre-personal period of the child, which is what is being dealt with now, the child is pre-egoic, and as a consequence is not aware that he or she is aware of the world. Moreover, as the child has not conceptualized the idea of awareness itself, he or she is only embedded in awareness. Too much anxiety at this time with such primitive psychological structures can obviously lead to massive psychological problems. Thus, in psychosis, the person *regresses* to this pre-egoic level of perception and thinking. Neurosis is actually only a step above that because it is still living in the world as if these pre-personal dynamics existed, that is, a world of magical thinking. With maturity or development the person masters magical thinking and is able to differentiate magical thinking and desire from the multiplicity and startling reverses in causality that characterize the phenomenon of the more subtle aspects in the material and energy world. It is the *integration* into higher realms of subtle, causal, and eventually ultimate and absolute domain that the trajectory of the informed ego is aimed. Paradoxically, as the ego approaches its original goal, the foundation of the ego sense must dissolve. A great mystic once said, "In order to find oneself one must first lose oneself." This search for our ultimate self, the self that transcends body, mind, form, and thought itself is rooted in our collective, biological, genetic, and psychic history.

H. S. Sullivan

It appears as though the conventional "I" sense is a mirage in the destiny of the human body-mind in its journey through infinity. Yet, in a paradoxical way, this same "I" sense, although radically changed, may be at the very root notion of infinity and its relatives, compassion and bliss. Harry Stack Sullivan (1953), as we have mentioned, building on the needs and equilibrium structures and rise of tension states, saw these as leading to the first rudimentary experiences of "I." As a child draws this gradual distinction of the experience of "I," several other things also begin to emerge in their experience. Sullivan points out that the child eventually begins to distinguish between two absolutes of experience, that of absolute tension (terror) and that of absolute euphoria. This euphoria is intimately related to the condition or experience of bliss, which is profoundly associated with the state of deep dreamless sleep in all of us. This bliss/euphoria mode goes underground in the waking and dream states but is sought by means of seeking happiness and fulfillment of different kinds.

It does not take a great seer to recognize that this description of "absolute tension" vs. "absolute euphoria" is actually another way of saying that early boundary formation emerges in the oscillation between *expansion* to boundless infinity, i.e., the primal sea of free energy or light itself, and *contraction* to a bounded, almost, collapsed state. That primal state has all the sublime and cataclysmically embedded tendencies that operated in the perinatal environment. Immense affective energies are repressed in order for the roots of "I" to arise. In other words, this emergent oscillation and fluctuation proceeds from an identification with formless, boundless, blissful light energy and radiance, to self-contracted, fearful, boundary-forming and ego-emergent processes. One goes from ecstatic to that bound consciousness that is in fear of dissolving back into its primal state. Yet there is the functional need to evolve some sense of boundary in order to survive and evolve effectively in the world one discovers that one has been cast into. In the ecstatic state (by the way, "ecstasy" literally means out of place or out of boundary) there is the intuitive recognition that great feeling, joy, and compassion suffuse the world process itself! This again lends more support to the Buddhist precept that compassion is structured into the very stuff of creation. While Sullivan did not explicitly say this, its formulation is implicit in his view.

According to Sullivan, the child begins to develop this relationship between euphoria and tension in an inverse way. That is to say, euphoria is related to body tension in an inverse relationship of $y = 1/x$. This is the very earliest stage or awareness of a patterning of primordial energy transformations that set the stage not only for other transpersonal and transegoic states but is also deeply embedded in our other interpersonal and family dynamics.

These first experiences of absolute tension and absolute euphoria and the vast matrix between them sets the stage for our experience of energy dynamics between family members and our other interpersonal relations, which are termed by the ego psychology school as object relations. I point out in addition that this whole field of involvement with "objects" is a field in which the relationship between oneself and others is very powerful, given that these others are family members, and that this occurs over literally thousands and thousands of hours with sometimes the same repeated pattern, i.e., the family unconscious matrix. When this flows harmoniously, a normal and healthy individual develops. When there are great degrees of difficulty in this early patterning of primordial energy stages, severe problems can result.

One of the most severe in this whole constellation is when the child is experiencing the difference between absolute tension and absolute euphoria in unwanted libidinal situations in the family, such as incest. This occurs in multiple personality development, which will be explored in a later chapter. Here the child has been so devastated by terror that it uses the most primitive mechanisms that it can to protect its psychic boundaries. This early splitting and splintering goes deep within the embedded and emergent nature of the potential unconscious. This early splintering may occur, but certainly not always because all levels of consciousness, including those that will emerge later and those in which we are perpetually embedded, are all in potentia at this early dawn of childhood experience. The levels of the subtle, causal, and other realms are here in potentia. With such a shattering experience of terror that has happened in multiple personalities, the splitting goes all the way into the potential realms of the emergent causal unconscious! As the limbs are twisted so grow the trees. With other syndromes of less terrifying magnitude, the pathology is less serious. The outline of exactly how this occurs is what follows in these chapters.

At each stage in development, regardless of what stage it is, the child must manage anxiety and the threat of loss of his/her objects or other loved beings. I want to emphasize here again that these "objects" are actually energy patterns ($E = mc^2$). Given that purely material fact, it is held that they are permutations of the transcendent intelligent energy that pervades all material and energy creation and is also the substratum that pervades psychological cognitive development as well. These objects, including the "object" of other personalities, are energy patterns. Energy patterns, as has been seen in the new physics, are not related to each other in terms of billiard balls in the world bouncing off each other's solid boundaries but rather in terms of interconnected, interfacing levels of influence, reflecting and enfolding each other. This realization dawns as a tangible reality in the higher stages of development. Physicists presently speak of the quantum interconnectedness of distant systems, the Buddhists quietly refer to "dependent origination."

A CLOSER LOOK AT THE SEPARATION-INDIVIDUATION PROCESS

It has been a long march from simple sensorimotor schemas and actions, on through to localization of body tensions and "I." Leaving that behind us for awhile, let us pick up again and braid the threads of Mahler's work in this oscillating field of individuation and cooperation. Mahler (1975) and others clinically surveyed this early phase of development when the child first really begins to consciously experience himself or herself as isolated and separate from the world. There are several subphases of this process which will be touched on. The subphases are called differentiation, practicing, rapprochement, and what is termed "on the way to libidinal object constancy." There is general observational agreement on this stage sequence. Others have slightly different perspectives but they are basically very similar.

Each stage in this sequence has imprinted in it this threat or fear of object loss. Again, "where there is other, there is fear." Each phase, it seems, seeks greater integration in the arduous trek up to the Absolute. So these two dynamisms of individuation, and subsequent re-integration from this perspective, function perpetually at every phase of development. It is an extremely emotional journey. The end point is the stabilization of the ego process and all its related functions.

Differentiation

Differentiation, in the sense of the child being able to know that there is some difference between what itself is and what itself is not, dawns at approximately four months. Look back at Chart 2.1. This is also the period of peak symbiosis with the mother. It reaches its peak at approximately seven to ten months. During this phase, the earlier mentioned reciprocal affect theorem of Harry Stack Sullivan can be seen to operate between the child and the mother. That is to say that when the mother smiles the child smiles and vice versa. Vice versa because the child also learns fear and terror at this period. No doubt you have seen this in your own children or younger siblings. It is also noted that the tension focus gradually shifts from the exclusive position of the body only for the child to that of mother-images and other sensory perceptions that slowly increase in its memory process. This is, of course, rooted in all human development and perhaps includes even animal development. It increasingly occurs with the child's waking hours. At this stage–and this is important–whatever the child experiences he or she identifies with. It is true that narcissism rules, as does the polarity between euphoria and tension. The child experiences in a dim way "I am that" but as yet has no distinct experience of "I" in order to know what "that" really is. The child begins to differentiate from the mother cognitively at roughly around seven to ten months and increases his or her visual object relationship with her. This is the first stage of real psychological autonomy.

Piaget (1952) points out that at this very early period the child is beginning to perform experiments with its body and coordinating the action systems of the body. This requires an awareness of body muscle tension and actions in various ways. After the use of repetition and a number of reflexes such as sucking, etc., in infancy, the child begins to assimilate external things and accommodate to his or her internal world. This is generally in response to the sense of either internal or external disequilibrium, but also occurs as a spontaneous and creative exploration and theory building about the environment. This leads to the first acquired adaptations and also increases the child's repertoire of reflex and repetitive patterns. Here is seen a greater association between inner meaning and external images. Piaget is quick to point out that this experience occurs with each sensory modality; taste, eyes, etc. Eventually more and more is coordinated between these particular organs of perception including the hands, and a greater sense of integration and equilibration occurs. When the child moves from these primary to more secondary circular reactions, then eventually the external environment becomes more and more integrated with functional needs. They seem to develop in a hierarchical fashion, but the lens of unfoldment also focuses some light. It is seen to develop through this whole period eventuating, of course, in object constancy.

Practicing

The second major period is *practicing*, according to Mahler and others. It generally occurs from seven or ten months to roughly 15 or 16 months. During this time the infant has evolved the ability to move away physically from the mother by locomotion. It is the first really prolonged period of separation. During this time the infant learns rapid body differentiation from the mother but also establishes a specific bond with her that cannot be replaced by anyone else. The parent is as sensitive to this conscious love affair as the child is, sometimes more so. There is a growth and functioning of the separate ego sense while near the mother. This is the source or era of what can be called the genesis of a "transitional object." The child periodically moves away from the mother at this time in order to master the new environment and satisfy the innate creative impulse to see new things. It is crucial to note here that during this back and forth behavior occurring during this period, the child returns to the mother for a kind of "emotional refueling" supplied by the mother's nearness and yet must move away from her again in this process of differentiation. Any supermarket anywhere in the world is teaming with these little scenes of practicing if you look carefully at mother-child patterns. This occurs repeatedly in a powerful family affective matrix. These energy transformations, which are termed "object" transformations, are in reality transformations of affects derived from patterns of interaction in the family! If the mother is overly anxious or fearful or has serious unresolved problems of her own, this implicates the dynamics of the child. This occurs regardless of the sex of the mothering one.

Here is where one can see the origin of the borderline personality styles. The borderline personality style is rooted at this period because there is indeed the emerging difficulty of ego separation and loss with all the potential danger involved in that and yet still the intuition of one's integration or connectedness or wholeness with the "significant other" in the process. This process is not only a psychological process but the actual emotional energy experienced by not only the child but the mother.

I remember in therapy one day seeing a borderline mother handling her 2-1/2 year old male child and the child asking the mother, as the child hid in the closet, if the mother could still see him. It took a great deal of therapeutic work to get this mother to say to her child that she could not see the child through the walls. She did not seem to understand that the child needed to feel separate from the mother and that her difficulty in doing this was related to her own boundary issues.

This subphase, of course, can be divided even more if one chooses to do so. There is, again, the polarity of seeking wholeness on one end and yet the sense and the need for separation on the other. This process of intuiting wholeness while working on separation can be seen reflected in a number of symbolic ways that included play, vocalizations, and so on. It is the period of the dawn of the formal ego in the world. Again this ego is not yet stabilized, arising as it initially did out of brief periods of body tensions and needs. However, later on in this period of seven to ten months, a transitional ego has emerged out of the flux of undifferentiated consciousness. In other words, the psychic system of the ego makes transitory use of fluctuating, functional, fleeting cognitive structures that later dissolve or change–what might be called "dissipating structures." These dissipating structures of the psychic system that give structural rise to the ego find and maintain their proper form, size, and strength in accordance with the particular needs of the organism over and above what the environmental stresses are on the psychic system. Oddly enough, the more experimentation and freedom of the psychic structure to develop, the more order and strength of the ego. Needs of the psychic system evolve naturally into harmonious functions. When the symmetry of the organism's history or past is broken by the emerging psychic system of the ego, creativity has emerged. This creativity has embedded in it new, higher orders. This is the cognitive trajectory of the unfolding ego that will eventually prepare a way for the Self. At this time, indeed, the ego is a ripple on the void of undifferentiated consciousness.

Rapprochement

The next phase is the phase of *rapprochement*. This phase is said to occur at the end of the period in which the child learns to sit upright and has enough locomotion to be able to move around freely. For most of us this is generally around the second full year of life. You may have noticed in your own child that during this period the child may experience and verbalize a number of negative attitudes. This is called the "terrible two's" and what is occurring here, clearly, is the little child establishing itself over and against what it is not. The child's frequent "no, no," has its counterpart in neti, neti; "I am not this, I am not that."

By this time, to your delight and occasional irritation, the child manifests a stable ego in the world. During this mutual period frustration increases and separation anxiety also increases. In a paradoxical way, the child, even more than a few months ago, requires more of the mother's attention than before. He, or she, because of separation anxiety, wants to fuse again with her to soothe his or her separation anxiety. The ego function constricts the psychic process and therein attempts to suck in the energy and imagery of the mothering one by the process of introjection. The borderline development is seen to occur here because there may be a number of mixed messages from the mother. The mother may be quite understandably irritated by the child's upsurge in demands after they seemed to be gradually diminishing. The mixed messages of the mother can make the rapprochement phase a very difficult and mixed subphase. The energy patterns of "my inner self" and other people on the outside can become very blurred and unstabilized. The emerging ego learns to handle boundary issues by alternating the psychic process between constriction and expansion of the affective energy matrix.

There is a close relationship between the child's experience of anxiety and psychophysical "tension" and the reassuring "attention" that the mothering one provides. This occurs in the family unconscious matrix, since most of this learning is outside of conscious awareness and occurs in the family environment. Mahler says quite clearly that, "In the rapprochement subphase . . . is the mainspring of man's eternal struggle against both fusion and isolation." This pattern is learned in the matrix of the family unconscious system and all future borderline patients touch upon this and *awaken it in other people* when this phenomenon occurs.

The borderline could be described as the style that oscillates between fusion and pseudo-autonomy. The borderline fears both loneliness and being "eaten" or engulfed by the world of blurred, oscillating boundaries. Its cousin, the narcissistic style, also has a blurred boundary, but its disposition is to "eat" the world and make it an extension of itself! The devaluation that arises for it is toward others since others could not be as important or central to its concerns. These two styles, however, are related to each other around this issue of boundary and critical self-other evaluations based on the management of this boundary.

The Way to Libidinal Object Constancy

Finally, the last subphase occurs and is called "On the Way to Libidinal Object Constancy." This phase is said to follow because childhood proper is said to occur now. The child is out of the infancy period. The work of Henry Stack Sullivan and Freud truly begins with this full stage of libidinal cathexis. You will remember that the child still conceives the world to be very alive and, at the same time, is in the process of learning from the socially sensitive ego that it is a separate island of consciousness in a great sea of unconsciousness. Slowly, the development of the ego begins to encroach upon the sense of "basic aliveness" perceived to exist throughout the universe. The child does a great disservice to itself in its need to control the vast surrounding environment. He or she withdraws the consciousness principle from it and limits this supreme process to specific others and himself. In the modern adult "scientific" way, have we not done the same thing in order to gain control over the vast environment? By making the other an "object" to our subjective "I" experience, we gain some mobility in the world of objects and form yet lose the perception of unqualified aliveness. The child's processes to fight anxiety are developing along with his or her power to deny, split, and dissociate (not-me) from the world. This dynamic obviously is repeated innumerable times in the family matrix and much learning occurs here both consciously and unconsciously. Depending upon the familial environment and the cultural setting and, of course, the child's own subtle predispositions, certain defenses to anxiety occur (Ackerman, 1957). The forms of defense in neurosis are rooted here in this family matrix. In Chart 2.3 can be seen the stages of ego development as generally agreed upon by most researchers in this area. Minor changes, of course, can be noted in the work of any particular researcher. In this chart is the correlation of insights from Loevinger (1966), Erikson (1963) and Werner's (1948) conception of personal-social development.

"Tension," "Attention," and Structure

It has been noted in this brief foray into human development that the child's development occurs in stages that overlap each other. It has also been seen that the development is in many ways self-organized with affect, cognitive structures, and other structures that pass away as greater and more inclusive structures come to replace, or unfold, and hierarchically integrate them. This is the observation of Piaget and just about every other developmental theorist. The two basic dynamic principles of all forms of self-organizing processes are observed here and at every stage of development. The system shows its capacity for self-renewal by continually integrating new data and materials while maintaining its functional integrity. It also demonstrates its arch or self-transcendence by creatively moving out beyond its previous mental and physical boundaries. This is the inherent teleos and cannot be reduced to simpler drives or contingencies of reinforcement.

In addition to these structures of affective and cognitive development, and the increasing need for integration and autonomy at each stage, there is also, at each stage, rooted and worked out an unfolding toward the Absolute. This can be perceived either in terms of seeking "higher balance" or more inclusive "self-consistency," etc. The basic insight remains, however, of a dynamic wholeness emerging at each stage. It was noted that "tension" and "attention" get locked or fixated by each stage, partly of necessity for development and also partly because it becomes associated and identified with that particular stage. Remember that the first periods of "awareness" arose out of tension states. Substantiated tensions dealt with by fluctuating, transitory structures over time give rise to the ego. The ego then attempts to substantiate and continue itself. Thus we have an ego arising primarily from out of tensions that then identifies with more sophisticated tensions. Therein arises *ten-*

CHART 2.3. Stages of Ego Development.

Stage	Dominant Processes and Concerns
Presocial and Symbiotic	Ego development is focused on differentiating "self from nonself." It has two substages. The first presocial stage sees the infant unable to distinguish between animate and inanimate; all is alive. The second stage of symbiotic processes sees the child strongly attached to the mother, unable to differentiate from her, although he can distinguish between her and the rest of the environment (see Mahler).
Impulsive and Need Driven	The child asserts his will in the world, verbalizes demands and becomes negativistic. He is a separate ego in the world; separate from mother. No real voluntary control over impulses yet. Learns shame. Hedonistic and exploitive of others who are objects of need satisfactions. No real grasp of rules yet. Things are "bad" because of punishment only. New sexual and aggressive feelings emerge.
Opportunistic	The child now becomes more independent and in control of impulses. He is still manipulative and exploitive and wants his way all the time. Rules are followed only because of what he can gain, no really internalized "moral" values.
Conformist	Rules are slowly internalized, society's dictates are followed simply because "rules are rules." As yet interpersonal rules are still in terms of needed actions and not yet feelings and motives. Reciprocity has emerged in their relationships, but still there is excessive concern for status, appearances and appropriateness to others (see Kohlberg).

sion and attention patterns at various stages in the process which attempt to order and reinforce the sense of the ego's own fragile existence. Ego, therefore, is ultimately an illusion built upon tensions or tension states built upon various degrees of terror and, in some degree, must always be threatened by the possibility of dissolution of boundaries either by terror/awe or bliss-euphoria, both

CHART 2.3. (continued)

Stage	Dominant Processes and Concerns
Conscientious	Interpersonal relations now become focused around feelings and motives, not only needed actions. The adolescent's own moral/ethical principles are asserted. He or she can conscientiously resist group pressure (see Kohlberg). One develops ideals and higher motivations by which one judges oneself (see Piaget).
Autonomy	Conscious concerns focus on "role differentiation, individuality, and self-fulfillment." Interdependence suffuses all relationships, with all also needing autonomy and self-respect. Tolerance of other viewpoints is valued. Conflicts are primarily moral and internalized (see Loevinger and Werner).
Integrated	A very high stage, feelings of "ego-integrity, not despair." Strivings for peace, self-actualization, reconciliation of earlier modes of conflict, transcendence of role definitions of self and others. Philosophical-religious concerns (see Loevinger, Maslow).
Transegoic	The first sustained encounter with or unfoldment of noetic or subtle experiences. Initial experiences of universal processes, psychic and numerous experiences. Concern with ultimate values and identity in the cosmos. Many other levels beyond the above unfold through development in a psychospiritual discipline (see Wilber, Aurobindo).

of which will dissolve the sense of the boundary! The psychotic evolves from the first, the mystic evolves from the second.

Yet, through all of these, an agency of experience appears to be gradually developing that seems to occur within the state of relative tension and euphoria. This agency of experience becomes more differentiated, obviously, with development and eventually becomes differentiated even from the tools and the functions of the functional ego at any particular stage. Gradually, however, it becomes clear that this agency of experience *contains or witnesses* experience, but is not experience itself. And in a curious sense, it does not develop, but rather the ego's capacity to recognize it develops. This agency of experience we will term the Self. It is that aspect of experience that *recognizes* or witnesses the underlying undivided wholeness of all things, and also the process of differentiation and integration that the ego must experience in the foray into egoic physical and mental experience.

This Self can also ontogenetically be seen to gradually involve itself in various stages of cognitive and emotional development. When this Self no longer requires these stages it disidentifies with them. Thus, through development, this Self which is evident in the most primitive stages, engages with the psychological structures needed at each stage and then disidentifies with them in order to pursue the innate process of transcendence. There are "basic structures," and there are "transitional structures" (Wilber, 1981). Here we take up again the developmental thread observed and spun by Wilber. The basic structures are those that *remain* after they emerge from the embedded or emergent aspect of the unconscious. These include the states of consciousness that are played upon in the family matrix that I have explored and also those seen in the yogic system of levels of consciousness. I say remain because once emerged, the person is always aware of them. They never recede totally into unconsciousness, and the person operates on them to some extent. The "transitional structures" are stage functional. That is to say that at a certain stage of development they are very appropriate and when the person transcends that stage they lose their influence on that person in many ways. An example of transitional structures are those early moral reasoning structures of Kohlberg. The chakras are a level or system of consciousness in which certain potential thought patterns and potential behavior patterns are embedded in potentia. These can be seen, of course, in personality styles (Rama et al., 1977) and in the family matrix. Wilber (1981) outlines each of these stages and those trans-egoic stages beyond those of the intact ego. Each stage includes a degree of involvement with mind, ego, and body until complete translation into the noetic milieu occurs. This happens, of course, only in those absolute and transcendent states in which the Void and the Absolute Consciousness are no longer seen to be paradoxical but rather to be a unity. I hope to eventually outline the cognitive structures that are conducive to these transegoic states.

The stages of development beyond the firmly established ego with appropriate self-esteem and security operations include that level of basic structure that Wilber calls the "Vision-logic." At this level, the Self identified with this level attempts to fulfill the highest aspirations and potentials it may possess. This often means egoic sacrifice or even dissolution. These include traditional modes of what Maslow called self-actualization and what some people would call the higher reaches of intelligence in the conventional sense.

> Welcome O Life! I go for the millionth time to seek the reality of experience, and to forge upon the smithy of my soul the uncreated conscious of my race.
>
> –Steven Dedalus
> (from *A Portrait of the Artist as a Young Man,* James Joyce)

It is a stage of unfoldment which seeks to integrate a vast new world using the most sophisticated cognitive structures of formal operations. It is still largely structured by the "tyranny of opposites," e.g., good vs. bad, us and them, some of which gets played out in social and family dynamics. However, a rich idealism and conscious search for universality has taken root by this time. A sense of energy and aliveness seems to infuse the world and yet feels connected to the very bodily experience of the adolescent. This is the current of living energy bathed in a largely libidinal context. At its best it fully exploits the new perceptual and cognitive capacity of the system and points toward an even more inclusive vision:

> The Truth apprehended by the Subconscious Psyche finds natural expression in Poetry; the Truth apprehended by the Intellect finds its natural expression in Science . . . On the poetic level of the Subconscious Psyche, the comprehensive vision in Prophecy; on the scientific level of the Intellect it is Metaphysics.
>
> –A. Toynbee (1956)
> *An Historian's Approach to Religion*

At its worst it falls into paranoia and egocentric grandiosity. If it does not seep into politics, or some other place where it becomes a social tragedy, it becomes merely the cultural-hormonal corollary of female PMS–PMMS (paranoid macho messianic sadism), the belief that the world is in mortal danger and that you alone have been anointed to save mankind and the world from impending destruction through your own extravagant displays of masculine power, ego, and aggression (Pittman, 1987). This is not totally tongue in cheek. If this seems farfetched, observe a popular action-type video and note the hero's cognitive and libidinal dynamics as he overcomes the villains from outer space, or the future, or some other place where the psychodrama of heroic youth can be played out.

This stage at its best, however, is the highest stage of what conventional moral development is in Kohlberg's system and the highest levels in Maslow's system of actualization. It is also the dawn of more transpersonal stages of development that occur in meditative practices and which contemporary Western psychology is only beginning to explore. Beyond vision-logic lie what could be termed subtle levels of consciousness. There are dynamics at this level which I will not explore in detail in this book. However, each level also is an intuition of wholeness and also an experience in differentiation within that wholeness. Beyond this is the realm that is involved with subtle mental impressions and subtle addictive experiences of bliss. Again this phase exists in potentia at the very dawn of the human's physical-psychological experience. We each experience this causal level at times when we are in deep sleep without dreaming and the body is full of bliss and wordless peace. The "subtle" occurs when we are having experiences of oneness and the intuition of archetypal processes but are still very much in communication with the conventional world. Of course, beyond the transcendence of the causal level are those of ultimate levels, in which there are very few words except the direct intuitive knowledge while in an awakened state of continual transcendence and experience of the radiant intelligent transcendental force that was the first intuition of our ancestors in the predawn of history.

THE ADOLESCENT FLUCTUATION

These subtle visions, ideals, and higher strivings all tend to really first come to the surface of self-consciousness in adolescence. Indeed, Piaget had pointed out some of the emerging conceptual schemas that underlie and support adolescence and its new ability to construct grand, although highly egocentric, systems of thought. The different streams of the developmental ascent we have focused on–the cognitive, the affective, and the noetic–begin to integrate in self-consciously creative ways during this often radically life-altering passage.

Of primal importance in late childhood and early adolescence is the powerful upsurge of vital energies of the physiological and overtly genital variety. This no doubt accounts for much of the "storm and stress" of this period in Western cultures. It is also at this juncture that "society" as an idea in the mind of the person begins to have a real effect through self-consciousness. An excessive concern for social appearance begins to dawn as well as a vastly increased sensitivity to roles, self-esteem issues, and physical appearance. For the first time, one's peers begin to consciously reflect the social organization that is becoming increasingly more important in the overall consideration of life-issues for the person (Hartup, 1970). The emergent conceptual powers of the young adolescent are now enlisted in the service of these new values, peer relationships, and increasing societal expectations.

It is also during this crucial passage that family and cultural patterns are self-consciously seen and reflected upon by the young mind. Social and class differences, which until now were simply the way it was, are slowly being evaluated in the light of other models. The effect of these differences in cultural, family, and racial background are seen by the adolescent as they struggle to integrate them in a working model and image of themselves (Hess, 1970). The emergent cognitive structures of concrete and then later formal operations are employed in this struggle to establish a stable ego. In this process, which includes ego expansion to previously unknown areas of identification and these more inclusive cognitive structures, grand new systems of morality and ethics make their appearance on the conscious stage.

Abstract ethical and moral systems that are self-validating emerge at some point from the earlier, merely socially informed ego structure. The judgement of what is right and wrong based on inner, and also universal, principles of moral reasoning take a central place in the adolescent's evolving world system (Hoffman, 1970; Kohlberg, 1963). It is as though the adolescent at this stage of moral reasoning intuitively senses an integration of the personal reflection and universal reflection in an almost holographic way. These values of the adolescent are sometimes markedly differentiated from the parent in order to be different from the parent. It is an improvement over the two year old's negativity of "not this, not that" in that the adolescent often affirms higher values in their egoic self-assertions. Again new religious beliefs and questions emerge from this expanded capacity to feel and conceptualize on a grand scale (Mussen, Conger, and Kagan, 1963; Kuhlen and Arnold, 1944).

All these new forces, the enormous leap in conceptual grasp, the flood into the body-mind of new psychophysiological and emotional energies, the expanded relativity of viewpoints in cultural, family and philosophical possibilities–all lead to a grand fluctuation in the system. New orders and structures rise and fall in the process. They emerge on the scene, organize behavior and more information, serve a purpose for a while, then dissipate. Some structures remain, and upon these structures the new identity slowly emerges. In dealing with the inadequate models of reality and ethics left over from childhood, a great new system is constructed. Adolescents seek, with the aid of their new cognitive structures, rarefied ideals and schemes of reality into which they seek to thrust their new highly energized faith and will power. Deeper, archetypal forces and primordial energies may be tapped at this stage. The "vision quest" of many non-Western societies is rooted here where the adolescent about to enter adult life must go out alone in the wilderness to seek a special "inner guide." In the West we are more likely to be highly verbal about the process and enter the previously mentioned phase known as "vision logic." In either case, all the forces, capacities, and emergent noetic urges integrate through a new fluctuation and synthesis into a higher order of complexity and self-vision.

Summary

In summary then, late childhood and early adolescence unfold around certain issues and dynamic forces. In that cross-over from childhood to early adolescence, the main preoccupation is with one's plans for society, peer relations, the new demands of that society and fears about being adequate for the task. Self-doubt is always there, reflected in physiological concerns, new strivings, and unsureness about the future. As the dynamic genital energies and body changes rush through the system, the new identity, drawing upon all its cognitive powers, must integrate the new roles it meets in a way unique to it.

> The integration now taking place in the form of ego identity is, as pointed out, more than the sum of the childhood identifications. It is the accrued experience of the ego's ability to integrate all identifications with the vicissitudes of the libido, with the aptitudes developed out of endowment, and with the opportunities offered in social roles. (Erickson, 1963)

When this fluctuation does not result in a stable, higher order complexity, we witness what is called "role confusion." If the situation intensifies and is accompanied by pervasive anxiety and depression, along with severe distress in sexual orientation, friendship patterns, or related areas for more than perhaps three or four months, then we have what is curiously called an "identity disorder."

Since the genital dynamism is out in the open by this age it must be integrated into this vast fluctuation and series of passing dissipating structures until a greater harmony and stability is established. The healthy ego's sense of boundary requires enough permeability so that interpersonal relationships and sexuality can be integrated into the balanced interactions of true intimacy. This is a true "communicative intimacy" based on mutuality of functioning in the areas of emotions, sexuality, self-esteem, and goals. If this does not arise, the system develops isolating, emotionally distancing styles and behaviors. The ego process constricts the life-force or subtle current of living energy that pervades the body-mind, and is most obviously identified with, but is not identical to, the sexual urge. This, of course, leads to all kinds of symptoms, from simple depressive isolation or acting out behavior to severe forms of psychosis and schizoid reaction patterns.

The family constellation is crucial here in the choice and expression of symptomatology (Ackerman, 1957; Lidz, 1958; Wynne, 1958). It is a common clinical observation that schizophrenics often have their first real "breakdown" at the beginning or the end of the adolescent maelstrom (Whitaker, 1975). Often it takes the form of florid, grandiose visions and bizarre ideas. It is infused with a failed form of vision logic or the visionary quest. The system of mutual defenses, shared family issues, and enfolded orders of powerful emotional relationships of this whole process is the dynamic field of the family unconscious.

Yet somehow most of us come through adolescence intact. Nobody emerges from adolescence without some perceived "scars" and unwanted episodes. For the most part, we integrate the numerous forces and fluctuations with our increased cognitive and affective range. Success in these social and interpersonal excursions opens the door to a deeper understanding of the noetic urge that lives and matures in these circumstances. Religion, philosophy, and higher science take on a newer, more personal meaning as we see the inadequacies of society and experience our ethical need to increase real justice and other ideals in the world. While egocentric in many respects, it is an age that opens and self-consciously synthesizes the noblest aspirations of body, mind, and higher cognition we have so far attained.

At the very edge of this stage, the underlying cognitive structures that helped give rise to the content and expressions of this stage, that is to say, the structures of formal operations, begin to go through another fluctuation. A newer stage of post-formal operations unfolds. It enables one to see beyond the shifting mirage of ever-increasing roles and relationships and targets what would initially be deemed the "essence" or "core" of identity. In this higher stage of adult cognition even the notion of a subtle, "inner core" of identity or self eventually is relinquished by the body-mind. The highly refined and self-reflecting system dissolves the idea of the SELF as any kind of entity with fixed boundaries or parameters. The ego becomes a process, not an entity or unchanging reality in itself. It is humorously realized as the sage Mahamuni Babaji says that "the ego has no form and existence of its own. It is really a ghost, but it can feed on any form it holds."

So now all the threads of development identified by Western psychology have been touched upon, from the cognitive lens of Werner and Piaget, to the emotional intricacies and vortexes of Freud, Sullivan, and Mahler. We saw that family behavior and socialization influences this process profoundly. We have focused primarily on the earliest stages, those of infancy to childhood, and briefly touched the emotional cognitive and noetic fluctuations of adolescence. Most of this is summarized on Charts 2.1, 2.2, and 2.3 where the stages and their constructions can be seen to mature and unfold out of a higher, teleological enfolded order. The braiding together of these diverse strands of cognitive, affective, and noetic development lead us to a fabric that partakes of all of these, yet is distinct from them. These lines of growth lead to those structures that open the door to what evolves beyond them. They usually arise in early adult development and lead to what are termed post-formal operations.

THE UNFOLDMENT OF POST-FORMAL OPERATIONS

A radical new epistemology unfolds in the higher cognitive stages. The cognitive structures that are permanent and also most conducive to these later states of consciousness generally emerge only after the highest stages of cognitive development outlined by Piaget. Piaget and others described what are termed *formal operational* structures (see Chart 2.2). In that stage of cognitive development, a linear concept of causality has emerged and is extraordinarily useful. Also the concept of *independent variables* and *closed boundaries* has unfolded. These and other notions have matured from the earlier stage called *concrete operations* (see Chart 2.2). However, a number of researchers who have studied the reasoning processes of creative adults and scientists have found that in addition to Piaget's stage of formal operational thinking, the mode that underlies present adult and good, but conventional, scientific thinking, there is a mode of thinking that appears to subsume and perhaps transcend the mode of formal operations.

Koplowitz (1984) shows how general systems thinking includes Piaget's model and then expands linear causality to embrace cyclical aspects of causality. Boundaries can be both open and closed in this network and so the causal network is made more subtle, intricate, and vastly expanded. Embedded in this is the tangible sense and concept of greater and greater unities. Piaget held that the search for equilibrium dominated the course of each stage. It is a model of biological and evolutionary development that has some limits in its scope. It is true, however, that Piaget's schema of assimilation and accommodation does obviously lead to higher orders of complexity and organization which is really, I sense, a form of hidden teleology. Recent researchers are even more overt in regard to this hidden intelligence and directionality.

The newer biology and evolutionary theories have recently explored breaks and arches beyond the stable state theories. This includes the work of Prigogine and others (Prigogine, 1984; Jantsch, 1980). This view expands the development of systems, not only those in biochemical processes but also in the higher life-force processes, to embrace processes not envisioned by Piaget or Werner or even Sullivan and Mahler. This includes symmetry breaking processes, "fluctuating" subsystems that lead to sudden higher but transient states of order called dissipative structures, and also frequent nonlinear processes that lead to qualitatively different processes and therein novel situations. Creativity appears rooted in evolutionary/developmental processes involving the life-force and appears as the impetus that transcends those structures, cognitive and otherwise, that arise during development. These conceptions, processes, and structures, including some we have not mentioned, e.g., "auto-catalysis," "far-from-equilibrium," etc., are not easily handled by the conventional cognitive structures of formal operational levels. It is the very essence of the creative process.

This new mode of thinking is more conducive to the present creative aspects of scientific thinking. As such the concepts of an all-pervasive space-time and causality, of vast interconnectedness and other aspects of both psi and the new physics of Einstein, Bohm, and others, are much more acceptable. Relativity and quantum mechanics, along with the holonomic approach, are all a function of these cognitive structures that emerge only after the advanced stage of formal operations.

Unity or unbroken wholeness are also a reflection of this new ability to see beyond overt contradictions. Klaus Riegel (1973) has noted that with formal operations there is the need for *noncontradictory* thinking as part of the way the world operates. Yet complementarity and the ability to "balance" cognitions is necessary in order to overcome this bias and move on to what Riegel calls "dialectic operations." Here the particle and wave nature of light can be seen to be complementary realities, both true. Thus, beyond the perception of duality is the recognition of ultimate unity. There are other examples of such post-formal operational thinking that provide the kind of cognitive structures conducive to the transegoic sense of unity. This work has been done by those already mentioned, also by J. D. Sinnott (1984), S. Benack (1984) and Alexander and Langer (1992).

Koplowitz (1984) outlines four central concepts and how they are transformed from the stage of formal operations to that of post-formal operations: in formal operations the nature of boundary formation is closed. Piaget had stressed that in formal operations the "separation of variables" and the schema of "all things being equal" was of guiding importance. The advances in general systems thinking have made it clear, however, that boundaries are functionally open in numerous processes and ultimately are an aspect that is *constructed* in an overall, grand unity.

The notion of separate variables also goes through a transformation. During formal operations, *independent* "discrete" variables are seen to relate to each other. They may multiply or bounce off of each other as in the old model of atomic interactions. Recent investigation of subatomic and even subquantum processes has made it abundantly clear that variables and identities are *interdependent* on innumerable levels.

The primary concept of a permanent object, so long worked for in the earliest days of childhood's sensorimotor period and finally stabilized during concrete and formal operations, gives way to the dizzying notion of objects with shifting or mutual identities. The wave/particle nature of light is an example. For decades this idea wrecked havoc with the logical intellects of the century's greatest physicists. Now it is common knowledge. Matter itself, issuing as it does from formless energy to form an object, is seen as a derivative aspect of the vastly interconnected universe of free energy.

Finally causality itself moves from linear to cyclical to, eventually, all pervasive. That is to say that in formal operations, actions are seen to result in other discrete actions. With the unfolding of post-formal operations, however, causality is seen to be multileveled and capable of effecting the initial cause in a somewhat cyclical manner. General systems thinking in the context of family psychopathology is only one example. Eventually however, causality, like space-time itself, is seen to pervade the universe. The dynamics of quantum interconnectedness, nonlocal causality and the unfolding-enfolded order of the holonomic universe are specific working examples of this process.

With the dawn of these post-formal operations the ego begins to truly recognize its own transience. This stage or process mode of cognition fully embraces multi-level meaning, linear, and non-linear causality, the wholeness of nature and of necessity its perpetually permeable boundaries (see Chart 2.2). Many of the most innovative modern theories are drawn from this mode of thinking. It sets the stage for a radical epistemology, a new way of knowing.

In biology, one finds general systems theory a major new way of thinking. Levels of causal influence are seen repeatedly. The interconnectedness of all aspects of this undivided whole movement gives rise to the possibility of nonlocal causality in physics as seen in Bell's theorem and the holonomic paradigm of David Bohm. The structural forms or facts of quantum mechanics are well known, but there are least eight different interpretations of these facts (Herbert, 1987). Mind is very supple at this juncture. The structures that foster or allow this mode of cognition are embedded or implicit in this level. Cybernetics is another example, as is the whole use of circularity in causality attribution in several diverse fields.

In the field of family therapy and family process, the present day Milan School's use of circular questioning to chart the family's unconscious communication patterns in order to open new cognitive and affective maps is another specific example of this process (Palazzoli et al., 1980). This tool is still evolving and will look very different in the years ahead. There are many other examples in this field that recognize the paradoxical and dialectical in family and system processes (Bopp and Weeks, 1984).

It is also an aspect of this level of cognition, as previously mentioned, that it can sustain apparent contradictory realities. Indeed, it seems to thrive on paradox and counter-paradox, as in the instance of the dual nature of light as particle and wave. However, it is also possible that the physicists' view of the material world as replete with *reversible* operations and laws, and the biologists' view of living systems as essentially *irreversible* processes, can exist balanced side by side. This essential aspect of post-formal operations is necessarily becoming a more normal mode in scientific thinking. This process is certainly not confined to science. Any great work of religion or art reflects this.

Despite all this, however, there remains a nagging disjuncture between what is observed in the process, and that which observes. Future scientific insights will reveal more data about the external world, but it will be data of content and not data of process unless a leap to identification with the object of study is made. Bateson was right when he stated that at a certain point ontology and epistemology become fused because the subject, in the process of knowing, becomes identified and fused with the object of knowing. In Yoga science, when perfected, it is called dhyana–where the subject in contemplation on the object becomes fused with it. In briefer experiences, it is felt as insight. In either temporal frame, the witness and what is witnessed enter a common ground and the common ground of matter and energy is light! In this way, the traditional "I" sense is eclipsed. This is the dawn of conscious, non-mental intelligence. It is the outer wave of a fountainhead of intelligence previously experienced only in flashes of insight and intuition. Until then, ego psychology legislates out the sublime.

In this mode, the boundaries of conventional relations are changed, renegotiated, and transformed, spontaneously. In this sphere of cognition the process of insight can go many ways. When the lower or previous chambers are clear, one experiences positive new perspectives on situations, etc. When the lower levels are not clear the insights are distorted and one experiences paranoid insight or other painful takes on an essential truth! It is a mode of cognition open to different directions. Needless to say, the psychoneurotic can endure this process only briefly because it profoundly disturbs the ego-sense. However, it is the trajectory that the psychoneurotic occasionally touches.

This mode of post-formal operations allows both paradox and non-paradox to dance gracefully, not limited by the usual dualistic conceptual categories and experiences. As such, certain types of insight are possible that would appear contradictory at another, more densely "mentalized" level. Take, for example, the Zen Koan–"Before I understood the Tao I felt as though I had lost my parents. After I understood the Tao I felt as though I had lost my parents." Notice the background and foreground emotional reversal and then eclipse by insight into wordless meaning. Another more practical example, based on the earlier Piagetian notion of actions as rudimentary in all intelligence, expresses this implicit transcendence of duality: "who sees inaction in action, and action in inaction . . . ." Or better yet this; "the understanding which knows action and inaction, what is to be feared and what is not to be feared, what binds and what frees . . . is pure intellect" i.e., Sattviki buddhi (Gita, XVIII.30). This experience of intelligence and insight is almost always accompanied by a decidedly pleasurable or blissful experience. This experience or boundaryless surrounding in a blissful web is of crucial importance in later development.

Suffice it to say here that the cognitive processes have become so supple that no particular form or structure of experience is held to be the "I" sense, since all form is seen as fleeting in some way. Form itself is identified with nature, while a more nonlocal or infinite and paradoxically empty but all encompassing source that gives rise to form is tacitly realized to be one with the witness of all this. "Form is emptiness, emptiness form." One plays with the various rhythms of form, anticipates and counter-points them, while not identifying exclusively with these forms. It is, in a sense, abstract rhythm. In rhythm we find the roots of mathematics, physics, and all geometry. The witness plays with these. "At the still point of the turning world" it too sees "action in inaction." The witness is all-pervasive, prior to and beyond all fleeting, conditional forms of nature, both explicate and implicate. The material-energetic universe is witnessed to take on and discard numerous forms and appearances in the "external" world. The cognitive mental flywheel is also more translucent and it becomes easier to see also its own names, forms, and different appearances. The Self we posit here, the all-pervading witness, transcends both notions of subtle "inner" and "outer." It transcends all pairs of cognitive dialectical opposites of the mental processes and thus opens to what is beyond name, form, and thought. It integrates *fully* with that intelligence that was prior to language, that wordlessly witnessed the dream state, that *continued to develop* in deep sleep through our waking development of all kinds, cognitive and egoic. It opens to the infinite, of which nature is a permutation and manifestation. Many other examples and cases can be cited. This disposition or perspective on matter-energy and cognitive modifications of the Self can be found in some philosophical works, notably the *Ashtavakra Gita*, the *Lankavatara Sutra* and the *Diamond Sutra*.

In all these cases, at the moment of realization, one has moved from the separate, alienated from the object "I" sense, and entered into a common ground with the object. This is the noetic domain and it becomes progressively less accessible to verbal language as the process deepens. Realization, again, *takes root* in this soil, but *it is not* this soil. The soil prepares the way.

This mode of operation will more and more come into the possession or plane of humankind. It is on the evolutionary arch, and many are breaking into this realm more each year. It is a necessary mode, and will give rise to numerous, heuristic scientific theories. The scientific theories will be mental by definition. The substratum or ground out of which they arise will come to be more and more a non-mental domain. Our survival as a species will depend upon it. With the nuclear threat we have become unstable adolescents with demi-god tools. The primitive perception of "us, not them" has not yet realized its essential inseparability with others. It still perceives others as discrete and therefore "where there is other there is fear."

This final stage of post-formal operations prepares the stage for noetic insight, intuition, and intelligence to come forth or descend into human processes. Like our ancient ancestors who by firelight sketched the herds and beasts on the cave walls, at the edge of all our insights into the external world will be our structures rooted deep in our inner world. The noetic is that first deep, sustained, conscious intuition that both inner and outer are of the same world. In this context, it is noteworthy to quote at length Sir Arthur Eddington on Relativity theory and the limits of scientific knowing (Eddington, 1978).

> . . . It is a knowledge of structural form and not knowledge of content. All through the physical world runs that unknown content, which must surely be the stuff of our consciousness.

> Here is a hint of aspects deep within the world of physics and yet unattainable by the methods of physics. And moreover we have found that where science has progressed the farthest, the mind has but regained from nature that which the mind has put into nature.

THE BIOLOGICAL SUBSTRATE OF COGNITION: THE BRAIN

It would be an oversight to go further without at least some mention of the neuromelanin nerve tract and the neural or brain correlates of the cognitive structures and processes outlined in this chapter. This neuromelanin tract, which has been intimately connected with the dynamics of human development since the earliest embryonic stages and which we have suggested is deeply implicated with evolutionary forces, is held by us to be a luminous current with a certain affinity to the process of biological superconductivity. By late adolescence and adulthood it has reached its fruition by leaps and stages of growth and has been fully integrated into cognitive, sensory, and noetic development. It is the background against which the seamless current of the life-force is perceived. Now we ask is there any current anatomical or electrophysiological evidence for these observed levels of cognitive growth and development? Is there any research that says these discrete and massive leaps in intelligence are reflected in on-going neurological processes in specific areas of the brain?

Well, to be sure, there definitely is! Studies showing the EEG or electroencephalograms of children and young adults bare witness to much of what has already been presented (Denton, 1987). Apparently there are growth cycles of four functional brain areas that strongly correspond to Piaget's stages of cognitive development in both brain hemispheres. These growth cycles or periods of fluctuation are followed by periods of stability and consolidation. W. Hudspeth and others located these discontinuous growth rates at four recording sites, representing the visual-spatial, the visual-auditory, the sensorimotor, and the frontal divisions of the brain. "It is significant that, with one exception, the total growth curve exhibits growth cycles at the exact ages Piaget has identified as sensorimotor (birth to 3 1/2 years), preoperational 3 1/2-7 years), formal operational (11-15 years), as well as a fifth, dialectic operations (15+ years)" (Denton, 1987). The last is the dawn of the post-formal operational stage.

The early sensorimotor stage sees 21% of its total development by the age of 3-1/2. At around 2-1/2 years there are changes in the growth rates of different areas of the brain. The visual-spatial system for instance sees about 12% of its overall development, the visual-auditory about 10%, and the frontal system about 11%.

In that second, or preoperational stage, age 3-1/2 to 7 years, the visual-spatial system reaches about 48% of full development, and the visual-auditory about 19%. The frontal system is thought to remain stable from 3 to 5 years, then increase to 16% of adult maturity. Similar developments were seen in the formal operational and dialectic operational (post-formal operations) periods. The actual localized skull bone growth, which precedes the growth of the soft brain tissue, has growth spurts at ages 1, 5, and 16.

This does not confine the growth of cognitive intelligence to brain size. It merely shows that there is a very strong correlation between the cycles and stages of cognitive development and our corresponding neurological development. As you might well imagine, just as the growth of the brain's hemispheres affect cognitive development, this growth process also affects the growth and integration of the emotions. It is not a simple task to separate biological and neural substrates from other lines of influence in development. Suffice it to say that it is probably not a matter simply of right brain vs. left brain and then integration, but also front-back (frontal lobes-occipital lobes) and bottom-top. Each has an integrative aspect to play in a total process through time and other events.

Some neuropsychologists (Tucker, 1984) believe the activation and arousal of emotions in any situation is related neurologically to the way each hemisphere is hooked up preferentially to specific regions below the cortex. Dense connections to the frontal lobes suggest it may actually activate what we do in the world through its denser connection to these deeper structures near the base of the brain, where the spinal cord domes into the skull. The right hemisphere may keep us aroused and aware through its own denser connection to the back, or posterior, and topmost areas of the brain.

Similar connections and possibilities of neural-affective interconnections have been suggested by Luria (1973). We will look at the way this process more intimately affects our control over subtle cognitive and motor processes when we explore the terrain of psychosomatic interactions in a later chapter. Suffice it to say here that the brain and its central nervous system or CNS appears to be an *active*, selective, and higher-order generating, purposeful system, as is our view of evolution. In fact it would seem to almost be pulled or teleologically informed by the force of evolution itself toward higher levels of order and complexity. Just as the mind's higher order cognitive processes can exert influence on the brain's EEG by certain disciplines, so it appears that the force and process of evolution, which is much greater than we presently know, can exert an influence on the evolving brain, CNS, and its branches. There is literally an "energy" moving through the process which we have hypothesized to be intimately related to the neuromelanin nerve tract.

We might add in this latter connection then how one can more easily see the relationship between this "energy" and how the accounts of "mystical" texts interrelate to the observations one can make about those numerous adolescent psychosexual dramas. It would seem that the biological need for an intensification of endrochronological and other factors in late puberty and early adult life may also be needed to keep this still developing brain literally nourished and nurtured. This "energy" may be partially supplied by the same unfolding sources that accelerate the other process, especially sexual energies. In those cases of "awakening Kundalini" and related psychospiritual crises, there is reportedly an initially strong increase or intensification of sexual energies that seem to be directed to the brain and consciousness, perhaps to nourish it in the wake of a vast opening or leap in consciousness. The ancients referred to this developing area in the brain as the Brahma-randhra or "Chamber of Brahma." The *fully* mature brain is thought to be prepared to maturationally encounter Kundalini in its late 30s and 40s. It is also the case that the neuromelanin nerve tract seems to accumulate melanin with age in certain areas of the brain, especially the locus coeruleus area at the top of this nerve tract that was mentioned in Chapter 1 on the luminous current. On every level, biologically, neurologically, and molecularly, the mind and brain are becoming progressively more oriented toward light. We will return to this again in future chapters. For now, let us return after this brief foray in neurology to the final stages of cognitive development, the stage of post-formal operations, and peer into what dawns beyond it.

POST-FORMAL OPERATIONS AND THE TRANSCENDENCE OF EXPERIENCE

With the final unfolding of post-formal operations, a radical epistemology has emerged into human consciousness. The categories of conceptualization have re-integrated such that marvelous new possibilities freely present themselves. Thinking constantly renews itself, then transcends what it has just given birth to. The new, wider orientation to boundary, causation, identity, and relationships makes possible the deeper grasp of nonlocal, enfolded orders and the vision to see these numerous events as arising out of that all pervasive, enfolded reality. These deeper notions of order will eventually lead far beyond the present day understanding of science, arching infinitely beyond the quantum-relativistic universe. It makes possible the transcendence of boundary experience itself.

Through post-formal operations, the illusion of separation is traversed by a higher intuition of emergent unity beyond and enfolding diversity. Insight into the process of unfolding experiences allows the witness to play into, and yet not be identified or bound to, any particular unfolding experience–mental, physical, or even psychic. The earlier cognitive processes of the body-mind tended to identify with the categories of space and time that dominate the waking state. However, at the "higher" cognitive unfoldment, the body-mind tends to use the categories of space, time, and conventional causality as tools. It begins to see itself as inhering in reality itself and the ego becomes a progressively more lucid and functional, but limited, tool. This is due to the more supple nature of the thought processes seeing beyond the mirage of shifting egoic identifications. The post adolescent cognitive differentiations are subsumed in a resplendent unity emerging from a more subtle order. The fusion of ontology and epistemology becomes functional and leads to the integration of the linear rational and the intuitive symbolic modes of cognition into the multileveled superational sphere of direct apprehension.

At some point, there is a bifurcation of thought processes and intelligence Vygotsky revealed that speech and thought were on separate lines before the formalization of language brought them together into a new marriage. Eventually language and thought merged and were embraced by pure intelligence. Now they separate again, the latter enfolding the former. In the case of all "objects," including thoughts, arising to the witness it is soon seen and tacitly realized that, as far as the subject is concerned, objects arise *to* it, then *in* it, and finally *as* it, when the "I" sense is fully transcended. This is not an *experience* of transcendence; it is the *transcendence of* experience.

This supple play with arising mental forms during post-formal operations gradually reveals intelligence to be less and less identified with any particular object or boundary or thought. This leads paradoxically to less and less conventional differentiation and boundary construction to a greater sense of intelligence beyond form pervading all forms. The discrete "I" sense is eclipsed in the formlessness of intelligence. It cannot be located anywhere specifically in the body-mind. It has become nonlocal. There is a less and less discrete expression of intelligence and an increasing realization of "I" and intelligence pervading and going beyond all forms, names, and contexts. "I" is required for boundary experience, for subject-object categorization; no boundary, no conventional "I." "I" and that emerge as paradoxically one. The poet is right when he realizes that "every point of view, every kind of knowledge and every kind of experience is limited and ignorant" (Schwartz, 1959).[1]

This is not simply poetry, it is at the heartbeat of scientific method and creativity! As the mind opens to this higher realm, it returns with new knowledge, new insights, and a profound respect for what is tangibly more inclusive than itself. When Bohr, Kekulé, Edison, and others gathered their logical and higher rational information together, they then focused on it as they let the mind drift with intuition into a kind of formless but conscious sleep. When they awoke they often had realized a solution to the problem! This meth-

1. I suspect that both cognitively and neurally this stage arises maturationally around age 40. When successfully navigated, the causal level of mind unfolds. However, when it fails, we enter what is called the "mid-life crisis."

od has been used for ages by creative minds in all areas. It has certain affinities to dhyana in meditation and the technique of Yoga-Nidra. In the methodology section we will explore this process in more detail, including its sister condition of lucid dreaming. It is a matter of consciously entering the realm of supra-rational intelligence–that unbound free consciousness–and then using the lens of one's own person or personhood to focus the light on a specific area. Our mind is the lens, light is free energy, consciousness, and intelligence.

In a most real sense, then, the transcendence of boundary is the transcendence of conventional "I" and experience. In the earliest sensorimotor stages, intelligence is purely biological, prior to conceptualization and language and *immanent* in the action schemas of the child and world. This is a world of matter and form where indeed $E = mc^2$. In the final stages of cognitive intelligence before formless intelligence, mind has become so supple that it tangibly sees and orients itself toward the literal *light* that is $E = mc^2$ immanent in all arising forms, appearances, and names. The ground of post-formal operations is formless intelligence and light suffused with the warm current of the life-force. "I" has become inherent, all-pervasive, and entered into that One without another. Beyond this point nothing rational or intelligible can be said.

THE INTERIOR OF BLISS

But all of this has not been evolved while we were awake. Throughout this span of increasingly waking state constructions of intelligence, from primitive ego on up through the finer gymnastics of the intellect, there has been an undercurrent as deep and wide as any of the conscious surface waters. Even the dreamscape, with its mirrors, leaps, and unexpected presentations, is sometimes flooded or oddly estranged from this undercurrent of little memory and even fewer names. This is the inner landscape of deep dreamless sleep, whose terrain is contoured by the current of bliss.

Sullivan had recognized it and its opposite in the dynamic interplay of absolute terror and euphoria. From the earliest days outside the womb the infant spends hours sleeping in its nest. This euphoria goes underground in waking development, only to be sought perpetually in the search for happiness, release, and the sense of well-being. Psychoanalysis, as usual, saw only one direction of the current, and that was always as regression to the womb or even earlier saline fascinations. Apparently there is *regression* in the service of the ego, but no *progression* in the service of that same ego! The Behaviorists saw even less, merely some operant excitement or localized pleasure. There is the good-breast, the bad-breast, etc., all forms of simple "object splitting" and, of course, the multifarious exposition of neurotic unconscious defenses to its appearance. Yet in each stage or situation spoken of throughout this commentary the presence of bliss has been felt through the agency of deep sleep.

Each stage of development includes waking, dreaming, and deep sleep. There is no doubt that with time and experience the waking ego goes through phases of development leading to a greater expression of intelligence and insight. Piaget, like Vygotsky, stressed that intelligence itself was prior to language and articulated symbols. A child's dreams become more complex as they mature, even though the "primitive" is always on the ledge of the dreamscape with its images, terrors, and shifting modes of reality and affect. The adult, too, experiences these modes, these junctures and jungles of feelings, familiarities, and fantastic creations. Adult dreams are also more symbolically, linguistically, and educationally rich than those of a child or even adolescent. However, the adult can also solve problems, consider situations, and even give birth to novel scientific creations/insights, by unraveling the dream in the waking state. Numerous scientific insights and artistic creations issue from the fluid image-affect world of the dream. Ideas here are not always edited away by waking mental limits and presuppositions. LaBerge (1985) and others point out that learning tasks that require concentration and the acquisition of new skills is followed by increased REM (rapid eye movements) dream-sleep. Learning new skills is certainly a manifestation of intelligence. The dreaming state therefore has its own evolution of intelligence.

Noetic or psychospiritual development is also reflected in the dream state. These phenomena range from the prophetic or relevatory dream, to the psi episode, lucid dreams and their potential, all the way up to the luminous "clear-light" dream. There is less of a "progression" here however than there is in the waking state's unfoldment of intelligence. The current of bliss permeates each of these from the ocean of deep dreamless sleep.

Dispensing with the bias toward reductionist thinking, it becomes possible then that deep dreamless sleep, too, may develop a form of intelligence, yet not be so "mental" in expression as the waking and dreaming conditions. Since deep sleep occurs in a regular fashion, it too may be developed and refined through all the stages of development. It is always there.

So what are we left with in regard to this zone of consciousness? It is a terrain that is the repository and guardian of that intelligence that was/is prior to language, symbols, and discrete sensory references. Piaget indicated that intelligence of a certain form was prior to language. At a slightly different angle, Vygotsky (1962) indicated that language and thought have different genetic roots, develop along different lines, and that in their phylogeny, thought and language have a prelinguistic and preintellectual phase respectively. Both agree that at around two years old, speech, autistic and social babble, begin to marry and serve intellect in the child. What is suggested in our present study is that at certain levels of cognition, language and intelligence *bifurcate again*! There is always a level of intelligence that never totally fuses with language and conceptualization. This intelligence pools in the cavern of deep, dreamless sleep.

This bliss/deep sleep or causal level is certainly intelligent. Its intelligence gets developed over time also, not by "thoughts" per se, but rather by the conscious exploration of the bliss current in life circumstances. This is a practice seen at the heart of many meditative disciplines. Its opposite, the states or conditions of terror, are also in evidence as witnessed by the clinical phenomena of night-terrors and nightmares. We will return to these and their connection to deep, dreamless sleep and potentially heteropsychic influence in the section on "sleep and the parasomnias" as we explore the multiple personality process.

It should be added that embedded at this level is the root sense of mind and that of "relationship" itself. It is a region of the most subtle mind that plays or engages the conceptual categories of space, time, and the arena of causality. It was a stream, this current of bliss, that existed before language and conscious gesture and is still the reservoir from which creative intuition pours. It is both the bedrock of mind and arches above the mind. It is the "Overmind" if you will. It is a level that can influence the experience of space, time, dimensionality, and other dynamics the mind gives form to as seen in the experimental techniques of lucid dreaming and/or Yoga-Nidra. The observer of the waking state is also the more subtle observer of the dream state. The dream state and its internal current of images can be influenced "from" the dreamless sleep stage, often referred to as the Causal mind or state. One can also self-consciously reflect in the dream state enough to flow into the Causal. Each is progressively enfolded into the other, waking into dream, dream into Causal. Beyond the Causal is the fourth stage, Turiya, which is simultaneously aware of the other three stages.

Earlier it was suggested that Sullivan's absolute euphoria was the first expression of it outside the womb. When the infant/child sleeps soundly, there is no mind, no boundary. A basic aliveness abounds that is parallel to the basic aliveness of the universe of life itself. The Buddhist witnesses compassion itself rooted in the universe. Yet we need not go that far to recognize this. For the adult in deep sleep without dreaming the mind seems to subside to its seed form. Its signature is bliss; our memory of it is blissful. Since no images, words or solid ideas clothe it as they do in the waking and dreaming conditions, we only know that we slept well. We easily acknowledge its blissful nature. And yet should danger be signaled by our sleeping child we will arise quickly and attend to it. Thus it is a strangely active stage, yet devoid of image or cognition as we generally know it.

The Vivekacudamani or *Crest-jewel of Discrimination* (1921) of the sage Sri Sankaracarya is an ancient exploration of these states. This masterpiece of the Advaita Vedanta tradition of exploration and methodological experimentation with these conditional experiences states quite clearly that:

> 170 In dreams, when there is no actual contact with the external world, the mind alone creates the whole universe consisting of the experiencer (subject), the experienced (object) and the experience (their coming into relation). Similarly, in the waking state also, there is no difference.

Therefore all this (phenomenal universe) is the projection of the mind.

208 The blissful sheath has its fullest play during profound sleep, while in the dreaming and waking states it has only a partial manifestation, occasioned by the sight (all sense-perception in the waking state or its memory in the dream state) of agreeable objects and so forth.

This condition of deep sleep without dreaming is thus very paradoxical to us. Having no words, images or firm ideas to express itself, and with only an affective and intuitive memory of it possible to waking and dreaming, it appears empty. Yet after this deep sleep without dreaming we wake up feeling refreshed, nourished. It feels full and alive in a very basic, non-verbal way. It is not an intense, localized pleasure, but a more diffuse, nonlocal condition of bliss. It is the finest sheath or level of the system. Occasionally immediately after orgasm, when the usual mental patterns are briefly oblated, this seemless bliss is evident. In deep relaxation it arises also. But these are sporadic expressions unless cultivated.

You may well ask just what the "cultivated" condition of bliss and consciousness looks like to the observer or meditator. How is the "I" process navigated or "resolved"? One of the more powerful ways among many is that found in the ancient Mahamudra tradition of the practice lineage. It suggests that:

> an inner sensation does not transcend the mind but arises within its realm. Like the sun's rays emerging through patches of clouds, the inner sensation of bliss, clarity or nondiscrimination fluctuates, rising high one moment, falling low the next, or remaining steady. If the meditation on inner sensation is maintained without the mind becoming attached to it, mental defilement [distractions, etc.] will clear away by itself and understanding will emerge. Understanding consists of an unceasing stream of the mind's luminous clarity, without the duality of appearance and thought, meditator and meditation. This is described as simultaneous realization and perfection.
>
> –Gampopa (in T. T. Namgyal 1512-1587), *Mahamudra*

If this discipline is practiced and perfected, then

> the meditator attains naked, unsupported awareness.
> This nondiscriminatory awareness is the meditation!
> By transcending the duality of meditation and meditator,
> External and internal realities,
> The meditating awareness dissolves itself
> Into its luminous clarity.
> Transcending the intellect,
> It is without the duality of equipose and postequipose.
> Such is the quintessence of mind.
>
> –Je Phagdru (in T.T. Namgyal)
> *Mahamudra*

It seems reasonable to conclude, from experience and non-reductionist reasoning, that the condition of bliss is inherent in us, that it occurs on a regular basis, and most importantly, also develops in intelligence through personal or ontogenetic development as do the waking, dreaming, and various ego states. It is a blissful, intelligent, and apparently non-mental condition. This reality, embedded in the human body-mind, will be a source of immense power and insight when cultivated through discipline, meditation, and intuition. It will someday provide an intimate laboratory for the most sublime of practices in an advanced humanity. We will return to this in the final chapters of methodology.

CONSCIOUSNESS AT DEATH

Previous chapters have focused on the psychology of the waking state, the dynamic influence of unconscious forces and both cognitive and emotional development over the early human life span. The current of living energy was always rooted in the body-mind since embryonic times and the potentially guiding influence of neuromelanin and its apparent capacity to absorb light and to conduct energy through the biosystem. Its intimate connection with the dynamics of light, intelligence, and development has made it our closest known association to the living mystery of evolution. We began with the subtleties of consciousness prior to birth and at birth itself. In order to round out a full human cycle it is natural that now we come to look at consciousness at death.

Since consciousness appears to be prior to birth and the "psychological birth" of the infant is *not* identical to the biological birth of the infant, we are now suggesting that the usual physical death of the human being, including an arrested heart and a flat EEG pattern, is also *not* identical to its psychological death. For support of this idea we again turn to research, both modern and ancient.

There is a long history of curious phenomena about conscious experiences of death, stretching back into antiquity. Ancient records and accounts of what occurs in the dying process are contained in elaborate mythology and writings. The oldest known psychological and religious-philosophical descriptions of this are found in the *Egyptian Book of the Dead* (Budge 1960). A more accurate translation of the text's title would be *Coming Forth By Day and the Going Forth By Night*. It goes back to perhaps 4000-5000 B.C.E. and forms the basis for many of the primal ideas encountered later in the Bible and Christianity. The notions of an ultimate moral judgement, of realms of experience in the underworld, of psychological and transpersonal dynamics, are all clearly delineated in this ancient Kemetic document. There, too, are described the dynamics of light, intelligence, and consciousness at death and beliefs about the beyond. As we mentioned in Chapter 1, this civilization was the first known sustained civilization which lasted, essentially unbroken, for 5000 years before Christ! They charted the stars, calculated and raised the pyramids, taught biological psychiatry, and were aware of the dynamic unconscious millennia before the European rediscovery of these phenomena. Their calendar was as accurate as our own to within hours a year and was in operation from 4236 B.C.E. on! Surely a civilization this sophisticated and preoccupied with death, mummification, and the destiny of the soul knew something of the psychology of death.

The Tibetan Book of the Dead or the *Bardo Thödol* is another ancient text in this area (Evans-Wentz, 1960). Divided into three parts, it deals with the subjective experience of death, dying, and the states beyond embodiment, as does its precursor the *Egyptian Book of the Dead*. The first part, the Chikhai Bardo, addresses the psychic processes happening at death. The second, or Chonyid Bardo, focuses on the peculiar dream state that is believed to arise right after death itself. Our psychological tendencies emerge in a unique dynamic unfoldment. The third, or Sidpa Bardo, turns its attention to the onset of re-birth tendencies and prenatal events. Both the Egyptian and Tibetan texts deal extensively with archetypal projections and experiences. The first arises from the Kemetic tradition, the second comes primarily from the Buddhist lineage. Both also specifically deal with the sense of an immeasurable, liberated, intelligent, and conscious light encountered at the dawn of death that appears to literally outshine all egoic limits and with the perception of light itself arising within and without the body-mind. Finally, and very importantly, both have extensive methods for the interaction and identification with this phenomenon of intelligent light.

The *Bhagavad-Gita* (Arnold, 1977) from the Hindu *Mahabharata* is still another reference to phenomena known to occur at the moment of death. It speaks extensively about the trajectory of the soul in the post-mortem condition. World literature is replete with descriptions that are a variation of these early cognitive, emotional, and psychospiritual "maps" of the territory. Psychical research of the nineteenth and early twentieth century was drawn to this area. Modern parapsychological research has catalogued the testimony of thousands who have experienced firsthand the expanded field of radical dynamics of this last of earthly phenomena (Osis, 1961; Guald, 1977; Tyrrell, 1942). It is a cross-cultural and transcultural phenomenon. But just what is the phenomenon?

The closest medical and scientific contact we have about the subjective experience of death comes from the study of *near-death experiences* or NDE research. Moody (1975, 1988), a physician, and others have provided us with a detailed and well-documented schema of these phenomena. Searching through the literature, both clinical and philosophical, he has come to outline ten special features of the NDE where a person has been certified as clinically dead but recalls upon resuscitation a number of patterned experiences.

First, people may not even know that they are perceived as dead to others, and often experience themselves *floating above* their own bodies. Here, fear and confusion may arise. They then may see other people who are still "alive" in the immediate environment doing various things such as crying or trying to medically resuscitate them.

Second, despite being in critical pain, when death occurs a great sense of peace, calm, and relief may sweep through their inner landscape. Pain evaporates, but consciousness does not.

Third, most people have an out-of-body experience, or OBE, where they are more removed from this physical body yet seem to retain some form or experience of a feeling or "energy body."

A fourth common phenomenon to arise is what is universally perceived as a "tunnel experience." It generally occurs after full separation from the physical body. Here a tunnel or portal opens to them and they are drawn or propelled into a great darkness. Sometimes a stairway image or perception will arise instead of a tunnel, but always the personal consciousness experiences itself to begin moving through this darkness and at the end of it often encounters a brilliant light. Some report vibration and others report accompanying sound. But in each variation this central theme remains.

A fifth experience common to NDE and a variation on the preceding experience is the encounter, once through the tunnel, of beings seemingly made of light. Not ordinary light, mind you, but a beautiful, intense light suffused with compassion and understanding. The light is brighter than usual and the beings of light are perceived as friends, family members, or lovers who have previously died. Often resuscitated people report what appears to be telepathic forms of communication in this experience. These beings are frequently pointing toward the next experience.

A sixth universal experience then dawns. It is the encounter with an immeasurably bright, intelligent, compassionate, and understanding Being of Light. The Christian "sees" Christ, the Buddhist perceives the Buddha, the Muslim experiences Allah, the Hindu encounters Krishna and, no doubt, the Kemetics found Osiris. The point here is that the person experiences a Being of Light whose magnitude is seemingly beyond comprehension. The particular image seems to be a product of cultural imagery, psychological predisposition, or spiritual practice, or Sadhana.

The seventh experience occurs when this Being of Light leads the person to a life review. Here, there is reported to be no actual physical environment, but rather a three-dimensional, expanded view and review of literally every single event in the person's life experience! It is outside of time and experienced in a detached way. Their actions in life in various permutations and enfoldments in the life of others are reviewed. The feeling is that love itself is the great teaching in life, the other is knowledge.

An eighth experience for many, but not all, is a sense of rising or expanding upwards. It may be to the heavens of one kind or another. It may be to some incalculably blissful level or condition. Some feel themselves rise up to the stars and beyond.

A ninth phenomenon commonly reported is the reluctance to return to this plane. NDEers are drawn back out of compassion for others. Some feel they were given a choice as to whether or not to return. Others feel some unfinished work needs to be completed for the sake of others.

A tenth experience or sub-experience within this overall experience is sometimes a flash forward sense into the future. The intuition of a vast, new dimension unfolds to some NDEers. After this, all NDEers move back to re-embodiment and the dense phenomena of the physical world.

Needless to say, this NDE is a life attitude changing experience for the person who has experienced it. It is a cross-cultural and transcultural phenomenon that occurs to both children and adults, atheists and believers in God, poets and hard-nosed experimental psychologists.

Sabom (1982) and other physicians have seen this phenomenon repeatedly in cases of cardiac arrest, surgery, and other medical emergencies. Moody (1988) and others have pointed out that these experiences cannot be reduced to some disorder of the nervous system. The NDE is not psychosis, schizophrenia, or mere hallucination. It is not the result of an organic brain disorder, or a CO_2 overload. Nor is it the revived memory of one's biological birth and movement through the birth canal. All these conditions do not express themselves in consciousness as an NDE for many clinical reasons. It is what it is, the dynamics of consciousness during the final stage of embodied life.

In essence, then, we suggest that consciousness is prior to physical birth, and at least briefly beyond clinical death. The relationship of mind and body arises in consciousness. Objects, events, persons, and places occur in this energy and information field. From our deepest thoughts to our most expansive feelings, consciousness will always be intimately associated with our most adventurous conception of light.

AN ALL TOO BRIEF SUMMARY

This chapter opened with the simple intention of braiding together affective, cognitive, and noetic lines of development and providing an overview of human development. We outlined the theories with their biases and primary visions. We began with consciousness prior to birth, then dwelled at birth, then walked through the contours and stages of development, cognitive and emotional, to end with the dynamics of consciousness at death. The triple ascent of mind, body, and the noetic was painted by scientific theories from this school and that. The contribution of cognitive developmental psychologists such as Piaget and others was drawn in to map out certain areas. Neurological development was briefly cited where necessary. Heinz Werner and the orthogenetic process provided a great poetic vision that is both scientific and aesthetic, yet limited at a certain point. Drawing freely from such work their depth of insight has illuminated the evolutionary way. In so many ways their weave held together the cognitive or mental sheath. The psychoanalytic viewpoint provided flesh, blood, and soma to the process of human development and helped balance a sometimes overly cognitive perception of things. It is the affective and energetic sheath. I have weaved them, I hope, into an acceptable fabric while describing the limits and biases of each. Several other researchers were most instrumental in the inner details of the human work.

Mahler has held a microscope over the first three years of life. Her detailing of the rollercoaster of autonomy and separation has been of great help. Her insight that human birth was not identical to human psychological birth helped us keep our mind open to the parallel notion that human clinical death is not identical to human mental or psychological death. The NDE is a real event.

Sullivan's deep insight/intuition of the bliss/terror rise of consciousness from the body tension zones has been invaluable in helping to see how awareness is so deeply rooted to the body sense of "I." Each of the above were brilliant, colorful threads that together were woven on the loom of the human developmental aspiration. At a specific point, however, each were pulled back by the reductionist cord. More or less each tried to explain the higher by the lower. The final efforts in this chapter attempted to alter this course.

Teleological processes were seen rooted in the score of this developmental music that humanity has played out over history, from today back to She-who-has-no-name on that ancient shore. The self-transcending dynamic that is evolution has not stopped in the present era. It is active and continues up through and beyond the "I" sense and more. All psychopathology syndromes cannot be completely reduced to earlier states and conditions. There can be the falling down into madness and there can be the opening upward to the noetic urge present in any human crisis. The clinician and the laymen need to distinguish one from the other; the clinician needs to know if they both occur together and then whether to treat them or refer them to others.

At the edge of formal operations one reaches the limits of conventional, intelligent, scientific thinking. Reigel and others peer over and map the still unclear level of that higher level of cognitive human functioning. It is perhaps pure discrimination, the blissful sheath, the seed and Causal mind in operation. It is a post-formal stage of operations where boundary is open and apparent contradiction tolerated since a higher organization and a new scheme of causality is implicated in the process. From General Systems thinking to non-local causality, a new matrix of influence and creative thinking is found. The ego or "I" sense becomes more and more tenuous. With insight and intuition, the noetic is born and flourishes. There are even times when the "I" sense is completely eclipsed, as in the flash instant of insight and the quiet corners of Yogic dhyana. The dawn of intelligent, conscious, non-mental processes has occurred. Its first deep wave is bliss. From this vantage the boundaryless, non-linear, and intuitive makes sense. The luminous current of the life-force becomes progressively more obvious at each unfolding stage in the process. The Zen Koan is at least accessible and one may even embrace and identify with the root-source, but always invisible, luminous current in which the "I" sense is arising.

The whole issue of "identity," be it localized around race, religion, culture, social status, or personalized combination of any of the numerous other labels, is always rooted in an identification and attachment not to the "I" process here, but an internalized image of ourselves. The loss or potential loss of this identity at any epoch in the psychosexual stages is rife with the sense of dissolution and unconsciousness. The model of limited, localized identity carries with it the fear of death and sometimes hope of a new life elsewhere.

In the latter part of this study a great emphasis will be placed on the cultivation of the real $E = mc^2$ insight into our intimate body and life. It is by cultivating post-formal perception and its energy dynamics along with the tangible sense of bliss and emptiness that a natural methodology will arise. When matter spontaneously arises from energy and we witness its endless modifications, we experience bliss and the unmanifest light prior to specific manifestations in nature. It is a most obvious practice.

Practical aspects will fall out of this. Newer, more heuristic science and knowledge flow from this plane. The witness is that which it seems and yet is always more. In one of its facets, which is high scientific thinking and religious or artistic insight, all kinds of theories and techniques are born and flourish. From circular causality, to non-linear actions, to the paradoxes of the quantum of action, all becomes recognized to be permutations of mind and nature. This would appear to be the edge of the human romance with the psyche. What sporadically took root eons ago continues today. It is a process and journey first known long ago by some distant lake-dweller newly reflecting on herself around a moody ancestral fire.

REFERENCES

Ackerman, N. W. *The Psychodynamics of Family Life*. Basic Books, New York, 1957.

Adler, T. "Even babies empathize, scientists find; but why?" *Monitor*, June 1990, p. 9.

Alexander, C. N. and Langer, E. J. (Eds) *Higher Stages of Human Development: Perspective on Adult Growth*. Oxford University Press, New York, 1992.

Arnold, E. (trans.) *The Song Celestial or Bhagavad-Gita*. Self-Realization Fellowship, Los Angeles, CA, 1977.

Aurobindo, S. *The Life Divine*, All India Press, Pondicherry, India, 1973.

Benack, S. "Postformal Epistemologies and the Growth of Empathy," Ibid, 1984.

Bopp, M. J. and Weeks, G. R. "Dialectical Metatheory in Family Therapy," *Family Process*, Vol. 23, 1984.

Brothers, L. "A biological perspective on empathy," *American Journal of Psychiatry*, 146:1, January 1989, pp. 10-19.

Budge, E. A. W. *The Book of the Dead: The Hieroglyphic Transcript of the Papyrus of ANI*, University Books, Secaucus, NJ, (1920) 1960.

Capra, F. "Modern Physics and Eastern Mysticism," Journey of Transpersonal Psychology, Vol. 1, 1975, pp. 20-40.

Chodorow, N. *The Reproduction of Mothering: Psychoanalysis and the Sociology of Gender*, Univ. of Calif. Press, Berkeley, CA, pp. 111-129, 1978.

Chomsky, N. *Aspects of the Theory of Syntax*, M.I.T. Press, Cambridge, MA 1965.

Denton, L. "EEGs bolster Piaget Theory," in *The APA Monitor*, August 1987, p. 27.

Eddington, A. *Space, Time and Gravitation*, University Press, Cambridge, 1978.

Ehrenwald, J. "Mother-Child Symbiosis: Cradle of ESP," *Psychoanalytic Review*, 58, 1971, 455-466.

Erikson, E. H. *Childhood and Society*. W. W. Norton, New York, 1963.

Evans-Wentz, W. Y. (Ed.) *The Tibetan Book of the Dead: Or The After-Death Experiences on the Bardo Plane*. Oxford University Press, London, (1927) 1960.

Fantz, R. "Pattern vision in newborn infants," *Science*, 140, 296-297, 1963.

Fodor, N. *The Search for the Beloved: A Clinical Investigation of the Trauma of Birth and Prenatal Condition*. University Books, New Hyde Park, New York, 1949.

Friedlander, B. Z. "Reception language development in infancy," *Merrill-Palmer Quarterly*, 16, 7-51, 1970.

Gauld, A. "Discarnate Survival," *Handbook of Parapsychology*, B. Wolman (Ed.), Van Nostrand Reinhold, Co., New York, 577-630, 1977.

Gesell, A. "The ontogenesis of infant behavior," in L. Carmichael (Ed.) *Manual of Child Psychology*, John Wiley & Sons, New York, 1946.

Gilligan, C. *In A Different Voice*, Harvard Univ. Press, Cambridge, MA, 1982.

Grof, S. *Beyond the Brain: Birth, Death and Transcendence in Psychotherapy*, SUNY Press, New York, 1985.

Hall, C. and Lindzey, G. *Theories of Personality*. J. Wiley & Sons, New York, 1978.

Hartup, W. W. "Peer interaction and social organization," in *Carmichael's Manual of Child Psychology* (Ed.-P.H. Mussen), J. Wiley & Sons, Inc., New York, 1970.

Herbert, N. *Quantum Reality: Beyond The New Physics*, Anchor Books, Garden City, NY, 1987.

Hess, R. D. "Social class and ethnic influences on socialization," in *Carmichael's Manual of Child Psychology*, ibid. pp. 457-558, 1970.

Hoffman, M. I. "Moral development," in *Carmichael's Manual of Child Psychology*, ibid, pp. 261-360, 1970.

Inhelder, B. and Piaget, J. *Early Growth of Logic in the Child: Classification and Seriation*, Harper and Row, New York, 1964.

Jantsch, E. *The Self-Organizing Universe: Scientific and Human Implications of the Emerging Paradigm of Evolution*. Pergamon Press, New York, 1980.

Kohlberg, L. "The development of children's orientations toward a moral order: I. Sequence in the development of moral thought." Vita Hym.; 1963.

Koplowitz, H. "A Projection Beyond Piaget's Formal-Operations Stage: A General System Stage and a Unitary Stage," in *Beyond Formal Operations: Late Adolescence and Adult Cognitive Development*. Praeger Press, New York, 1984.

Kuhlen, R. G., and Arnold, M. "Age differences in religious beliefs and problems during adolescence," *Journal of Genetic Psychology*, 65, 1944, pp. 291-300.

LaBerge, S. *Lucid Dreaming*, J. P. Tarcher, Boston, MA, 1985.

Langer, J. *Theories of Development*. Holt, Rinehart and Winston, Inc., NY, 1969.

Lewin, B. D. "Education or the guest for omniscience," *Journal of the American Psychoanalytic Assoc.*, 6:389-412, 1958.

Lidz, T. "The intrafamilial environment of the schizophrenia patient: VI The transmission of irrationality," *AMA Archives of Neurological Psychiatry*, 79, 1958, 305-316.

Loevinger, J. "The meaning and measurement of ego development," *American Psychologist*, 21, 1966, 195-206.

Luria, R. A. *The Working Brain*, Basic Books, Inc., New York, 1973.

MacFarlane, J. "Olfaction in the development of social preference in the human neonate," *Parent-infant Interaction*, M. Hofer, Ed., Amsterdam: Elsevier, 1975.

MacLean, P. *Cerebral Evolution and Emotional Processes: New Findings on the Striatial Complex*, Academy of Science, New York 1970.

MacLean, P. *The Triune Brain, Emotion and Scientific Basis in the Neurosciences*, F. P. Schmitt, Ed., Rockerfeller Univ. Press, New York, 1970.

Mahler, M. S., Pine, F., and Bergman, A. *The Psychological Birth of the Human Infant: Symbiosis and Individuation*. Basic Books, Inc., New York, 1975.

Moody, R. A. *Life after Life*. Mockingbird Books, Covington, GA, 1975.

Moody, R. A. *The Light Beyond*, Bantam Books, New York, 1988.

Mussen, P. H., Conger, J. J. and Kagan, J. "Psychology of the Adolescent," *Child Development and Personality*, Harper and Row, New York, 1963.

Namgyal, T. T. (trans. by L. P. LhaLungpa) *Mahamudra: The Quintessence of Mind and Meditation*, Shambhala Publications, Boston, MA, 1986, pp. 352 and 361.

Newsweek, "Science Section," March 12, 1984, p. 76.

Osis, K. *Deathbed Observations by Physicians and Nurses*, Parapsychology Foundation, New York, 1961.

Palazzoli, S., Boscolo, M., Cecchin, G., Prata, G. "Hypothesizing-Circularity-Neutrality: Three Guidelines for the Conductor of the Session," *Family Process*, Vol. 19, No. 1, 1980.

Peerbolte, L. "Prenatal Dynamics," in *Psychic Energy*. Amsterdam, Holland: Service Pub., 1975.

Piaget, J. *The Construction of Reality in the Child*. Basic Books, New York, 1954.

Piaget, J. *Six Psychological Studies*. Vintage Books (Random House), New York, 1968.

Piaget, J. *The Origins of Intelligence in Children*. New York: International Universities Press, 1952.

Pittman, F. *Family Networker* article. April 1987, pp. 77.

PPPANA (The Pre and Peri-Natal Psychology Association of North America) 2162 Ingleside Avenue, Macon, GA 31204.

Pribram, K. "Non-locality and Localization: A Review of the Place of the Holographic Hypothesis of Brain Function in Perception and Memory." Preprint for the 10th ICUS, November, 1981.

Pribram, K. *Language of the Brain*. Prentice Hall, Englewood Cliffs, NJ, 1971.

Prigogine, I. *Order Out of Chaos: Man's New Dialogue with Nature*. Bantam Books, New York, 1984.

Rama, S., Ballantine, R., and Ajaya, S. *Yoga and Psychotherapy: The Evolution of Consciousness*. Himalayan Press, Honesdale, PA, 1977.

Rank, O. *The Trauma of Birth*. Harcourt Brace, New York, 1929.

Riegel, K. F. "Dialectical Operations: The Final Period of Cognitive Development" in *Human Development*, 1973, *16*, 346-370.

Sabom, M. B. *Recollections of Death: A Medical Investigation*, Harper and Row, New York, 1982.

Sankaracarya, S. *Vivekacudamani or Crest-Jewel of Discrimination*, Indian Press, 93A Lenin Sarani, Calcutta, India (1921). Translated by Swami Madhavananda.

Schwartz, D. *Sumer Knowledge: Selected Poems*, New Directions, New York, 1959.

Sinnott, J. D. "Postformal Reasoning: The Relativistic Stage," in *Beyond Formal Operations: Late Adolescence and Adult Cognitive Development*. Praeger Press, New York, 1984.

Stern, D. N. *The Interpersonal World of the Infant: A View from Psychoanalysis and Development Psychology*, Basic Books, Inc., New York, 1985.

Sullivan, H. S. *The Interpersonal Theory of Psychiatry*. W. W. Norton, New York, 1953.

Toynbee, A. *An Historian's Approach to Religion*, Oxford Univ. Press, London, 1956.

Tucker, D. M. and Williamson, P. A. "Asymmetric neural control systems in human self-regulation." *Psychological Review*, Vol. 91, 1984, pp. 185-215.

Tyrell, G. N. W. *Apparitions*, Macmillan Press, New York, 1942.

Vygotsky, L. S. *Thought and Language*. The M.I.T. Press, Cambridge, MA, 1962.

Werner, H. *Comparative Psychology of Mental Development*. International Universities Press, New York, 1948.

Werner, H. and Kaplan, B. *Symbol formation*. J. Wiley & Sons, New York, 1963.

Whitaker, C. A. "The symptomatic adolescent-an AWOL family member," in *The Adolescent in Group and Family Therapy*, M. Sugar (Ed.). Brunner/Mazel, New York, 1975, pp. 202-215.

Wilber, K. *The Atman Project: A Transpersonal View of Human Development*. Theosophical Publishing House, Wheaton, Ill., 1980.

Wilber, K. "Ontogenetic Development: Two Fundamental Patterns," *Journal of Transpersonal Psychology*, 13:1, 1981, 33-58.

Wolff, P. H. "The causes, controls and organization of behavior in the neonate," *Psychological Issues*, 5, 17, 1966.

Wynne, L. "Pseudomutuality in the family relations of schizophrenics," *Psychiatry*, 21, 1958, 205-220.

SECTION II.
THE FAMILY OF SYNDROMES/ THE SCATTERED LIGHT

He continually sees the Real Self, who studies to unify philosophy, and the teacher's explanations, with the facts of his own consciousness.

–Yogavasishtha

Personalism invades the material as well as the spiritual . . . the trees and the mountains have always possessed essences. We do not have to make absolute distinctions between mind and matter, form and substance, ourselves and the world. The Self in the center of the world, animating it and making it living and personal.

–Molefi K. Asante

Chapter 3

The Borderline Personality: Syndrome or Paradigm Anomaly

AN EVERYDAY PORTRAIT THROUGH THE CLINICAL LENS

> the inability of this committee to make a firm distinction between a mystical state and a psychopathological state may be due, in part at least, to more fundamental theoretical problems in psychiatry.
>
> –from the committee on Psychiatry and Religion
> for the Group for the Advancement of Psychiatry

> . . . to erect a self boundary or barrier, and hold a separate-identity feeling *against* the prior wholeness, not only involves illusion, it requires a constant expenditure of energy, a perpetual contracting or restricting activity. This . . . is the primal repression.
>
> –K. Wilber
> *The Atman Project*

In the pulse and flow of civilization, evolution has taken many a curious step. Despite the apparent differences in climate and national tribes or race, humankind at this stage issues primarily from the same genetic roots *Homo sapiens sapiens*, that arose and thrived in East Africa unwritten millennia ago. There are differences in wealth, power, and survival. There are differences in values and in the perception of death. Wars bleed us apart; commerce and compassion bind us together. Given the electronics of global intercommunication, we are all children of the nuclear threat. Doubtless no such idea crossed the panorama of our early heroine by the lake. Her concerns were much simpler, the store of food, the fear of the leopard, the rippling reflection of the night stars in the water.

Yet, She-who-has-no-name and her progeny laced and scattered their seed all over the earth. Some have become generals, nurses, and spies. Some have been farmers and poets, shoemakers and musicians. Each is a psyche, a system of individual needs, peculiarities, and a unique history. Language and symbol have multiplied the individual's grid of reality through science, religion and every experience this side of death. Some of these fragments of families have wandered into the labyrinth of an unstable consciousness. Some seek help, others recover or completely decompensate. When so many appear in the cave of the shaman or in the office of the psychotherapist, a pulse can be taken on the collective psyche they partially reflect. Here is a collage of a reminiscent example.

You know her, and yet, she has always been difficult to grasp. In your interaction with each other, she often seems to be very intensely involved and committed, but then can very quickly change her emotional and psychological feeling about the situation, such that at another time she seems very aloof, putting distance between the two of you. This occurs often in your relationship and, odd as this may seem, somehow your relationship continues over time. Frequently, she is impulsive and unpredictable in her behavior. She may even occasionally hurt herself. Her mood swings from seemingly normal to feeling very depressed, or at other times, inappropriate in intense anger with an apparent lack of control. You may have the sense that there is some profound identity crisis lurking below the surface, but again, you cannot quite put your finger on it because she is so slippery and difficult to grasp. Moreover, the tonality of your relationship does not seem to be peculiar to you, since other people that you know who also know her indicate this about the way she deals with people. In fact, you might even have noticed in some very small way that she reminds you of yourself at certain unpleasant times in your life.

What was just described is not an isolated episode in the life career of a person, but a coherent pattern of instability in interpersonal relationships over time. I am describing the characteristics of the so-called "borderline" personality. It is also sometimes called borderline syndrome or borderline functioning. I am speaking of it here very generally as a borderline personality. One of the most striking characteristics of this style or kind of individual is the often rather intense relationships that they may develop with other people, often including frequent, impulsive, and unpredictable behavior. There are mood swings at times from feeling normal to feeling down or dysphoric, again with sometimes inappropriate expression or lack of control over anger. The intuition that you may have about this person perpetually experiencing a profound identity disturbance is perceptive. The focus of that crisis may be around gender identification, racial identification, or some other form of identification, but the primary dynamic is a sense of *intense oscillation* between what they identify with and then disidentify with. The affective-ideational dynamic is one from isolation, to fusion, to reactive isolation, to desperate refusion. Back and forth round and round they go. There is often difficulty with being alone, since being alone brings about intense feelings of emptiness that seem unbearable.

The psychotherapist, particularly the individual and family therapist, can note a number of things about this person's way of managing and navigating vital affective and cognitive energies that move in the living current that pervades the body-mind. They can note the labile, rapid transferences that occur with this client and also their own difficult countertransferences with this client. In fact, the difficulties in countertransference for the therapist are one more sign of the "borderline" functioning of the individual. Countertransference refers to that web of associations and feelings that are stimulated by the patient in the therapist. To some therapists, the whole style and situation may seem more like a poor personality organizational problem itself rather than a particular personality syndrome. This points out the difficulty in perception on the part of the clinical and psychotherapy community regarding this kind of process.

It appears that the "borderline" personality operates primarily in the "boundary" between supposedly separate psyches and personalities. The dynamically experienced world of these people is a world of persons in conflict or union with other persons. There is nothing here about abstract energy, etc.; it is a deeply *personalized* plans for better or worse. Psychologically speaking, it is not so much "what" is the matter with you but rather "who" is the matter with you. This can be readily seen in the two actual clinical cases presented near the end of this chapter. Before that, however, there are other issues to be considered.

The other difficulty with this so-called "borderline" syndrome or personality pattern is that certain aspects of this stabilized pattern can readily be seen in other psychological categories including schizotypal, narcissistic, hysteronic, antisocial, and other styles. This borderline style is a very, very difficult creature to catch with a firm label. This, again, is actually one of its defining characteristics. The strong transference and countertransference reactions on the part of both client and therapist are noted not only in individual, couple, and family therapy, but even by hospital staff when confronted with this style of interpersonal relationships (Brown, 1980). Very quickly the matrix of "who, them, you and me" becomes energized. In addition to this constant alternating between what appears through the dualistic clinical lens to be dependence and independence, or the even earlier individuation and separation struggles mentioned in the chapter on development, Mahler (1972; 1975) and others (Blanck and Blanck, 1974) point out that this style will even occasionally give way to a frank psychotic episode. Awesome events and forces become highly personalized around perceptions of boundary, identification, and either positive or negative engulfment fantasies. In a very real way, the borderline personality has in germ form nearly all other personality styles embedded within it.

Other clinical processes may later develop out of what appears initially as borderline functioning. This includes the psychosomatic complications all the way to the extreme loss of all boundaries seen in brief psychotic situations.

Well, just what are those boundaries that seem so permeable at times between the borderline and others? What are the processes that account for this style? Clearly, the psychodynamic lens focuses a great deal of light on this pattern and by reduction to earlier conditions helps explain much of what is seen. Yet a complete reductionism seems to throw the baby out with the bath water, to overlook what the borderline may tacitly accept and see of the real world.

THE PRIMITIVE PROCESSES

After a brief clinical evaluation and history taking, the psychotherapist will hopefully register several things about the functioning dynamics of this particular pattern. This personality style has been labeled in the psychological literature in a number of different ways. The labels used have ranged from preschizophrenic personality structure, to psychotic characters, to pseudoneurotic schizophrenia and several others (Kernberg, 1967). At the present time there are a number of different theories about this seemingly unstable, yet self-perpetuating, personality pattern. However, there are two basic theories from which all the others seem to be derivations. The first is by Kernberg (1967), the second by Kohut (1971). Let us look at the first.

This approach arises from an object-relations model, a school of ego psychology. This ego psychological model itself is derived from even earlier psychoanalytic investigations, insight and perceptions. In this model, all of the above behavior describing and attributed to the borderline personality can be readily observed by the clinician and perceptive layman. In addition to this, Kernberg notices that the borderline personality very often will develop what is called a "transference psychosis," as opposed to a "transference neurosis," with the therapist. This is because under prolonged or acute stress there may be brief psychotic episodes in this borderline functioning syndrome. The borderline, remember, is not able to repress unwanted imagery and psychic energy in the manner of the psychoneurotic individual. As such, the borderline is closer to the psychotic configuration and may give in to that process at times. This will be demonstrated by actual clinical cases later in this chapter.

One of the key aspects of this borderline functioning is that the ego development of the individual is usually sufficient enough to keep a certain degree of reality testing operative such that they are not always hospitalized with an overt psychotic disorder. Kernberg also noticed in great detail the amount of primitive psychological "splitting" processes in the borderline syndrome. This is in keeping with the previous observations by Mahler (1972, 1975) highlighted in Chapter 2. However, Kernberg is not in complete agreement with Mahler's hypothesis. For Kernberg, it is oral conflicts that are the genesis of borderline functioning. This is believed to be so because of the borderline's relative fragmentation and discontinuity in intimate and interpersonal relationships. Constant, deep relationships are not possible. While the individual may experience him/herself as intact, the basic oral issues are experienced in a highly conflicted way, e.g., fear of abandonment, dependency, impotent dependent rage, object constancy, and permeable boundaries in interpersonal relationships. Because of this, the later capacities to stabilize the anal and Oedipal periods are weakened. Mahler, however, takes a different view.

In Mahler's scheme, during the first four critical subphases of differentiation and individuation in the early months and years there occurs a constant normal oscillation between the needs for separation and individuation and the concomitant needs for nurturance, security, and union with the mothering person. During this early period, the child seeks increasingly more gratification from what is perceived to be external sources, but rooted in that very experience of an external source of satisfaction is the fear that that same source may be taken away. "Where there is other, there is fear."

It is also noted by Kernberg and others at this early stage that there are very primitive projection mechanisms executed by the psyche and its rudimentary, nascent ego. In the Advaita Vedanta tradition of Eastern introspection, this projecting power is referred to as the Viksepa-Sakti of the Rajas tendency, or gunas.

In the adult borderline, the therapist or close friend can observe a significant degree of free-floating anxiety that does not appear to be bound to anything or any apparent symptom in particular. Along with this is seen a low degree of impulse control. Primitive psychological splitting and projective or dis-owning processes continue to operate. Closer observation reveals that there is a gradual blurring of self and object images for the borderline syndrome. This, from an object-relations model, is an indication of ego weakness. Out of this perpetual sense of ego weakness will emerge what is called a "regressive refusion of self and object" in which the boundaries of the ego continue to blur with those "significant others" around them. This, of course, is rampant in what passes for their intimate relationships. It should be noted here that this development occurs in a matrix of family relationships, most of which are unconscious and, in many ways, binding. The person at this stage is deeply embedded in the psychological and affective matrix of the family, and from this crucible learns in a deeply structured sense the pathways of energy transformations for all subjective, objective, and interpersonal relationships. The dynamics of the Family Unconscious matrix are thus deeply interwoven in the fabric.

Since for the human psyche "where there is other, there is fear," this fear of loss of object relations creates a sense of terror and reactionary clinging on the part of the merging ego. Remember the process of polarity between absolute tension and absolute euphoria that Sullivan observed and postulated in infants. Against that background, the sense of increasing periods of awareness, later termed ego states, occurs. They arise out of momentary states of body tension and are therein always tenuous. Because of the constant fear of losing this emerging island of awareness in the unknown, fearful, vast ocean of "other," anger and frustration emerge.

> Vicious circles involving projection of aggression and reintrojection of aggressively determined object and self-images are the major factor in development in both psychosis and borderline personality organization. In a psychosis their main effect is regressive refusion of self and object images; in the case of the borderline personality organization, what predominates is not refusion between self and object images, but an intensification and pathological fixation of splitting processes. (Kernberg, 1967)

It can be seen how the emergence and perpetual presence of frustration, hostility, and fear of others can be played out in the theater of borderline personality development all the way from the early stages of individuation and separation as enumerated by Mahler and others in Chapter 2 to the attempted level of adaptive human functioning in the adult world. Whether this is initiated even earlier, such as during the oral stage, is not really substantiated. Maybe, maybe. Certainly the actual observable behavior can be seen in the era of individuation-separation after the oral stage.

This process can be traced back observationally to the period of separation and individuation at four months and then all the way up to three years. Throughout this stage, the trajectory of psychological splitting take many forms. Some of these early forms of psychological splitting are listed here: (1) *primitive idealizations* of good vs. bad images, e.g., the good-breast vs. bad-breast, etc.; (2) early *projective identification* of good self and bad self with these particular images; (3) the polarity that develops between the sense of omnipotence and at the same time the potential sense of *devaluation* because of the threatened loss of the object. All these lead to a pathology of object relationships that is in the transformational grammar of our psychic energy.

These dysfunctional splitting and defensive processes can be seen in adult disorders, particularly in what has been described as the borderline personality. A manifestation of this style is seen in anorexia nervosa in which there is a disturbance of self and its reflection or mirror in significant others (Rizzuto, Peterson, and Reed, 1981). In anorexia nervosa there is a disturbance of the sense of self reflected through shared unconscious family dynamics and imagery on the most profound levels. This, of course, is a "borderline" or shared psychic boundary problem between family members.

You may have noticed that the above formulation of the borderline personality, coming as it does from the object-relations approach, comes from psychoanalytic views, is based on certain assumptions about the structure of reality that may not be operative given the new perspective of undivided wholeness. The new world view, in physics and biology, of interconnectedness and undivided wholeness sees an essential unity between the affective/psychological, physiological, subtle, and the neurological levels. Specifically, you may have noticed that the implicit doctrine of "epistemological loneliness" or ultimate skin and ego-bound, self-conscious isolation inevitably arises out of this formulation in which the development of a separate ego is seen as the goal of development. Epistemological loneliness or subtle narcissistic isolation and the assumption that the world is basically an intricate mechanical marvel as opposed to a matrix of undivided wholeness, of interconnection, make some of the assumptions of the psychoanalytic perspective seem tenuous. The object-relations and psychoanalytic lens does not account for the documented psi events that occur in the cradle. It does not even really account for the less intense, but more predominate, process of "reciprocal affect" between mother and child as enumerated by Harry

Stack Sullivan (1953). It does not account for recent empirical studies of early empathy development in infants and children. The object-relations and ego psychological models are incisive tools when dealing with high and mid-level ego development, but they fall woefully short by assuming that the development of an autonomous well-balanced ego is the ultimate goal of human development.

Ego psychological and psychoanalytic tenets have led us to the correct perception that the borderline personality functioning lies somewhere between the "low of psychotic disintegration and the medium high of neurotic stabilization." However the theory does not effectively deal with undivided wholeness in the material and psychic and psychological planes of interaction. It looks as if it is a *tacit wholeness* that the borderline senses that is generally denied by the adult world and seen as only and purely regressive thinking by the psychodynamic orthodoxy. Yet, the rest of modern science says this tacit, energetic interconnectedness is a reality!

The late nineteenth century assumptions about energy dynamics that are the pillars of psychoanalysis and object-relations are woefully inadequate in terms of the current tenets and findings in the new physics and what is well known and well documented in parapsychological research, not to mention the testimony of mystics throughout the ages. The object-relations and ego psychological models are useful, but limited, tools and frames of reference. They appear to rely too much on the notion of "boundary" as a *barrier* at the expense of boundary as a sustaining contact and exchange or permeable process with the world. This inculcates the illusion of separation in the relations of self, other, and things that arise in experience.

There is another approach that opens a different set of doors through which to peer at this syndrome. In some sense, it is more economical in description and does not fall totally prey to the reductionist bias. This is the somewhat revisionist approach of Hans Kohut. I say revisionist because both Kernberg and Kohut are offshoots of the psychoanalytic tree and, in a sense, are dealing with a crisis in psychoanalysis itself. That paradigm crisis is about the range and actual permeability of boundary, self-processes, unconscious phenomena and the different "dynamics" of fields vs. entities.

Kohut, in his book, *The Analysis of Self* (1971) presents the borderline constellation quite differently from the object-relations school. In this approach, the overall pattern of borderline behavior is looked at and generally perceived to be a kind of "narcissistic personality disturbance." From this perspective, the personality is seen to be *arrested* in development at a place where cohesive, grandiose self and cohesive idealized objects have come into existence. They have come into existence, become fused and the new psyche invests these objects with its own narcissistic libido or energy. Yes, the infant has separate objects in its world, but these objects are merely differentiated parts of itself. These transitional objects are called self-objects and they represent the first real steps in the emergence of a cohesive self. Because of this cohesion, apparently, a stable narcissistic transference is possible. However, also, the fragile ego's fear of annihilation and regressive fragmentation is defended against successfully by the shields of avoidance, dissociation, and isolation. These two possibilities go back and forth creating the process of oscillation already referred to. Affectively speaking, shame, low self-esteem and other such intrapsychic feelings and experiences predominate.

Kohut also sees the preponderance of primitive psychological splitting of the world even in that most early pre-ego or autistic and symbiotic period referred to by Mahler. The radical difference here in Kohut's model is that "self" is not seen to be located in the psychoanalytic framework. Rather, the self is seen as a superordinate structure within the mind itself, since it is thought to be cathexed or charged with instinctual energy and endures through time. It is not a function of the ego.

The self is seen to be an autonomous process. Kohut, as a therapist, notices the tremendous transference problems of the patient and the countertransference problems of the therapist. In terms of technique, the therapist at times needs to tolerate a sense of "impotence" when traditional therapeutic moves are not effective with this client. The borderline personality, in the countertransference situation, touches upon the therapist's own prior experience of affective and psychological embeddedness in his or her own family of origin, and this is constantly reactivated by this borderline syndrome in the therapist. This is why it is such a difficult problem for the therapist to treat. The therapist from the conventional clinical point of view is falsely assuming a genuine separateness, and the borderline client is indicating that there is no real or ultimate separateness from one another. It is his or her poorly managed individual interpretation of *our* collective delusion of discrete selves or persons that he or she is suffering from. He or she will pretend to be separate in order to attempt to enter into the consensually accepted and conventional world, but will fail in intimate situations and become panicked by the fear of the loss of the tenuous "I" sense. Here is seen the much talked about fear of engulfment.

The dysfunctional pattern of regressive narcissism that Kohut sees is actually those powerful "object" libidinal, *affective* ties to scattered images of family members. The dynamics involve a matrix of energy transformations in a field of shared imagery, identifications and cathexis. The oscillations are between and within these fields which unfold other fields in their operation. It is a web of relations that reflect, amplify, and infuse each other in both a literal and figurative sense. Here one comes face to face with that powerful shared, unconscious, affective matrix and ideational pattern that is termed the family unconscious. Remember that the material and psychic world is of one full, whole undivided movement, that a current of living energy can be directly experienced to run through and suffuse or enfold all the objects of the world. The normal adult overlooks or egoicly represses this living interconnectedness in order to remain a separate adult ego. The borderline has not forgotten or totally repressed this prior canvas of experience, yet manages the situation poorly.

While Kohut has seemingly improved upon the notion of the self as autonomous from the ego, he still would appear to make the common error found in the psychoanalytic paradigm. It seems as though Kohut confuses the self, which observes, with the contents of the observation. Therein Kohut's "self" becomes another concept or permutation of the mind with a psychic structure and a specific localization in the system. In the present study there has been a localization of the ego that arises from conditions of body tension, etc., but no localization of the Self at all! Indeed, the door is open to the possibility that the Self is non-local by nature. Here is Kohut in detail on this matter:

> The self is a structure within the mind since (a) it is cathected with instinctual energy and (b) it has continuity in time, i.e., it is enduring. Being a psychic structure, the self has, furthermore, also a psychic location. To be more specific, various–and frequently inconsistent–self representations are present not only in the id, the ego and the superego, but also within a single agency of the mind. There may, for example, exist contradictory conscious and preconscious self-representations . . . side by side, occupying either delimited loci within the realm of the ego or sectorial positions of that realm of the psyche in which id and ego form a continuum. The self then, quite analogous to the representations of objects, is a content of the mental apparatus.

The reader is asked to notice how the contents or foreground is the focus, while the enveloping, seamless background of awareness itself is ignored here. This is a subtle but significant difference in frameworks. The former is discrete, localized, and the object of frozen energy. The latter is continuous, non-local and a field of interconnected relations in which the concept of separateness is alien, or at best an abstraction and limiting case.

RECAPITULATION AND ANOTHER VIEW OF NARCISSISM

The epistemological and energetic processes that both object-relations psychology, emerging as it does from psychoanalytic theory, and the self-psychology of Kohut and others share many basic assumptions. Both assume (1) That borderline functioning has its origin in the early oral phase of development and that the later dynamics and behavior seen by Mahler in the autonomy-separation phase is a reflection of the earlier oral conflict. Perhaps, perhaps. But this is conjecture about the oral stage, whereas the actual behavior and affect is observable in the later development. (2) A primarily intrapsychic model of the world is assumed which denies the common psychological ground or field of influence as primary, a field of influence which is readily noted in parapsychological research, many other branches of science, and the field of family therapy.

(3) The energy assumptions of both Kohut's model and the other object-relations models are not in keeping, in particular, with modern psychics, biology, and certain areas of neuroscience. In particular, "objects" are not entities, billiard balls, or even fine atoms, but rather are "fields of influence" and thus the *assumptions about energy dynamics* must be radically re-evaluated. These include the intuitions and assumptions about autonomy itself. Given the reality of undivided wholeness, the interconnectedness of the quantum field, the interconnectedness of the affective-ideational field in the family and numerous such research findings, including an experimental lineage of introspective experiential traditions, it becomes increasingly clear that there are limitations now being experienced by the models so far offered to explain the dynamics of the borderline syndrome. (4) The ego psychological model and the self-system of Kohut may not be comfortable with the recent research discovery that compassion may be primary and innate (*Newsweek*, April 12, 1984) within the individual and that conflict itself may be a *secondary modification*, a derivative, of this primary and personalized empathic linkage between human infants and their significant others.

The Mahayana Buddhists maintain that the whole world psychically and physically is rooted in compassion and a basic "aliveness." This basic sense of aliveness may come to be regarded as the source of the actually experienced, vital sense of "narcissistic" energy when it is involved in personality dynamics. That is to say, this real, "basic aliveness" in the world is seen, in a dualistic clinical framework, to become "narcissism" when the all-pervasive conscious energy becomes extremely localized in the body-mind by the constriction of the ego around certain experiences. The child is born into empathy and compassion. The ego must learn it. Kohut and others posit that a basic empathy is a primal need, but this is seen as essentially walled off within the emerging ego sense. I am suggesting that empathy is native to the field of shared consciousness and is only later localized in seemingly separate, conscious personalities! Recall that the infant asleep is without mind and in a blissful state. The state has no boundaries. In our adult deep sleep, with no dreaming, mind is in its blissful, seed condition. There is no boundary between its bliss and the condition of unbound nature or basic aliveness. Bliss is by nature non-local and we participate in it, not the other way around! Hello, Copernicus.

From the object-relations and psychoanalytic models, all regressive behavior is just that. It can be nothing else because there is no admission of anything above and beyond the well-functioning, autonomous, internally-balanced ego and nothing below it but primitive disorganization and fear. There is no teleology, and all trans-egoic states are instinctually and reflexively reduced to pre-egoic states. All that is not ego is a form of regression. The transcendental trajectory is reduced to the saline sac. This confusion between pre-egoic states and trans-egoic states is a fundamental one and must be grasped if one is to differentiate between a true "spiritual emergency" and its much greater preponderant cousin, frank psychosis and psychological disturbance. The former moves to seeing that basic aliveness is an unfolding world, the latter sees the yawning of death and disintegration.

THE BACKDROP OF WHOLENESS

If one is open to the possibility that the psychological and psychic field is a field of interconnecting influences that exists, operates and influences us in profound ways from the very beginning of life, then we can begin to see the following scenario. We begin to see that since there is no absolute autonomy but only degrees of wholeness, then the personality organization itself becomes a process of psychic localization, of degrees of differentiation and stabilization within this overall field of material/energetic and psychic process. It is a matter of localizations in a vast field and not a core, or some ultimate "inner," condition. In this perspective, the boundaries become even more permeable and as such open the borderline disposition to heteropsychic influence at various times. This oscillation between fusion and individuation, this back and forth between what resembles like dependency and autonomy, is taken in a very different light. Undivided wholeness is the reality the borderline tangibly feels but manages so poorly. The deepest psychic structures of the borderline do not repress the ego dissolving memory and experience of prior, real fusion. The source of both life and death come toward the ill-prepared ego that wants merely to perpetuate its frozen self-image of itself. Intimacy is potential dissolution and the messenger of psychic death.

The above, of course, is the terror and catastrophe of the psychoneurotic borderline who ultimately fears "the other" and ego-death. Contrast this with the mystic or transcendental process in which there is ultimate faith in the luminous reality and vaster benevolence of "the other."

Dissolver of Sugar

Dissolver of sugar, dissolve me,
if this is the time.
Do it gently with a touch of hand, or a look.
Every morning I wait at dawn. That's when it happened
before.
Or do it suddenly like an execution. How else
can I get ready for death.

You breathe without a body like a spark.
You grieve, and I begin to feel lighter.
You keep me away with your arm
but the keeping away is pulling me in.

–Rumi (*Quatrain* #3019)

At each stage, the perennial intuition of the Absolute is dealt with by the ego and the more independent agency of the self in Kohut's system. The present perception of the self is very different. It is not an intrapsychic, but rather transpsychic, model. The self that is posited here is the luminous substructure, the resonate heart of that self-regulating, radiant transcendental life-force which has been postulated throughout this book to be the bedrock and source, not only of the material world, but of mind and attention itself. In the psychotherapeutic process of transference and, particularly, countertransference, as it stimulates the level of borderline functioning in the therapist, a parallel process is brought into the fore and recognized to be actually a common field. In this common field, the clinician can make a functional deferential diagnosis between the borderline and the narcissistic personality. The former tends to experience tenuous boundaries and the latter, blurred. One fears engulfment by the world, the other feels the world is merely an extension of itself. Finally, the numerous psi experiences in borderline types of personalities have been noted by many therapists (Ehrenwald, 1948). These practitioners note numerous times, from even a psychoanalytic perspective, that there are certain holes or anomalies in the clinical perspective concerning the boundaries of the borderline patient.

I generally agree with Mahler that the borderline personality development occurs, is given its initial impetus, during that period of autonomy and separation, particularly the rapprochement phase that she refers to brilliantly. It is during those stages of roughly four months to three years that a number of profound psychological changes occur, all of which are embedded in the family matrix. I also tend to be more sympathetic with others (Masterson and Rinsley, 1980) who, while agreeing that the borderline development begins here, also suggest that the really narcissistic style has its origin in the earlier practicing stage of this autonomy-separation process. In the prior practicing stage, the little self is *triumphant* in the world, not retreating from it and anxiety as you see in the later rapprochement phase. I wholeheartedly agree that splitting occurs as a psychological function, but much of this splitting occurs before the ego itself is capable of doing the splitting! In other words, there appears to be a certain pre-egoic splitting that is being done by an agency that is not the established ego! For the present time I will refer to this simply as the psychic entity.

It was offered earlier in chapter two that the ego, indeed, does arise from initial bodily states of tension in the way that Harry Stack Sullivan enumerated. With this rise and subsequent stabilization of tension there also arises a subtle but constant fear of dissolution, that is to say, fear of object and self-object loss. These gradually increasing periods of ego awareness arising out of body tensions and the grasping primitive egoic attention upon these experiences reinforces the fear of object loss and the intuitive recognition that the ego itself is but a tenuous, fleeting experience. The ego itself is intuited to be a transient phenomenon clutching at other transient phenomena. Out of this body tension process, a sense of stabilized "I" or ego does arise, but it is based totally upon the sense of contraction and freezing of attention, or the psychic lens of "I," upon certain zones and areas in the body through the process of memory and development. Then it is off flying in the shared world. Successful actions executed on the environment support this early perception and success. Later, if the discriminating ego or "I" sense attempts to localize itself in a mental or physical process it only discovers upon reflection that it is ultimately not substantial but actually empty. Ah Crow!

> To hatch a crow, a black rainbow
> Bent in emptiness
> over emptiness
> But flying.
>
> –Ted Hughes, *Crow,* 1971

Emerging along with this different conception of borderline functioning is also the notion that an "object" is an energy field and all energy fields are interconnected with each other in a very real way! This includes not only matter-energy fields but also psychic influence through various fields. The view advanced here is that each stage of both cognitive and emotional/affective development is seeking not only a balance of intrapsychic and other forces at that stage, but stabilization, such that inborn processes of transcendence towards the Absolute can be nurtured. I agree with Wilber (1981) that some of these cognitive and affective structures are basic and some of them are transient and pass after they have been dealt with, disidentified with, and no longer serve a functional purpose. Both Kohut and Kernberg assume that the borderline's "inner self" is ultimately a separate aspect from other selves, that is to say, other selves of other people. I offer that the Self is the same Self of all self-organizing principles. With a field of undivided wholeness, all separation into discrete categories is functional, but certainly not absolute. In the perspective of Kohut and Kernberg there arise, of necessity, the notions of real isolation and separateness and the defenses arising to defend that ultimate separateness. I am with Wilber and others who assert that the fear of union is our primary repression. Undivided wholeness, if not understood, is a threat to the separate self-sense. It is a series of great waves and storms around the tiny, just emerged island of "I."

Stand back for a moment and wordlessly watch the "I." You see an illusory ego emerging, becoming frightened of its own sense of transcience, hopelessly clutching onto passing phenomena in an attempt to reassure itself of its own existence. This is the primary source of illness, this clinging to transient phenomena in an attempt to internally stabilize one's self in order to deal effectively with the external world. At a much later stage of development, even both these notions of an internal and an external world are transcended or subsumed by the tangible notion of intelligent undivided wholeness.

From this perspective, the transference and countertransference process in psychotherapy points up the observation that the borderline personality, given its effect on therapists and our conceptual difficulties with it, is indeed an anomaly in our own psychological paradigm of psychic atomism, determinism, and narcissistic isolation. When you see the borderline personality from this new perspective, as intuiting real, undivided wholeness from a very early period, it becomes a personality not completely given into the ego's denial of its basic connectedness to all else. It has recognized the basic aliveness and personalism and essence of objects, others and natural forces. This does not deny that the ego needs to deal effectively in the internal and external world of the child. If this is not done, anxiety arises which then demands more egoic manipulations to control it. A vicious circle. The child's real world includes experimenting with the body and actions in the environment, gaining gratification by being able to get what it wants in the world, and also organizing experience and various experiential tensions within that greater field. The child's oscillation in its involvement with others is the natural intuitive recognition of the flow and identification of self with the self of others. Sometimes the two of you have been fused, sometimes not. On an ultimate level, these selves are identical, yet as we deal in the world of form and object, there is a functional but necessary pseudo-separation in order to effect the development of the "I" in its human expression. It seems to be the peculiar aspect of human development. This back and forth flow within the borderline and other pathological conditions occurs in a psychological and psychic energy field that also gets stabilized, fixated, and acted out in numerous other relationships. This is stabilized in the network of those all powerful early family relationships, and is naturally carried into other families and social situations. This is not unique to family members and the psychotherapist;

people in mental health professions working on hospital staffs have also recognized this process between borderline personalities and staff. It would seem that borderline personalities, in their involvement with us, touch upon that level of embedded shared consciousness that we all intuitively know and aspire toward, but generally deny by way of the hegemony of the ego.

There are anomalies in the clinical literature that the borderline syndrome amplifies. These are the belief in psychological atomism, mechanism, and other assumptions of a dying paradigm. These will be seen as particularly weak when it comes to explaining and exploring the more esoteric kinds of personality problems, such as the multiple personality, the psi experience, and so forth. In the case of multiple personality, the psychological splitting was so early, so intense and sometimes so pre-egoic, that a deep, shared, embedded unconscious is warped or fragmented at the very beginning and that fragmentation reaches into all the worlds of the developing person. That degree of splitting reaches deep into the shared unconscious in addition to the developing individual unconscious. It seems that on the deepest levels of the unconscious, many worlds exist that are kept out of awareness for reasons of psychological survival. The functioning borderline personality seems to be able to stay just above that level of embeddedness in which the world loses its differentiation and many worlds are possible. However, the multiple personality and the paranoid, in different ways, succumb to this perspective in their peculiar processes.

CASE STUDIES OF BORDERLINE FUNCTIONING

Case 1

At this juncture I would like to present two cases taken from my clinical practice. They are both borderline syndromes and will satisfy many of the conditions previously spoken of concerning borderline functioning.

> Sandra X. is a patient in her mid-thirties who presented in crisis after Thanksgiving to the therapist. She would initially

speak only by phone for fear of being seen in the office by someone she knew. Her voice was desperate and it was very difficult to get her to come to the office after her third call. She would not use her real name until she came face to face with the therapist and preferred the phone name of Joan.

The initial phase of the work was crisis intervention and structuring the weeks at work and home. She was quite paranoid in ideation, but seemed to trust me. Her anxiety level was extremely high and she nearly passed out on several occasions. In addition to alcohol abuse, she had several psychosomatic problems and was seized by anxiety in the middle of the day at times. She constantly felt that her colleagues would find out her secret and she would be fired and humiliated.

As therapy progressed the crisis of losing control decreased weekly. This took six months! It was during this time that the patient spoke at length about her family and husband at the therapist's encouragement. When faced with anxiety welling up, she would dissociate briefly in the session with a depersonalization experience. It was during one of these periods that the therapist realized that the patient was re-living painful experiences in the past.

With probing and encouragement from the therapist through her denial and desires to leave therapy for awhile, she eventually indirectly revealed a history of physical and sexual abuse in the home. During periods of depersonalization at home she would physically hurt herself in fantasy-imitation of earlier situations. She claimed the pain helped her focus. The therapist discussed her case with his colleagues in the field and received some valuable feedback on the management of borderline personality styles.

The patient's dissociation was re-framed as avoidance of the therapist and a most gentle confrontation ensued. Periods of extremely low self-esteem, despite a graduate degree and professional position, oscillation about how close to get to the therapist and fear of impulsive action and loss of control predominated the sessions. Guilt and depression were everywhere in abundance.

As a way to control her numerous anxiety attacks and depersonalization, the therapist taught the patient diaphramatic breathing and other body-mind procedures to control anxiety. It was re-framed as a method of higher order control over the system. After two months this procedure worked. She stopped physically abusing herself because the breathing made her aware of the pain, since it short-circuited the dissociation she had practiced. She had been stabilized and the third phase of therapy began.

Many hours were spent in exploration of her family of origin. Her identifications with her parents were intensely focused on negative images, especially her mother, who she felt had been excessively abusive. During this period, we also worked on her divorce form her clearly sociopathic husband, who had abandoned her for another woman months ago. Her losses were real and deep. She continued to periodically threaten suicide, but the therapist now did not believe her. Some weeks she felt okay at best, other weeks she felt she was about to lose it all. Feelings of guilt were excessive and easily displayed. A breakthrough occurred when she fully admitted her rage at her abusive mother and her mother did not die!

The therapist used the positive transference and skillfully used humor to manage her occasional negative transference. At times the therapist felt helpless to help her beyond empathic support and insight. This was part of the countertransference and the therapist needed to tolerate a sense of "impotence." Near the latter part of therapy, as she began to recompensate, matters of religion and "why" this all happened to her came up. To her surprise, the therapist encouraged her religious studies and prayer and suggested that she deepen her relaxation before her prayers. The pranayama or breathing exercises had helped her gain some control and balance earlier, so what did she have to lose?

Eventually her prayer and sense of inner balance came together. Her suicidal threats ceased, except near the termination phase. In a manipulation of the therapist, she threatened it. He confronted her with a gentle anger and told her he still cared for her. She could handle that balance now, something she

> could not do before. There were no more such events and therapy was gradually tapered off. The case took two years to treat. She eventually made real peace with her two parents after her anger was acknowledged and she was able to "forgive them." This process of forgiveness and decreased attention on the knot of pain was coordinated with her daily practice of pranayama as proscribed in therapy. Therapy ended on good terms and she moved to another area of the country.

With this patient, the clinician witnesses many of the processes identified with borderline functioning. In addition to the well-documented oscillation between fusion and differentiation, there is also the presence of many other symptoms of related psychological disorders. This also is characteristic of the borderline process, this multi-symptomatology. Beyond the activation of a period of that sense of helplessness as part of the therapist's countertransference, there is the mutual ground of the boundary between therapist and patient which oscillates for both of them. Finally, the history of abusive treatment in situations of trust and empathy was played out by the patient's symptom of self-abuse. The therapist employed the positive transference of the patient's "object splitting" into good therapist-bad therapist and let the patient control the oscillating distance with the bad-therapist image/affect. The breathing was used to help the patient tangibly feel the life-current and to flow with it until she intuitively felt that this current is always and will always be there, prior to her ego or "I" sense. This involved having the patient experience this current in many different situations as they naturally arose in her life, e.g., in the midst of a panic attack, in prayer, in the control of her stress-related disorders of the GI tract, etc. At times, in a session, it was helpful to explore this current "philosophically" by engaging the patient in an exploration of this current as operative not only when she was awake, but also as always being there in dreaming and deep sleep. At moments of peace she began to feel that this current of living, embracing energy was her inner friend and not an evil force that wanted to swallow her, thus requiring her to psychophysically and emotionally to contract and hold on tight in order to survive.

Case 2

This next case history concerns Deborah X., a 25-year-old single mother of a 2-1/2-year-old son. When she self-referred to the therapist who worked with families, she was extremely anxious, chaotic and rambling in speech, disorganized in appearance and not quite clear about why she was there. She said she recently had trouble concentrating.

The first session was simply one of structure and crisis intervention. The therapist made concrete plans for the next session and asked her to do some simple tasks. The therapist saw her in the next few days for only a brief time in order to make contact more obvious. Because of her obvious distress, the therapist was aware of doing more than usual to engage her.

During the next few sessions, the work focused on structure for her in her daily life. In a very behavioral way, the therapist structured her time. It was also necessary to structure her private work time as a typist since her difficulty in concentrating on anything made her time less efficient when at work or in the classroom. The therapist gently suggested that her inner world or organization was reflected in her external world. She accepted this and all seemed to be going well for the initial stages of therapy. She exhibited no paranoid or suicidal ideation, but was quite depressed, anxious, and confused. The therapist thought of her as a case of depressive reaction or possibly a system in the process of decomposition. Then the situation changed abruptly.

Just as the therapist was feeling what a great job had been done in "saving" this person on the edge of psychic disorganization, she abruptly cancelled two sessions in a row. When she returned on the third visit, she had no explanation other than she felt she didn't need therapy any more. Yet she had returned this time. Apparently her "structure" for keeping things organized had not remained as strong as the first few weeks and she needed more. The therapist told himself something vague about approach-avoidance and intimacy, but didn't really explore it. He returned to structure building again.

As therapy progressed over the next few sessions, she became more coherent and expressive, but often the sense of confusion and depression dominated the sessions. Oceans of empathy on the part of the therapist were only briefly helpful, just enough, it seemed, for her to get by on. As she got better again the therapist took more delight in her improvement. Then abruptly she cancelled the next two sessions but returned a month later in crisis again. The therapist was aware of liking this person in many ways, but was also beginning to feel a little inadequate in helping her since there was repetition here. The therapist took the case to his colleagues for a presentation. After their consultation the therapist realized that he had a borderline functioning individual on his hands. There was the oscillation between intimacy/structure/empathy and the need to not become dependent on the therapist. There was also the confusion of thinking processes, the anxious and depressive atmosphere of her presentation at times, and the therapist's higher than usual effort to engage her because he really liked her. Here is when the uncovering phase of therapy began.

One of the consultations was to gently present the issue of control in therapy. She was overtly and explicitly given the control of when she felt therapy was good and when she needed "distance." This was done over many sessions with the therapist reflecting on the process as it occurred. She responded well to this. When her next series of cancellations occurred and the new crisis arose, it was around her 2-1/2-year-old son. By this time the patient experienced only minor organization problems in school and at work.

Her son was an attractive boy, energetic and willful, yet essentially friendly and responded well to therapy. He had issued from a previous brief relationship. Marriage never seriously arose. The son, she said, would never obey her and she felt helpless at times to control him. As a reaction to this she often felt depressed, tearful, and inadequate. The two were quite affectionate with each other, however.

The mother-son sessions were spent in simple structural and behavioral control measures. The techniques were effective when she carried them out at home and in the community. A good deal of the time the therapist worked on her family of origin, the effect of the early departure of her father from her home, and the vague sense of relationships between her other family members and herself. This occurred with the child in the office sometimes, which afforded the therapist an opportunity to have her draw parallels to her own family. Several times the therapist worked with her dreams as they revealed her relationships in waking life. Family dreams were often of disengaged or vague people with a fluid boundary process. Some of her dreams were about her son.

During one session about six months into treatment a powerful family pattern emerged. Her son was hiding in a coat closet partially hidden from view in the office. As family matters were discussed her son kept asking if she could still see him as he hid from her view. She kept saying, yes, she could even though clearly neither she nor the therapist could see him.

It dawned on the therapist to reflect on this as a process of necessary differentiation for her son. He needed to feel separate from her, and this game of hide and seek was an expression of this developmental process. She became tearful as she spoke of her fear that he would leave (abandon!) her and that she would be alone. The therapist worked on this and the many other new associations to her father and family that this incident brought up. After this period, there were no more abrupt cancellations or fears of losing control of herself, her son, or school.

The final phase of treatment began as she began to transfer her ability to tolerate intimacy and structure to other areas of her life. The work was focused on her expanding social, interpersonal, and work life. Her social life encompassed a certain Eastern religious group noted for their emphasis on world brother/sisterhood and peace. She was encouraged to spend more social time with them. The therapist indicated a positive disposition to spirituality and stated that she may learn to integrate all aspects of her life if she continued to develop herself in whatever way she felt was good. The therapist recognized not only her psychological and social aspects, but that her spiritual side was equally important. She was surprised and felt good about this. With time she grew more sophisticated with religious/philosophical issues.

During one of these social meetings, she met a young man and began a long relationship. Since it was the termination phase of treatment, the therapist encouraged her to trust herself and enjoy the situation. The inner world reflects and draws much from the external world, was stressed to her by every method, e.g., gentle confrontation, dream analysis, absurd humor and self-disclosure. Therapy finally ended about 15 months after it began. She had fallen in love, was experiencing a sense of inner and outer balance, and was aware of her tendency toward "boundary" problems in intimate situations.

In both cases presented above on borderline functioning, the clinician first moved toward structure building to secure boundaries. Only later was work focused toward the tasks of differentiation, insight, and integration. Each type or level of organization elicits a strategically different type of intervention.

SUMMARY

I began this foray into borderline personality functioning with a simple description of this elusive creature. As it turns out, they live amongst us freely, are quite visible, and reflect much of our own less intense oscillating uncertainty in periods of acute distress. However, where we may experience a period of anxious oscillation between alternatives or persons, the borderline has adjusted and stabilized this seemingly unstable process. What are the developmental age details again?

This borderline organization appears to arise initially during the early subphase of individuation and autonomy so well described by Mahler. At the other end, the final rapprochement phase, between 15 and 36 months, seems to be crucial. Kohut and Kernberg believe that the process begins even earlier in the oral phase, but to be honest with you, seeing is believing, and the clinician does not really actually see it until the later autonomy-separation phase. Sullivan, from a different perspective, indicated the gradual rise of body-tension states into transient ego states with their attendant fears and needs for control. In Mahler, Sullivan, Kohut, and Kernberg, there are abundant descriptions of primitive psychological processes, especially those of splitting and projection.

For Mahler and most others, there is general agreement that the child moves from the initial stage of autism (0-2 months) through to the symbiotic phase (2-5 months), on to the rapids of the Separation-Individuation period (5-36 months). That crucial phase has three real subphases. There is the progressive differentiation of body image, tactile sense, and the dawn of the separate self sense. This occurs perhaps from 5 to 9 months. Refer to Chart 2.1 in Chapter 2 on development. These theorists assume the great anxiety to be re-engulfment, since the child has only recently evolved beyond the symbiotic phase where psychological fusion or merger is predominant. Note the need and relationship here between body-tension, the rise of transient ego states and muscle control. After the differentiation period is the practicing period between 10 and 14 months or so. The emerging ego is triumphant in the wider environment at this point. Here there is movement, you recall, toward and away from the mother. There also quickly arises the need to "re-fuel" after separation. This was played out in both clinical cases I described, especially the second case, in the need for repeated doses of structure. It is also a crucial time for family unconscious processes of shared imagery, affect and ideation, and the mirroring of each other in the deep structure patterning of functional self-other processes. The psychoanalytic movement has a copyright on the term "psychodynamic." I would only add here that in the shared field of family unconscious relations traditional boundary notions are crossed, identities often shared, and such "dynamics" as projective identification occasionally take on a different meaning. The process of "projective identification" is seen as a necessarily limited, sometimes neurotic, contraction in the shared psychic field of that greater reality of projective localization in which the "I" sees itself in the schema of reality at all levels.

The third leg of the crucial subphase is rapprochement proper at 15 to 36 months, where awareness of separation from mother, and also sometimes an increasing need for her, occur together. This can sometimes be annoying. The great anxiety here, it seems to me, is around potentially mixed parental messages and the child's fear of abandonment and subsequent depression. If the poor creature can navigate this far, then after this comes that stage of childhood proper where there is object constancy, an arising firm ego and all that comes with it. This new phase includes such goodies as castration anxiety, potential loss of self-esteem, gender identity, etc., a great welcome mat! Oh yes, there is also creativity, and simply, joy.

The defensive structure development of this era runs like this. First there is simple autistic withdrawal. At the symbiotic phase, there is regressive refusion with primitive introjection and projection, i.e., taking in and spitting out all the stuff of life. With the three real subphases of the separation-individuation phase, the principle psychological process is splitting, although the other psychological processes also are employed. After that, one can be on the way to developing a mature ego or a neurotic structure, but both require a sense of egoic mastery of internal and external reality.

Throughout this process of development I have attempted to show that in addition to a cognitive affective scheme evolving, there was also the pull toward the Absolute through the inherent evolutionary and Self unfolding process. The Self process, not the self of Kohut, but the Self of all self-organizing processes in operation, identifies with the cognitive, affective, and developing ego structures where appropriate and then must dis-identify when necessary to progress to the next stage. This evolves well until the transient, arising ego itself recognizes itself to be a limited, functional, and not absolute structure or tool and thus must pass away as other structures have. This process is most easily understood using the cognitive developmental structures of post-formal operations. The ego itself is recognized to be a transient, dissipative structure that gives rise to higher, more stable and subtle structures in its evolution. When this occurs in a balanced way there is a natural transcendence. When it does not, under the press and pull of life exigencies, there is regression.

I have attempted to place the data and argument within the context of a newer understanding of psychic and material energy dynamics whose terms are wholeness and interconnectedness. This is presented as opposed to the models of atomism, reductionism, and biological determinism. I have emphasized the observation and belief that borderline personalities tacitly and tangibly experience that authentic undivided wholeness which has no absolute boundaries of affect, ideation, and causation, but that their tools for management of these functional boundaries is poor. They have not fully accepted the illusory foundation of the arising ego, which must first define itself in terms of what it is not! In this particular way, the borderline is a failed mystic drawn by the higher trajectory of evolution, yet unstable and constricted at the foundation.[1]

Where appropriate, I have stressed the formative influence of the family unconscious and its shared matrix of affect, ideation, and energetic patterning. This is more conducive to the episodes of psi and early spontaneous empathy that arise and, also, it seems more congruent with the world views of seers and introspective scientists that have abounded since our earliest racial memory. This empathy is not a creation of the ego, but, rather, is a derivative of the compassion that is embedded in the world of consciousness itself. This compassion is innate, I feel, and is localized from a vast non-local source that is the universe itself. This is the suggestive outcome of recent studies in childhood empathy development and the testimony of nearly 2500 years of uninterrupted Mahayana Buddhist practice. Finally, the functional, but limited, scope of the ego was seen as arising primarily from body-tension zones, becoming more sophisticated and abstract, but always founded on an unstable sense of isolation, fear of other, dualism, and the threat of eventual dissolution. The ego resists this by all defensive means available to the process, e.g., splitting, denial, and hopeless grasping. Yet even this ego in its quiet moments can recognize (re-cognize) a current of living energy in its own body-mind. It may deny this basic current

---

1. In this sense, the serious borderline condition of anorexia nervosa of many females, beyond the neurotic manipulations, the numerous social and cultural pressures, the distorted somatic perceptions and the injured self-image, would appear to reflect a desire to be in total control of the emotional/vital/somatic world by way of control of food and nurturance. It is really the desire for the "pure body" or divya sarira. References to this are found in P. Yogananda's *Autobiography of a Yogi* in reference to a female practitioner, Giri Baua, who supposedly learned to live on sunlight alone! In young men there is often observed the desire to be pure "intellect" or mind without body. This is particularly the case with some young physicists and mathematicians. In both cases, the adolescent psychological distortion in this will to purity is perhaps a fleeting glimpse of higher processes in evolution. For the young girl, it is the vision of the pure body or divya sarira; for the adolescent boy, it is the pure scientific mind and intellect or rtambhara prajna.

of aliveness in the rest of the world by sophisticated intellectual abstraction, but it cannot deny its own direct experience. This current, this intelligent, luminous, flowing life-force threads through every stage of development. Its conscious development is the dim recognition of the Absolute in energetic terms.

The eye is now turned to another personality syndrome that is very common and is also intimately involved in the intuitive recognition of the unity of all phenomena, the intimation of the Absolute and, at the same time, the frantic clutching of the ego to passing differentiating experience. In the next case of the obsessive-compulsive, we focus our attention specifically on the frantic egoic attachment to ideas, rituals, and behavior in an attempt to hold on to an illusory world that terrifies, and paradoxically, reinforces the subtle sense of this transient, vulnerable, and illusionary ego.

REFERENCES

Blanck, G. and Blanck, R. *Ego Psychology: Theory and Practice*, Columbia University Press, New York and London, 1974.

Brown, L. J., "Staff countertransference reactions in the hospital treatment of borderline patients," *Psychiatry*, Vol. 43.

Ehrenwald, J., *Telepathy and Medical Psychology*, W. W. Norton & Co., New York, 1948.

Hughes, T. *Crow*, Harper and Row, New York, 1971.

Kernberg, O. "Borderline personality organization," *Journal of the American Psychoanalytic Association*, 15:641-685, 1967.

Kohut, H., *The Analysis of the Self*, International Universities Press, New York, 1971.

Mahler, M. S., "On the first three subphases of the separation-individual process," *International Journal of Psychoanalysis*, Vol. 53, 333-338, 1972.

Mahler, M. S., Pine, F. and Bergman, A. *The Psychological Birth of the Human Infant: Symbiosis and Individuation*, Basic Books, Inc., New York, 1975.

Masterson, J. F. and Rinsley, D. B. "The borderline syndrome: The role of the mother in the genesis and psychic structure of the borderline personality." In R. F. Lax, et al. (eds.), *Rapprochement: The Critical Subphase of Separation-Individuation*, 229-329, Jason Aronson, New York, 1980.

Moyne, J. and Barks, C. (translations) *OPEN SECRET: Versions of RUMI*, Threshold Books, p. 70, Putney, VT, 1984.

Newsweek, "Raising Children Who Care," Science Section, April 12, 1984, p. 76.

Rizzuto, A. M., Peterson, R. K. and Reed, M., "The Pathological Sense of Self in Anorexia Nervosa," *Psychiatric Clinics of North America*, Vol. 4, No. 3, December 1981, pp. 471-487.

Rumi, J. *Open Secret*, (translated by) J. Moyne and C. Barks, Threshold Books, Putney, VT, 1984.
Sullivan, H. S., *The Interpersonal Theory of Psychiatry*, W. W. Norton & Co., New York, 1953.
Wilber, K. "Ontogenetic Development: Two Fundamental Patterns," *Journal of Transpersonal Psychology*, 13:1, 33-58, 1981.
Yogananda, P. *Autobiography of a Yogi*, Self-Realization Fellowship, Los Angeles, CA, 1946.

Chapter 4

The Obsessive-Compulsive Personality: The Failed Compromise

THE YOU-NAME-IT-AHOLIC

I had a childhood that was mercifully brief,
I grew up in a state of disbelief.
I started to think too much,
When I was twelve going on thirteen,
Me and girls from St. Augustine,
Up in the mezzanine Thinking about God,
Maybe I think too much.

–Paul Simon
Song from *Hearts and Bones*

Out of all her progeny, our ancient skillful mother would be most intrigued by her modern offspring in the nervous, clever, time-pressured city dweller.

He probably works at a job similar to yours, but he is much, much cleaner and more orderly about it. He is certainly regulated and on time. Periodically, however, he seems to procrastinate endlessly. When you got to know him you found out a few things about him that were, at the very least, unexpected. He is an interesting sort of fellow, so you watch in different situations. He has demonstrated that he has a number of persistent and recurring ideas, thoughts, and internal images, sometimes even strong feelings and impulses that he says do not feel as if they really belong to him. Very often they are rather repulsive to him even though you may not see why. In addition to that seemingly jumbled but recurrent series of ideas and associations, he often seems to be following very specific private rules of some kind. They do not seem to be an end in themselves. Too often these behaviors seem more designed to control or prevent some sort of catastrophic event that might somehow occur now or in the future. However, they are not momentary, fairly moderate recurring thoughts such as leaving the house for a vacation and double checking the locks, stove-off, heat down, and calling the neighbors, etc. The acts seem to be almost continuous, and performed more from some state of internal drivenness coupled with the desire to forestall something else rather than from what appear to be requirements in the regular environment.

This person you work with, who has observed this in himself, is very intelligent and sometimes realizes that it does not make much sense. He doesn't draw much pleasure from it. But it does seem to provide some sort of strange and acceptable psychic soothing or tension release. One of the less attractive qualities about him is his seemingly endless concern with the morality of situations. He is always looking for the "right" and "wrong" of things, the "shoulds" and "oughts." Despite that, he is dogmatic and more than a little over-controlling when set loose in a situation. Even when playing, he has got to be "right."

One day you find out that some of his more intense preoccupations or concerns have to do with thoughts of killing someone or being contaminated by something! These recurrent thoughts and sometimes seemingly driven behaviors at their worst times turn into extreme checking, touching, and watching things, even excessive washing of his hands; "out, out, damned spot." Whenever you try to tell him to slow it down he attempts to do so, but then his internal pressure and anxiety level increases even more and the situation somehow seems to get worse. For this thought-junkie, so vicious a circle leads to more struggle in mental quicksand.

The above individual is what the literature would call an obsessive-compulsive personality or a personality with an obsessive-compulsive neurosis. It depends on your clinical point of view. The pattern of repetitive, obsessive, and compulsive behaviors is what is paramount in this social and intrapsychic picture. In this descriptive emphasis, in addition to noting the obsessive or recurrent images and ideas in the compulsive behaviors, you can easily notice a preponderance of anxiety and the potential for bottomless depression. In the very worst situations, true phobic avoidance of certain kinds of situations that are associated with the content of these odd obsessions will arise. You surmise that these have a great deal to do with fears of contamination, of hurting others, etc. It is suggested in the clinical literature that this disorder usually begins in adolescence but may also begin, at times, in childhood. Oddly enough, despite the pain and pressure the person is under, he often will not need hospitalization and, indeed, may become very stabilized for the rest of his life in this particular set of frozen ideas, associations, rituals, and behaviors.

When this person enters the office of the clinician, often the therapist will feel almost overwhelmed by the sheer amount of data that the individual produces concerning his or her particular problem. As this flow of information continues in the following sessions, more and more of this material surfaces. The clinician begins to develop a sense of the subtle, intrapsychic, and interpersonal styles and defenses that this individual has developed over time to control the *flow* and *current* of events in his/her inner and external life. Hints of massive denial and the capacity to suppress go very deep into the individual's inner landscape, and matrix of energy transformations. Eventually the intrapsychic defensive pattern of intellectualization accompanied by an ego-orchestrated emotional isolation will emerge in the clinical picture. The clinician's good history-taking will reveal the increasing loss of real spontaneity and feeling for life accompanied by affective or emotional contraction and shallowness. Here is clearly seen the "freezing," or constriction, of emotions in the excessive denial of any spontaneous feelings. Spontaneous feelings, in particular, appear to be defended against since they are experienced as unacceptable impulses welling up or invading this individual.

Watching over these defenses is a shrew-eyed vigilant ego. The ego's beaconlight of attention appears to be constantly scanning the horizon for danger and threats to its existence, an existence that, as pointed out earlier, has its origins in transient body-mind tension states in need of regulation. A great deal of the body-mind's psychic energy is directed by this vigilant system. Therefore, in addition to the continual stream of ideas, images, and impulses, more of which are experienced in a repetitive, unspontaneous, and marginally acceptable way, there are compulsive behaviors felt to magically prevent future harm and at the same time help the individual to control the intense internal states that threaten to erupt over and over. These behaviors reveal the defensive mechanisms primarily of denial, intellectualization with emotional isolation, and a general contraction or freezing of the life-current or basic aliveness that has been mentioned so often. Curiously enough, this obsessive character often enters into shared psychic systems, such as marriage, with someone who seems the opposite and in whom the person can project a certain basic and needed, but disowned, aliveness. This couple will oscillate back and forth in the "I only think you only feel" model of relationships. This, of course, is your All-American obsessive/hysteric marriage (Barnett, 1971).

When talking with this person or style you often have the strong sense that he or she is not really listening to you at all! This person's own internal agenda keeps popping up. Forget original thinking. This person seems to be unable to free attention long enough to hear you out. Oh, he or she can pay great attention to details, sure, but they are details that reflect individual concerns and habits. So, in a sense, attention is intense, but it is also intensely and narrowly focused. Thus, in many contexts, it is adaptive, such as in technical matters, and is thereby reinforced. When thereby reinforced, it becomes stronger!

This pattern has an internal reflection–one of pressure being built up inside. After awhile, this sense of internal pressure and psychic energy becomes the norm and is sought out in other theaters. This internal pressure feels necessary, but not necessarily his or hers. In other words, all the "shoulds": recurrent behaviors, internal images and thoughts, seem to take on a life of their own and feel as if they reflect some greater, higher order or morality. If attention is not held strictly to the task, if behavior and emotion stray too close to the unwanted feelings, the forbidden zone, then chaos is possible, including its ocean of depression. This bottomless possibility must be controlled at all costs! Many of the behaviors, rituals, thoughts, and so forth are enlisted to defend against and control the emergence of this terrifying crisis.

It seems and feels to me that this fear of loss of control is what defines this personality pattern perhaps more than any other. It is a fear of losing control that seems to be rooted in the fear of the dissolution of the ego based upon a subtle memory and dim insight that the ego itself is an illusory, arising "object." In an attempt to protect oneself against that dissolution, the primitive psychic apparatus mounts repeated efforts to snap-shot or freeze the emotions and life-force as they flow. The emotional and psychophysiological technology for doing this is by contracting the ego upon feelings and feeling states of the body-mind and therein attempting to bleed them of life energy therein, hopefully, controlling them. This strategy attempts to solidify, and thus deny, the transience and impermanence of all phenomena. From this perspective, the genuine life-force, often experienced at times as a flow of basic aliveness and psychic energy, is constantly interrupted by the defenses and attempts to control this natural, positive, and undeniable force. It gives rise to numerous psychosomatic symptoms. I have discussed this flow of life-current from the point of view of direct perception in Chapter 1. Near the end of this chapter, I will include more clinical cases of the process.

THE FREUDIAN INSIGHT: ANALITY, FEAR, AND REPETITION

The Freudian beacon is a brilliant light in the subterranean consciousness. It has intricately elucidated how the obsessive act serves to express unconscious motives and desires that, of course, are not acceptable to the rational and socially proper mind. As a consequence, there is a symbolic distortion of the motives and substitute gratification of them expressed by way of these obsessive acts. It was Freud's observation that these obsessive acts generally develop from rituals even in early childhood. These rituals, of course, are "security operations" or defenses from the Sullivanian point of view. Out of this observation of obsessive acts generally deriving from rituals, Freud (1939) came upon what he termed the "repetition-compulsion." For Freud, the

> principle of a repetition-compulsion in the unconscious mind [is] based upon instinctual activity and probably inherent in

> the very nature of the instinct–a principle powerful enough to overrule the pleasure principle, lending to certain aspects of the mind their demonic character, and still very clearly expressed in the tendencies of small children; a principle, too, which is responsible for a part of the course taken by the analysis of neurotic patients.

This repetition-compulsion dynamic is seen in the behavior of the obsessive-compulsive personality. As his understanding of the obsessive-compulsive personality neurosis deepened, Freud seemed to feel that these defenses or psychic energy transformations were really defenses against libidinal demands of the Oedipus complex resulting from the associated fear of castration in men. Remember, this is mostly going on at an unconscious level. As a consequence of it proceeding on an unconscious level, and therefore not totally under the control of the "reality principle," magical thinking could occur. In magical thinking there is a great deal of "undoing" of things. This ritualized doing and undoing of behavior appears to balance and defend the ego in a seemingly hostile world. The system attempts a balance between what are termed instinctual and counter-instinctual forces. Repression, as a psychological force, is active and makes possible this neurotic pattern. The poor borderline did not make it far enough in development to be capable of successful repression. This repression allows the "balance" to become a stable pattern in the system. I point out here, however, that it also nourishes the sense of egoic isolation and the need to feel in control of one's tenuous boundaries lest one dissolve and be absorbed in a hostile world. Too often the resulting stabilization merely allows the ego to remain on the fearful verge of dissolution.

Later, Freud saw these obsessive-compulsive rituals and Oedipal dynamics as constituting the essence of all religious seeking in life. That was an ambitious but gross misunderstanding of the Divine intuition. Throughout his life, Freud was fascinated, on and off, by the occult, admitted to telepathy, and yet was suspicious of the "oceanic" feelings. Talk about denial and oscillation!

The Freudian view outlined very quickly above would seem to cover a great deal of territory. However, Freud seems to overlook the social and familial ways that defenses are actually *learned,* not only unconsciously, but in direct observation of the personality patterns of significant others. We are referring to the learning of defenses to anxiety that occurs in the family matrix. This has been highlighted by Ackerman (1957) in his monumental work, *The Psychodynamics of Family Life*. The enfolding field of the *Family Unconscious* has also been explored, and this probes the influence of deep structure family patterns and dynamics upon the choice of symptoms. The choice of symptoms is not totally an intrapsychic matter, but is also an interpersonal process and, I would suggest further, a matter of collective, enfolded, and shared consciousness among significant family members over time.

Otto Fenichel (1945) in his summary gem, *The Psychoanalytic Theory of Neurosis*, approached the obsessive-compulsive pattern by extending the Freudian lens. Fenichel pointed out that these obsessions appear to be derivatives. In other words, they appear to ward off, by association, the other ideas that are related to them with psychic energy in the system. They keep the "real issues" far away from the anxious ego. Notice here the psychically interconnected boundary between those contents that are acceptable to the ego and those that must be walled off by defensive maneuvers because of their charged association to other, more undesired contents. "Boundary" needs to be thought of as permeable, not a barrier, since at some level of consciousness the acceptable and unacceptable touch each other. In the Freudian landscape it is the territory of the preconscious. As a consequence of this clinical observation, it appears that while repression proper appears to be basic to hysteria, the obsessive-compulsive personality uses repression *and* other defenses, such as doing and undoing, to maintain a sense of egoic balance and control of situations. Whereas repression alone is seen to be the primary symptom in hysteria, repression, other security operations, and inter-psychic defenses are seen to be used in the obsessive-compulsive disorder. The compulsion itself is seen to be a compromise, an attempted balance formulation of the ego. The compromise is between the impulse to perform a certain act and the psychic energy used to deny that act. Their minutely oscillating compromise formation is the obsessive-compulsive style. The process is interpersonal or externalized in the obsessive-hysteric marriage. Issues of emotional control and the need for order *and* emotionality in both partners oscillates back and forth. Each reflects what the other both needs and fears! (Martin, 1976). This again is a common coupling style, and I will return to it shortly.

Naturally, conflict is at the very root of the obsessive-compulsive behavior pattern. I would like to note here, for this reason and future reasons, that the behaviors of the obsessive-compulsive, particularly the compulsive and ritualistic aspects, appear to me to be highly associated with early toilet training with its accompanying *bowel tension* and *relaxation energies*. I am noting here that the obsessive-compulsive behavior pattern is powerfully involved or cathexed to toilet training, as Freud pointed out in reference to "anal eroticism" processes, and that particularly bowel function, is established in the early family matrix. This occurs largely *before* the Oedipal period of libidinal cathexis and other more focused sexual goals. This is partially in a pre-verbal and pre-logical time! Because it is both barely-verbal and pre-logical, it is, to a large extent, pre-egoic. This is difficult to spotlight because at around two years old, when toilet training becomes a powerful issue in many families and societies, the child is also establishing, through negative identification, his or her own nascent identity as an ego in the world. It is, therefore, a very libidinally powerful and conflicted time. As a consequence of this, of course, a great emphasis is placed upon the control processes that emerge from this period. These dualities, differentiations, and primitive splittings often develop ambivalence in the direction of excessive cleanliness versus the fear of contamination or poison. I sense that a great deal of orderliness, neatness, and body-tension control is a defense against an oceanic expansive or boundless euphoria with its threat of ego dissolution.

It needs to be emphasized here that during this period, when body sphincter and motor training is for the first time consciously necessary, anal retentive tendencies or anal expulsive tendencies can develop. These are both *intimately* associated with the *conductivity of vital energies in the body*.[1] In other words, the control of the anal sphincter is the first zone of the body to come under necessary control *all the time* by the organism. The oral sphincter is, indeed,

1. The control of subtle energies in the body, particularly in Kundalini Yoga, is done through certain internal physical locks or bandas. The one at the base of the spine is extremely important and is termed Mulabanda.

first nourished and stimulated by an external agent, specifically the mothering one, and there are, of course, sucking reflexes, etc., that develop into the more organized behavioral scheme that Piaget outlined. However, the oral sucking reflex does not need to be consciously learned or to be kept closed over time. This must be done, however, with the anal sphincter. As a consequence, it seems that this is the first place in which there is a constant holding onto and perhaps at times, choking off, of a basic flow of life-energies that were discussed in the first chapter. It can be seen how the relatively successful application of obsessive-compulsive behaviors and patterns can reinforce the egoic sense of isolation. The experience of isolation, of being on a separate island at sea, gives rise to a number of other psychological defense patterns. These psychological defense patterns against powerful impulses are very often transformed by the unconscious mind into their opposites. These opposites can be seen in the behavior and intrapsychic processes of displacement and reaction formation.

The earlier mentioned borderline personality is positioned "between" the psychoneurotic constellations, e.g., obsessive-compulsive style, paranoid style, etc., and the psychotic style. This again is because the psychoneurotic family, which includes the obsessive-compulsive, is capable of psychological repression. They may replace one obsession with another throughout life, but in each case the force of repression is at work. In many instances it looks as though the obsessive-compulsive is defending against the borderline style or functioning with its potentially psychologically dissolving loss of boundaries. This rigid attention process and boundary formation by the obsessive-compulsive does lend a measure of cohesion and inner security to the system. However, squeezing out a new or deep feeling from them is conflicted and exceedingly difficult. It reminds one of a case of psychic hemorrhoids.

Many of us have noticed that the obsessive-compulsive individual is often very attractive to and attracted by the more hysterical personality pattern. Very often these lead to a stabilized interpersonal couple. If one looks at the psyche of the obsessive-compulsive, one will note that there is a strong desire on the part of the obsessive-compulsive for order and control on all levels. By entering into this kind of relationship and pattern, the emotionally expressive and "loose" hysteric can find the order he/she senses is needed but disowns in him/herself. The mutual projective processes find balance in the other. In the individual obsessive-compulsive, a desire for a certain balance or what is called "symmetry compulsion" can be seen. These, again, are all various ways of attempting to control the constant and inevitable flow of life-energy, often experienced as psychic energy or vital energy, that I have suggested is a universal reflection of the absolute, transcendental, and expansive life-force.

THE FAMILY THEATER

I have borrowed where it seems appropriate from different observations in different perspectives. I have not emphasized the familial learning approach, but this can be subsumed under the patterns outlined by Ackerman and Taub-Bynum. This is to say that a great deal of modeling and learning of intrapsychic and interpersonal defensive patterns occurs within the family matrix. This occurs whether or not the family is perceived as a collection of intrapsychic influences, or whether one accepts the implications of a shared unconscious which is reflected in the family unconscious. A common family theater example is the parent who, under his/her own pressure to exert control in a world or social environment that is perceived to be hostile, bonds tightly with the child with anxiety and worry. This is supposedly for the child's welfare, but actually masks the parent's fear and anxiety. This is a common binding process and sets in motion a deep psychic process that the child learns as a way of handling anxiety. In any case, the result of early family learning and reinforcement is of paramount importance to the formation of intrapersonal and interpersonal psychic energy transformations.

Many of the defenses outlined above are easily seen to be operative in the obsessive-compulsive pattern. In particular is the use of psychic compromise in symptom formation for the egoic control of anxiety. This anxiety, however, appears not only to spawn another face of the desire to control it that is always partially frustrated, but on another level seems to reflect a sense of perpetual anxiety on the part of the ego that is concerned with its own continuous survival. Paranoid ideation is implicit in the picture, and if the obsessive-compulsive defenses break down, the paranoid usually walks into the room.

Expressed in a different way, the obsessive-compulsive behavior style anxiously begins in the early family matrix usually associated with toilet training. Freud does deal with this but only in passing in terms of the influence of family members. It is emphasized here that the family teaching, conscious and unconscious, concerning the flow and control of bodily tensions and energies is deeply rooted. This is a highly personalized and implicate matrix of whos: we, they, and them. It is the local and extended family theater of subjects and subjectivity. These later deeply influence physical and psychic boundary formation in the way that the energy currents are controlled. Remember, one is dealing with the flow of "energy fields," not "objects" separate and only externally related to each other. It, seems therefore, that the life-force, often experienced as psychic energy, is often frozen in the obsessive-compulsive pattern related to early training concerning the bowel functions and the flow of energy through the system. How this is handled has profound effects upon the personality's actual behavioral patterns and energy transformations.

The contrast between excessive orderliness and that hidden impulse or desire to "mess up" has already been alluded to. This obsessive-compulsive style, like other styles at every other stage of development, seeks a certain "balance" of forces in the system. This is an attempt to stabilize a system. However, from this new perspective, the fall comes when the system is overly stabilized and the energies for transcendence for that particular stage are frozen or overly constricted by the ego. The system does not seem to be able to free attention and respond creatively to novel situations that would lead to more information sharing and higher levels of complexity and stability. The psychic bureaucracy is stiff and outdated by new contingencies. The system of psychological images and affects has become fixated upon by the ego in a series of repetitive, frozen patterns. In tight emotional expression and other ways it exacerbates its case of psychic hemorrhoids.

It looks something like this: The ego perpetually contracts upon a feeling, attempting to own and control the feeling and, as a consequence, since only partially owning and controlling, senses failure therein increasing its own anxiety. This leads to a subtle, increased sense of loss of control and therein arises the compensatory need for even more vigilance and defenses, creating a vicious circle. It is a vicious circle, but it is also something that can be stabilized over time. This is why the obsessive-compulsive pattern very often does not turn up in the therapeutic situation. When it does show up, it is of an extreme kind, or else the style is reflected in other symptoms, e.g., insomnia, psychosomatic symptoms, etc. In making this assessment and perception I am operating from the position that the ego arises initially from a series of states of bodily tension that awareness focuses or localizes around. The perception of the present work is that it is the ego's delusion of its own permanence, and yet its tacit recognition on the level of intuition that this is indeed "bad faith," that the ego itself really is transient, that leads to the fear of dissolution and the compensatory use and search for contracting mechanisms to create and perpetuate a sense of security. The obsessive-compulsive is continually bailing water out of a sinking ship. It seems that the initial delusion of the ego is developmentally and situationally necessary. The difficulty comes when the ego attempts to cling or grasp at the intuited, recognized, flowing reality of psychological, physiological, and life-current energy. This is the specialized way that the obsessive deals with the threat of ego death, that is to say, the *excessive* use of words, images, and ideas in repetitive, frozen patterns. This is how he or she, at the basis of his/her disorder, is radically different from the borderline personality, who defends against the same ultimate reality, but uses different defenses. Both intuit undivided wholeness, both defend in different ways against that wholeness.

We have noticed the obsessive-compulsive pattern has a prior history of "relief" of internal pressure and anxiety by the use of these symptoms. Indeed the ego's vigilant attempt at control by words, images and ideas in frozen associations does indeed provide some anxiety reduction. It, therefore, adds a secondary gain to the system. This was pointed out by not only Sullivan, but also Freud. Any social learning theorist will suggest the same, but use different languages to point that out (Ullmann and Krasner, 1969). All of the above is accepted with some major changes and additions, plus a good deal of reframing, to include the stage appropriate seeking of transcendence in the Absolute, which is believed to be rooted in our very nature.

SOME OTHER NOTIONS

Obviously this obsessive-compulsive fellow has a lot of internal activity going on that requires a great expenditure of psychic energy. He is rarely relaxed, given his constricted attention and high level of body tension. To be sure, one appreciates a little of this compulsive attention to detail if he is one's physician, pharmacist, or engineer. One wants a nurse or technician who is very careful and attentive. It is only when he slips off the deep end that a serious problem arises. Until that time, he has much to offer. At times his behavior may inadvertently throw light on some of the more hidden areas of the psyche.

The obsessive-compulsive's use of language and words appears to go somewhat deeper than the psychodynamic observations presented earlier. It appears that the use of images, words, and repeated ideas in frozen patterns is a tacit recognition that the phenomenal world itself, both the waking and dreaming states, is really a world primarily of sensory perceptions, images, ideas, and *patterns* of perception. It is a truth of the transient phenomenal world, but is intuitively not true of the nature of the transcendental life-energy that the individual is experientially rooted in. A transcendental life-energy that the individual intuits is, itself, prior to and deeper than the particular associations that a person may have to that energy flow at any particular point. Also, other egos seem to experience a flow of energy even though their descriptions are different. The ideas, images and other productions of the conscious and the unconscious appear themselves to be egoic modifications and transformations of this radiant, transcendental life-current. The obsessive-compulsive ego's rigid defenses appear more and more to be a panicky fist hurled into the abyss.

It is almost as though the obsessive-compulsive's thoughts become entrained or locked in an overarching energy pattern that is greater than the individual principle of consciousness itself and the person cannot break loose. The successful meditative practice begins to reveal these thoughts to seemingly have a life and dynamism of their own at times!

The obsessive-compulsive mental pattern is not only woven of these thoughts, images, and ideas, but also of behavior in a pattern of energy transformations that appears to be fixated in at least three ways: First of all, it appears that the obsessive-compulsive, on some tacit level, actually *believes* in the magical control of reality by words as the child does at a certain stage of development. This includes the positive and the negative aspects of words. A positive aspect of words creates certain things in the imagination that are very entertaining for various needs of the child. It also corresponds to the primitive and magical logic of "if thine eye offend thee, pluck it out." It is a very primitive and magical thinking level of mentation that Werner and Piaget have extensively investigated.

This kind of primitive thinking, of course, is not special to the child or to that involved in the cognitive-affective style of the obsessive-compulsives. It can also be seen in the logic of most dreams, sometimes in the special logic of schizophrenics, and other such phenomena. It is *similar* to what is called the Von Domarus principle in the study of primitive or paleological thought patterns in schizophrenia (Arieti, 1969). In the Von Domarus principle whereas the normal adult accepts identity only upon the basis of identical subjects and employs Aristotelian logic, the primitive paleologican accepts identity based upon identical predicates. Without getting too involved in this primitive process and becoming too obsessional myself, I simply say here that for the child and for these primitive mental processes, and also sometimes for certain patterns of logic in the obsessive-compulsive, what appears to the mature adult to be a separate explicate level symbol of the object is not really a symbol to this child or patient. Rather it is, indeed, a duplication of the real object or the power itself. There is a primitive, real fusion of object, symbol, and name. This level amplifies the power of thought which is related to Freud's "omnipotence of thought." It stems from an imperfectly seen but intuitively recognized subtle implicate energetic level relationship between an object or image and the vibrational dynamics that correspond to it. It is the basis of what is called the real science of mantra in the East. At a certain level of meditational practice, the level of contemplation or dhyana, the mind fuses with the object of knowing and the dynamics of the process unfold in and through the knower.

This process of deep identification with the object also occurs at a level that is in many ways unstable, pre-verbal and, therefore, subject to what Harry Stack Sullivan would characterize as "paratactic distortions." It involves somewhat autistic and non-rational thinking from a contemporary perspective but yet this irrational thinking, this magical abode exists in the consensually validated world. So very much of what we actually *do* in the everyday cultural, family, and social moment-to-moment world is based on unreflective imagery, fluid associations, and shared myths!

Secondly, the phenomenal universe is tacitly recognized by the obsessive-compulsive to be transient. This type of primary anxiety for the ego is experienced as the possibility of dissolution and death. Thence, again, obviously arises the need of the ego to contract and hold onto this fleeting experience in order to avoid that terror and ultimate assault on its integrity. In the consensually validated world of interpersonal, social and cultural relations, the obsessive-compulsive also realizes the power of words, images, and ideas to affect relations with significant others. Significant others include not only the family members, but also one's socio-economic compatriots, working peers, the boss, etc. One has only to look at powerful speakers and thinkers in the world to recognize the true power of words and ideas. This part of their thinking is not an illusion, it is rather their over-evaluation of it that leads into difficulty in the case of the overly intellectualized obsessive-compulsive. Also the fact that they rarely offer any new ideas, but only old ideas in a frozen pattern also contributes to the disorder.

On the third level, the obsessive-compulsive's involvement with words and language appears to actually and genuinely reflect and intuit the elevating vision that words and images do possess. This is rarely seen in full blossom in the obsessive-compulsive because their habitual restricting of the flow of the life-current. However, this does flower in the words of artists, particularly in poets and writers. The poet or artist harnesses words, images and, sometimes, compulsive behaviors to harness the life-force such that they eventually transcend the symptomatology. The obsessive-compulsive, however, merely uses words, images and behavioral patterns to obscure the light and flow of conscious energy. Indeed, one must learn the scales of the piano well in order to be relatively free later in that function so that one can spontaneously create melody, rhythm, and music.

Lastly, I sense that on the deepest level of the mind, the obsessive-compulsive personality intuits that the world is literally rhythm and *vibration* and to control or integrate with this primary vibration is a goal of life. The obsessive-compulsive, obviously, is many steps away from this. He may, as Jung suggested, use a certain form of ritual, rigid religious dogma and practices, to actually defend against a religious experience! However, rooted in all this is the actual sense of the science of vibration. This, again, in yoga science is recognized as the science of mantra. It is also the fountainhead that lies behind music. I have already cited research before how various physically measurable sounds can manifest themselves on the psychological and psychic plane (Jenny, 1975). These include replicative demonstrations of the effects of sound to create images in the material world. There seems to be a convergence on the deepest level between the obsessive-compulsive attempt at freezing the natural vital rhythm and vibration of life and the true sciences of sound and vibration. Here one can see the many currents toward the same source condition and realization, and that source condition and realization is the recognition that "in the beginning was the Word."

RECAPITULATION

It appears that the obsessive-compulsive seems to genuinely intuit the "perfection" of his or her idealized self-regulating processes on all levels, including that of consciousness; in other words, of his/her own real Self. Like all other beings, this person moves naturally toward this Self in cognitive/affective development. The fall, however, appears to be associated with the excessive egoic contraction and fixation upon these particular arising words, feelings, intuitions, and ideas. This leads to a freezing of attention and ritualized patterns of thoughts, energies, and behavioral responses in an attempt to control this whole undivided vibratory matrix. By attempting to contract and control the feeling it gives the illusion of the ego being in charge of this whole process, and indeed it does provide some illusory degree of control over the flow of phenomena. However, in the process, usually a process affected very early in childhood, a condition arises in which there is a perpetual freezing of *tension* in the body and *attention* in the mind. Note the concomitant freezing of bodily tension states and a psychological freezing of attention in various modalities. Both are attempts to control the internal and external phenomenal world. In the final chapter on methodology this subtle process and observation will be crystallized in clinical practice. Suffice it to say here that too often these individuals excessively fear death and flee its symbolic expressions to an extraordinary degree. The root delusion of the obsessive-compulsive is that he or she can, by these numerous defenses, both intrapsychic and interpersonal, control the flow of internal and external reality, both of which are reflected in the current of the life-force. Hopefully, this helps avoid human suffering, as they hold a precise stopwatch in the face of eternity.

The clinician observes that very often the themes of power, dominance, and submission are involved in this particular obsessive-compulsive patterning. These, of course, are learned in the early family matrix where issues of unequal power distribution are of necessity dealt with. Rama (1977) and others have outlined the personality patterns that seem to be associated with certain states of consciousness. They associate the issues of power and control, of dominance and submission, with what is termed the third chakra level in the yogic system. This is a basic structure that has emerged, not a transient structure (Wilber, 1981). In Eastern traditions, the third chakra is usually associated with vital energy, power, and the capacity of the mind to deal in the world. It is physically located slightly below the navel area, the area that in acupuncture theory and practice is the focus of immense ki energies. These energies are not limited here, though. Much of this vital energy and life-current can be seen to be highly associated with the heart and also the previously mentioned base of the spine in terms of the learning to perpetually close the anal sphincter with the increasing ego control and body motility. This whole process creates a pulse or rhythmic pattern over this current of living energy and certain possibilities occur. Perhaps a metaphor would be helpful.

Doubtless, the constant beating of the heart in various emotional situations and in various degrees of frequency led to the first productions of music in the human individual and tribe. This basic sense of repetitiveness led eventually to observing the cycles and repetitions in nature and to the sense of needing to repeat things in nature in the tribal and religious rituals. These recurrent rituals and rhythms can be naturally soothing and give one some sense of prediction, control over, and communion with vast nature by imitating and introjecting nature's patterns. The difference, however, is that in the repetitive patterns of music, after a basic recognized pattern is established, there are orderly and *creative* permutations upon this basic rhythm. The rhythm may even change to another creative pattern. In the obsessive-compulsive there is merely the repetition of outlived patterns that provide only a small degree of security. This small degree of security, however, seems to be better than the greater fear of no security boundaries and thus no ego at all.

I have noticed in cases of successful therapy with obsessive-compulsives (these are few cases indeed), that with the gradual release of ego tensions, the symptoms are gradually overcome. Ego tensions result in perpetual states of body tension leading to what Reich called body and character armor. With the gradual release of ego tension, there is less tension in the body and less frozen attention in the mind. This can be done in therapy *only* if the body is also brought into treatment. Thus some intense affective and behavioral work is necessary. There is an increase in the creative flow of associations in successful therapy. These associations are not limited to an association and merely its direct opposite, but a freeing up such that many other associations *unfold* from a source or seed idea. At first, of course, there is an increase in associations that are connected with hostile and disowned ideas, impulses and affects. With acceptance, these fears are eventually overcome and transcended and attention becomes free. Tension becomes less.

Many particular manifestations of body armor and psychological body tension states can be seen in the work of Alfred Lowen. This is built upon Reich's pioneering work. Lowen (1971) clearly outlines how a decrease in body tension and a freeing of mental attention leads to a return to equanimity and a harmonious identification with the body. As one begins to re-identify with the spontaneously arising body-sense, there is a decrease in obsessive identification with the productions and conflicts of the transitory internalized and highly overintellectualized ego. A sense of primary ontological security, of basic trust in the universe, returns to the body-mind. There is a re-establishment of faith based upon an actual and direct perception of the flow of the transcendental life-current. It gradually becomes more and more obvious that the various thoughts, images, and ideas are indeed permutations of that one transcendental and transformational matrix of life-energy that is intuited to underlie, be the substratum of, and to pervade, all material and energy creation.

It seems the obsessive-compulsive individual is as fearful of both the loosening of the "top" of the mind as he or she is of the "bottom" of the system. "As above, so below" is twisted by the fear of dissolution such that the compromise is a psychospiritual contraction upon the life-force such that all prior and antecedent intuitions and influences are blocked off from the system. Sri Aurobindo repeatedly warned that on the spiritual journey both the higher and the lower open in the greater integration of the consciousness. This often occurs in intense life situations and psychotherapy.

CASE HISTORIES

Case History 1

Joseph X., a 24-year-old single white male junior executive was referred to a biofeedback clinician by his physician. He was referred for several reasons, including a series of GI tract disturbances, insomnia, anxiety attacks, and inability to relax.

During the clinical assessment it became clear that, while the patient was very intelligent, he tended to barely hold in his social anger. It would arise each morning as he headed to a fairly high-stress job. At work, he was constantly preparing to deal with a crisis that somebody had. Between awaking in the morning and walking into his office he would develop stomach and lower GI problems. At night he would think about what had happened over and over and therein create insomnia for half the night. His full panic attacks were few, but he always felt he had to hold on tight or he would lose control of it all.

Treatment focused on symptom control and reduction with only minimal psychological interpretations. The clinician dealt with the internal emotional and psychological issues of anger, family similarities in symptom patterns, and the need to be assertive instead of anxious. However, it was humorously reflected to the patient many times that merely long verbal exploration of psychological defenses would be like a pig in quicksand.

Instead, he was treated with biofeedback for his overt symptoms and instructed in the ways of pranayama or breath control to feel the flow of the life-current in his breathing. The judgmental process, which was severe, was hired to watch his thought spread wider apart as he relaxed more deeply. Soon he was able to apply the process of body-mind relaxation and then watching the circus of thoughts to other situations. His sex life improved immediately and his overt symptoms ended, including insomnia.

The more subtle work then occurred by the therapist humorously opening areas of possible anger in the client. Anger, resentment, fear, and other emotions were encouraged to be given some "air-time." Whenever they arose in the context of the session, the patient, who was attached to the EMG of biofeedback, was gently directed toward the correlation drawn between states of body-tension, his emotional tension, and the lack of free attention in his system. Humor often arose spontaneously. With time he achieved even deeper states of relaxation when he identified with the current of energy arising in his system. He was able to intuit that this stream of energy was always operative, whether his ego was aware or not, and that he could increase this blissful flow at will. The reinforcement was symptom relief and a more lighthearted approach to work, sex, and reality.

The next case involves a similar process.

The patient was a 35-year-old white gay male, Robert X. This patient had been in therapy previously and was himself a mental health professional. He was referred by another mental health professional who had some countertransference problems with the patient's gay orientation.

The patient often presented himself as excessively neat, polite, and verbally expressive. The initial problem was one of career choice. The patient would oscillate between choices and procrastinate on all fronts. He reported that his apartment was either very neat or a mess. He had many friends but had difficulty in his intimate relationships.

As therapy progressed, it emerged that there was another side to his orderliness. He often visited sexually explosive situations for "relief" when he was very lonely. He hid this from his friends in a secretive, compulsive way. He also had numerous concerns about food.

Finally, he could not seem to balance his need for intimacy and sexuality with his conservative religious orientation. He oscillated between the male bathrooms and the seminary.

Treatment concentrated around the above issues. A positive transference allowed therapy to deepen, so soon he and the clinician were dealing with issues of trust, depression, obsessive isolation, and fear. His family of origin was explored in great depth, including his primary process memory of the secret pact he had with his mother. Much of her own illness was reflected in him. The therapist reframed his escapes to the bathrooms as the avoidance of relationship and encouraged him to tolerate his anxiety. The therapist humorously suggested that his anxiety would not kill or dissolve him. His strong inclination toward some religious values was harnessed and the therapist pushed him to express them through relationships.

For over 9 months he presented with weekly crises, often crises in obsessive detail. The clinician openly confronted his obsessive style as a defense to affect and *change.* This angered him but also spoke directly to him. When he became vague on issues the therapist reflected that he was taking a strategy to avoid choice and perpetuate his suffering. He had to bury his long deceased mother once and for all.

When, after several very tearful sessions, he saw this, his symptoms decreased. The therapist encouraged his religious

> pursuits in relationships and soon he had two longer than usual love relationships over the next year. It was emphasized that he needed to structure his affective insight into behavioral change. This involved a new sense of openness and forgiveness, a releasing of painful history as a process of identification.

In these cases, the clinician uses interpretation of resistances and uncovering of earlier data in the interventions. The "identity" problem is treated differently from that in the earlier borderline situations. The client is capable of more reflection and tolerance of anxiety.

SUMMARY

This chapter opened with a portrait of what is called today the obsessive-compulsive personality or syndrome. Some general behavioral and cognitive-affective patterns were described and these were related to early ego development with its attendant arising tension states.

It was observed that the various symptoms and modifications of this personality style were in various ways attempts to control the current of the life-force. Hopefully, it was seen how the contraction of the ego around certain experiences, the clinging to the illusion of permanence and control in the midst of the real social/biological requirements of body energy control, lead to this process. The style of control is seen to be directly communicated in the family matrix, both consciously and unconsciously, along with all the other attendant anxieties. These experiences were first intensified around anal functions.

Later, I extended the range of this syndrome to reflect how it too has embedded in its process a press toward the Absolute, yet clinically reveals only fragments and derivative symptoms of failed balance and transcendence. Two cases in which this is partially reflected were presented as clinical case studies.

Therapy, in various forms, must always include the body and some intense affective and behavioral change. The whole symptomology arises as an attempt to hold *even more tightly* to ego tension states. These ego tension states include not only the physical tension of musculature, or in character armor, but also affective tension and the active fixation or freezing of attention, all of which is done to defend against the sense of egoic dissolution in the flowing current of the living transcendental force.

REFERENCES

Ackerman, N. *The Psychodynamics of Family Life*, Basic Books, New York, 1957.

Arieti, S. "Special logic of schizophrenia and other types of autistic thought," *The Study of Abnormal Behavior*, edited by Zax and Strictler (1948) 1969.

Barnett, J. "Narcissism and depending in the obsessive-hysteric marriage," *Family Process*, 10:75-83, 1971.

Fenichel, O. *The Psychoanalytic Theory of Neurosis*, W. W. Norton & Co., New York, 1945.

Freud, S. *Moses and Monotheism*, New York, Alfred Knopf, Inc., 1939.

Jenny, H. *Cymatics: Structure and Dynamics of Waves and Vibrations*, Vol. 1, New York, Schocken, 1975.

Lowen, A. *Language of the Body*, Macmillan, New York, 1971.

Martin, P. *A Marital Therapy Manual*, Brunner/Mazel Publishers, New York, 1976.

Rama, S., Ballentine, R., and Ajaya, S. *Yoga and Psychotherapy: The Evolution of Consciousness*, Himalayan Publishers, Honesdale, Pennsylvania, 1977.

Taub-Bynum, E. B. *The Family Unconscious: "An Invisible Bond,"* Quest Books, Wheaton, Illinois, 1984.

Ullman, L. P. and Krasner, L. *A Psychological Approach to Abnormal Behavior*, Prentice-Hall, Inc., Englewood Cliffs, New Jersey, 1969.

Wilber, K. "Ontogenetic Development: Two Fundamental Patterns," *Journal of Transpersonal Psychology*, 13:1, 33-58, 1981.

Chapter 5

Paranoia: The Fist in the Abyss

EGOCENTRICITY AND THE FLIGHT FROM BLAME

To see eternity in a grain of sand.

–W. Blake

The projecting power, through the aid of the veiling power, connects a man with the siren of an egoistic idea, and distracts him through the attributes of that.

–Sri Sankarcarya

Now it gets strange. In youth you knew him to be a very energetic person. He was ambitious, capable. However, sometimes he was also very stubborn, often defensive. Even then you noted an unwillingness on his part to compromise. Power always loomed up as one of his motives. Still he seemed to get along with most people. Many times his ambition and style were very adaptive to the situation. He was, as you observed, very argumentative, and at times would get into a hassle with you over seemingly nothing. In every situation, however, he would always try to avoid blame. He was very suspicious of your loyalty after you had an argument. You had heard that in his love relationships he was intensely jealous at times. Very bright, however, he remained one of your friends. In every new situation in which you and he were in, or else just by himself, he would always be looking for the supposedly "real" meaning of the situation. He was on the lookout for hidden motives, usually found it very difficult to relax, and often felt tense and was preparing for his counterattack. Eventually, this began to bother you more and more. Perhaps you remember mumbling under your breath about him being a weird guy, or even a bastard. He remained affectively restricted in relationships while you grew to be more and more involved with other people. Your relationship gradually diminished. Over time he appeared colder and colder. In some way or another you realize that you were never really very close.

The above may be a rather large, and perhaps overly expanded, picture of the "paranoid" person, but reflects a common pattern. This pattern is a form of paranoia. Paranoia in the clinical literature is not as streamlined and clearly focused as therapists would like to think. One can see evidences of paranoid ideation without there being a completely paranoid syndrome operative. Under a great deal of stress for a prolonged period of time, most of us are given to thinking styles that attempt to find out the "real" meaning and intricate balance of things going on. However, when offered information that disproves our hypothesis, we can usually change our mind. The paranoid has a great deal of difficulty doing this. It is as though all meaning in the world falls into a subtle orbit around him. In the actual so-called paranoid personality disorder, there is some paranoid ideation, but there is no actual delusional material. In actual practice, the paranoid style may appear clinically nonspecific and emerge across numerous syndromes, from organic to schizophrenic, to affective, on to paranoid proper. There are a number of things, however, that do seem to characterize this general psychobehavioral pattern.

There is generally recognized to be a pervasive, unwarranted suspiciousness of others accompanied by a sense of always expecting trickery, or even harm, from others. A hypervigilance is seen in this kind of personality pattern. The person continually scans the environment for signs of threat so that they can take precautions. The attention is narrowly focused around issues of survival, power, and possible ways of being hurt. They tend to be very jealous individuals. It has been noted that psychophysiologically they often experience themselves to be very tense, not being able to relax or feel relatively safe and unguarded (Shapiro, 1965). A great deal of psychic energy and attention is focused in a constant and tense search for confirmation of prearranged ideas. Often there is a loss of a generalized context in which these very events are to happen even though the paranoid is exquisitely sensitive to interpersonal relations. Issues become highly *personalized* and are focused around the dynamics of loyalty, betrayal, and the psychological dynamic of projection in their energized matrix of who, them, me, and us.

One of the central processes recognized in paranoia is the avoidance of blame. There is a constant looking for hidden motives and special meanings, a hypersensitivity to criticism, and a stance that is always ready to go on the counterattack. By this maneuver, the vigilant ego has legislated away a great deal of warm affect. These people are often experienced as rather calculating and cold. This particular feature they share with the obsessive-compulsive personality, who when they further decompensate, often reflect symptoms like those of the paranoid (Menninger, 1963). For the paranoid, however, there is always great concern around issues of power.

There is a concomitant avoidance of any true intimacy in this style or syndrome. The avoidance of intimacy is very connected with the sense of fearfulness concerning the boundaries of the personality. This also is shared with the obsessive-compulsive. However, there is also a process about the paranoid that is quite distinct from other syndromes. It is the presence of an exaggerated need for self-importance and importance in the eyes of others.

Under periods of prolonged stress, this paranoid process can emerge and manifest in its various forms across many syndromes from paranoid schizophrenia, where the thought processes are really delusional and frozen, all the way over to the pure paranoid personality transversing the whole circus of different symptoms and patterns in between. Their clinical presentation usually includes a progressive misinterpretation of other people's motives, different stimuli in the environment taking on a peculiar or menacing intention and a gradual calculus of self-referential signs and meanings that are impossible to disprove. During periods of acute stress, it is possible for the paranoid style to: manifest psychotic symptoms in the visual mode; experience the arising of an intricate play of delusions around certain themes; experience the emergence of highly personalized "ideas of reference," in which individuals perceive other individuals to be constantly talking about them; and have very irrational and phobic reactions to places, people, and situations. All of these paranoid colored patterns, of course, are weaved together in a very systematized, and apparently logical, manner. Logical, that is, if you do not look too closely at the paranoid's underlying assumptions. Always the assumptions have to do with the personal egoic integrity of the organism. One can see that paranoia manifests in a number of different, categorically distinct, but in reality rather interweaving, clinical ways.

FROM THE STREAMS OF SULLIVAN AND FREUD

Freud contended in his *Psychopathology of Everyday Life* (1901) that

> the most striking characteristic of symptom-formation in paranoia is the process which deserves the name of *projection*. An internal perception is suppressed, and instead its content, after undergoing a certain degree of distortion, enters consciousness in the form of external perception.

In a later work dealing with the persecution symptomatology in paranoia, Freud also noted that

> the sufferer takes a particular way of defending himself against an unduly strong homosexual attachment to a given person, with the result that the person he once loved most is changed into a persecutor and then becomes the object of aggressive and often dangerous impulses on the part of the patient.

Freud thought that here we have grounds for interposing an intermediate phase in which the love is transformed into hate (*Ego and Id*, Freud, 1923). This obviously is an example in Freudian terms of the energy transformation involved in object relations. Freud noted the affects in the psychic mechanisms involved in the transformation of this particular energy matrix. He noted the psychic energy process of cathexis with its initial homosexual desire. The assumption then, of course, is that homosexuality will be defended against.

This is generally true, but not always true. Not all paranoia, I believe, is associated with homosexual desire or the gay life-style. In Freud's day it may have been, but in this day and age this is not the case. Homosexuals or gays may become paranoid *after* they discover how society and family feel about their orientation!

Freud also noted the intense degree of *hostility* and the need to psychologically *deny* or defend against this hostility in this syndrome. Freud brilliantly recognized the projection process of the individuals inner world onto the outside world such that the perception appears to come from the outside and the internal ego is therein substantiated in the sense of being solid and not full of unacceptable impulses. This brilliant, if somewhat societally limited, understanding of paranoia came out of Freud's famous Dr. Schreber case. The patient saw "telepathic" mysterious rays coming from the sun, a symbolic representative, in Freud's understanding, of the power of Dr. Schreber's physician, Dr. Flechsig. Here the interpretation is placed within an intrapsychic model, such that it is hypothesized that the patient is hypersensitive, indeed, but he is hypersensitive to his own autopsychic influence and not heteropsychic influence. However, this is precisely the point in which there may be a hole or a breech in the Freudian tenet. Numerous observations testify that a patient, in addition to having a great deal of sensitivity to autopsychic influences, also experiences a great deal of social, interpersonal, and familial influences. This is mildly the case when the person with some paranoid tendencies is involved in a somewhat uncomfortable social situation. The person I am labeling paranoid is uncomfortable in his or her relationships with others. This tends to generate, by reciprocal affect, a sense of uncomfortableness on the part of others. The patient may then genuinely perceive the uncomfortableness of others and project or confuse his own hostility with that of others. As I said earlier, the paranoid style as a clinical syndrome is extraordinarily sensitive to interpersonal relationships. Remember, this individual is constantly on the lookout to confirm his or her ideas of others being hostile or manipulative of them. Often, in social and personal situations, they honestly perceive the social and interpersonal truth which no one else may really want to admit for social politeness or family intimacy-boundary reasons. There are a number of recorded instances in which investigators of this area have noted paranormal episodes involving certain phases in the paranoid syndrome. I will present these later in this chapter.

Harry Stack Sullivan (1953) noticed much of what Freud had concerning this particular constellation of behavior and psychic energy patterns. However, Sullivan had his own perspective. Sullivan paid a great deal more attention to the interpersonal dynamics of the psyche, whereas Freud paid more attention to the intrapsychic dynamics of the psyche. Sullivan felt that

> the person who approached pure paranoia would be one who, as an adequate way of handling his difficulties, transferred out of his awareness any feeling of blame in any connection. Since one cannot transfer blame to interstellar space, it is transferred onto persons making up the environment. Anyone competent enough to accomplish this must necessarily also have some explanation of why the environment is so peculiarly vicious, and the net result is very highly systematized delusions of persecution and grandeur. And I may add that the nearer one gets to the pole of pure paranoia, the more obviously the grandeur becomes an explanation for why one should be so persecuted.

The reader is asked to note here, again, the lack of blame in this particular pattern. While there are always signs of persecution depending on the particular conditional state of paranoia, there may or may not be elaborate delusions. That is to say that in paranoid schizophrenia there are delusions, whereas in the paranoid personality proper there are no delusions. It was Harry Stack Sullivan's feeling that in paranoia, the persecution distortion comes first and the grandiose explanations second. I see them arising together, dialectical and reciprocal. They are, in a sense, polar and compensatory with each other. The condition of *blame* and the *deep humiliation* of shame lead to the sense of being unworthy, which is a manifestation and reinforcement of critically low self-esteem. It may be feared as the bottomless pit to be avoided at all costs, lest perhaps the whole self disappear! It was Sullivan's view that most of the defenses of the psyche are geared toward what he called "security operations, psychic transformations of energy designed to protect the integrity and the self-esteem of the self system." These obviously include the primitive and more advanced projective mechanisms of the ego proper and also the early projective splitting in the pre-egoic phases.

Sullivan believed that paranoia always began in the rudimentary schizophrenic process. He felt this way because in the schizophrenic process there is a great deal of primitive referential thinking that has been experienced extensively in early childhood. For various reasons, this style of thinking is reactivated under stress with concomitant reactivation of tremendous amounts of anxiety. This self-referential process is largely composed of elements derived from presyntactic periods in the child's development which is that period of autonomy and individuation outlined by Mahler and others that was addressed in Chapter 2. These are early presyntactic or preverbal experiences and therefore paratactic distortions occur in what is called a "not-me" type of experience. These "not-me" experiences are different from the "good-me" and "bad-me." The "not-me" is more associated with things that are so frightening, primitive, and dangerous that they must be kept completely out of awareness by security operations. This is because they are fraught with such terrifying anxiety. They are the polar opposite of absolute euphoria in Sullivan's system and, therefore, are the mental stuff of absolute terror.

I draw your attention to the process of inner boundary formations between these different, primitive experiences. At such a low level, the process is very fluid. The nascent ego must quickly learn to swim, or at least, not sink in this sea of powerful needs, fears, and affects. Yet, even if the ego learns to float on this surface, it must not lose attention or it will drown.

These primitive images and affective energies survive in the "night terror" that occasionally an anxious individual or multiple personality will have. These night terrors are worse than nightmares which have more to do with an unfortunate or unpleasant situation or fear. In nightmares, the images of fear, etc., are actually seen in the dream process. In the night-terror the fear is so totally terrifying that it must be kept outside of awareness, completely repressed. It is in this general zone of "not-me" that the early paranoid self-referential processes mentioned by Sullivan are seen to be rooted. In this condition, the world is easily misinterpreted. In particular, there is a great deal of misinterpreting social cues and situations. When those misinterpretations are incorporated into personalized delusions, they are always delusions of one being hurt or taken advantage of in some particular way by someone or some group. The integrity of the ego and self-esteem must be protected from these overtly or covertly hostile sources. It is not so much a case of "what" is the matter with me, but rather "who" is the matter with me. This along with projection is the central mental or cognitive-affective stance in this particular dynamic. This attitude or disposition toward life and its field of relationships becomes stabilized over time. The paranoid delusion, once it has frozen or "crystallized" is like a powerful new Gestalt or energy pattern. Ushered in by the liberating "Ah ha" experience of solving some hidden clue in the interpersonal field, its new order resists change or fluctuation in its form.

Clearly, the way the young psyche perceives the defensive-adaptive mechanisms of the generalized family matrix they are embedded in has a profound effect upon what particular adaptive psychic defenses they may or may not evolve (Ackerman, 1957). Very often these paratactic distortions occur in the pre-egoic period. Should it become stabilized during the later family patterning period by various vectors of unconscious learning from significant others, etc., it can become a major personality style through adolescence and the adult years. It is characterized by the behavior and thinking processes that have been outlined in this chapter.

Often when this particular personality pattern establishes causal premises in the course of regular life events the motivations and causes are misinterpreted according to the paratactic distortions outlined above. Social and interpersonal confusion and hostility occur. This leads to an initial decrease in self-esteem. Quickly, however, the "unjust" meaning of the situation is uncovered by the paranoid, which is then reinforcing because it removes some anxiety. However, the patient later discovers, as the mind seeks to open to greater and more inclusive wholes, that this was only part of a larger conspiracy, and therefore they must be on the lookout again. It is a sort of intrapsychic, intermittent reinforcement of an illusory image/meaning yet hostile transitional object.

THE PARANOID PROCESS IN THE BODY

Unlike Freud, Sullivan did see the learning of such psychodynamics as the avoidance of blame, etc, occurring in a family matrix (1953). Sullivan had grasped, after peering into the family of origin of these individuals, that they were often the scapegoats in their family. That is to say, often the family used them to project on to and catch the family's blame for various difficulties. The individual became very sensitized to the experiences of blame. Everyone shared in this process from their own unique angle. He also became very sensitive to the presence, or even the approach, of anything that would bring on the kind of blame which leads to more shame, humiliation, and low self-esteem. Thus the vigilant ego. The constant and repetitive patterns of learning in this family pattern, both unconscious and conscious, lead to deeply embedded family unconscious influences and the evolution in that system through time of subtle energy fields within the family matrix. It is in this matrix that a shared consciousness, based upon mutual association, behavior, and affective and reciprocal feelings, is generated. There are shared delusions of couples termed "Folie a Deux." These can occur between dyads and, in many instances, can spread to families (Wikler, 1980).

On a socio-political level, of course, this is a well-known dynamic. Hitler used the projection of blame and contrasting "I am purity" theme quite well in Nazi Germany as shown in Reich's psychocultural study, *The Mass Psychology of Fascism* (1946). Again, all the projection outward of personal and even cultural blame is largely based on the primitive, but occasionally more sophisticated, projective mechanism of the psyche. In paranoia, this is done primarily to remove any sense of blame from the internal world and to project, to disown, to throw out that blame to the external world. Thus one is pure and the other is dirty, etc. I would like to point out here that this projection process of blame also very neatly abstracts the ego from the world process and reinforces alienated, dualistic perception.

David Shapiro, in his book *Neurotic Styles* (1965), draws the body into numerous and sometimes interweaving patterns of defense. This paranoid syndrome manifests in a number of different disorders, all the way from antisocial personalities, through genuine paranoid schizophrenia, to paranoid personality disorder, to the more common excessive stresses of normal life. The evidence of paranoid style can be seen in all of these in more or less degree. Shapiro focuses on the intense restricted attention and the lack of tenderness in the paranoid style. He also stresses the great increase in muscle tension and hyper-intentionality of these individuals. This *muscle tension* and *continued mental attention* in the condition of hyper-intentionality leads to chronic hypertonus or somatic tension of the voluntary musculature. Wilhelm Reich had captured and systematized it in his monumental work, *Character Analysis* (1949), terming it a form of character armor. This has been extended by his followers such as Alfred Lowen. From there it has spread to many other body/mind therapies. So, in a sense, the argument that mind influences body and vice-versa has not only been won, but has triumphed. The psychic influences on the body, the personality, and the musculature in contemporary psychotherapy are known to be profound and pervasive. Shapiro intricately paints the paranoid individual's excessive concern with autonomy in an antagonistic external world. Shapiro even feels that his fragile sense of autonomy in an antagonistic external world occurs as a bedrock and is prior to the projections of the paranoid. My view, however, is that the projective splitting of the paranoid is in itself a rather primitive psychic apparatus and was operative before the particular paranoid constellation amplified its usage. Regardless of that, most clinicians agree that the primitive mechanisms of projection have been captured in the paranoid syndrome more than any other style.

Shapiro brilliantly articulated the similarity and relationship of the paranoid syndrome to the obsessive-compulsive syndrome. He states that

> paranoid and obsessive-compulsive conditions [in an individual] are an outstanding condition of such an association. It is well known, for instance, how often the pre-morbid background of a paranoid decompensation will turn out to be an obsessive-compulsive and, particularly, an obsessional character. Even more convincing evidence of a close affinity between the two conditions is offered by the existence of certain borderline psychotic states, sometimes described as over-ideational pre(paranoid) schizophrenic states, in which obses-

> sional and paranoid features seem to intermingle and to shade into one another. In such conditions, it is difficult, for example, to say whether the elaborate intellectualizing that is one of the most conspicuous features of this state should be regarded as obsessional or paranoid. The diagnostic labels themselves are of little importance; what is interesting is the similarity of form that such a puzzle and such a gradual transition indicates.

Shapiro then makes the observation that "under whatever the conditions are that produce such changes, when an obsessive-compulsive person does decompensate severely, it is quite likely to be in a paranoid direction." This same systematic progression is the direction of decompensation that has been portrayed by Menninger (1963) in *The Vital Balance*. The destructive paranoid picture of a collapsing world often emerges when the obsessive-compulsive rituals break down and other attempts to avoid terrifying and debilitating anxiety fail. When they do, frank, primitive projective mechanisms involved in paranoia emerge.

I suggest that the reader note when the frozen energy patterns, the tense musculature of the body, and the frozen attention of the mind that are observed in the obsessive-compulsive processes break down, there will appear to be dangerous holes in the system at that time. These holes in the fabric of the obsessive-compulsive veil allow in the irritating grime of anxiety. Further along, as the paranoid decompensation progresses, it would appear that the ego attempts to *explain* these holes and rushes of anxiety into the system. These are explained on the basis of at times fanciful and other times slightly misinterpreted, yet socially and psychologically relevant, data. With the flood into the system of data breaking through the defenses of the obsessive-compulsive ritualizing and binding of anxiety, with the breach in the wall, so to speak, the paranoid is on red-alert–busily scrutinizing and attempting to put things back together before it is too late. This can become a stabilized pattern, as can the obsessive-compulsive style. The seeming increase in creativity on the part of the paranoid, in terms of interpretation of data, is on the one hand true in the sense of more "unusual" things being produced. However, they have often grossly misinterpreted the situation and even approach the bizarre. Thus there is a mixture of creativity and truth, but this truth is so misinterpreted as to distort the original truth. Whereas the obsessive-compulsive has frozen tension and attention on small technical details, thoughts, images, etc., the paranoid is looking for the hidden clue that will unwrap the big picture. At this level, the paranoid senses the real, meaningful, undivided whole of reality. This is the will to higher wholes, information processing and harmony or Maat gone awry. The paranoid style seeks desperately to understand the increasing flux and flow of the world process through some sort of insight into the meaning of the situation and then to approach it by *mentalization*. He forgets that it is more a process of *realization*[1] of the world process, which is not primarily a mental-egoic process at all. There is often an experience of enormous psychological, psychic, and creative energy flooding the system. In some cases it is referred to as feeling hypomanic. In either case it is a certain "high."

The paranoid has some real experience of expansive, non-local causality and influence in the world on all levels but cannot sustain it without the sense of dissolution arising. He arches toward the absolute but fears the empty. The artist is particularly vulnerable to this. Both the obsessive-compulsive and the paranoid are intrigued by, and fearful of, the realms of experience. These two styles, paranoid and obsessive-compulsive, are simply different ways of dealing with the same, real possibility and intuition of ego death. However, they are two different transformations in defensive apparatus in the process. When the obsessive-compulsive ritualizations and defenses break down, the more primitive process of paranoid projection, denial and splitting arises.

THE BOOMERANG OF FEAR

Most of the above has arisen primarily from intrapsychic and interpersonal models. Where appropriate, I have augmented the story

1. Whether your intuition leads you to focused inner attention in meditation, as in most Yogas, or to complete external attention, such as Vipassana meditation, the practitioner moves toward complete absorption in the process and therein the transcendence of all notions of "inner" and "outer" or external. Both paths reach beyond mental understanding and necessitate flowing, nondual realization and identification with the world process on all levels.

with the hopefully more inclusive paradigm of subtle interconnectedness and undivided wholeness on all levels. I have also left out certain data that does not neatly fit into either one of those first two perspectives and yet is very real data confirmed by clinicians through the years. The first one left out has to do with Freud's original inferences about "thought transference." This dread and fear of thought transference, of someone being able to read and thus invade one's mind, is one of the other prominent features of paranoia that many clinicians have observed. Freud had originally noted the "omnipotence of thought" in all narcissism. That is to say, the paranoid has the feeling and the sense that his or her thoughts can be felt by other people. From an intrapsychic point of view, of course, this is not possible. From an interpersonal point of view, and even from an object relations point of view, this is also not possible. However, from the point of view of a shared and collective affective-ideational matrix or interconnectedness, this is possible. This would presuppose a different system of energy dynamics being operative as opposed to those that involve fantasies of ultimate separation. This would open the doors to systems that allow other types of affective, ideational, and energetic processes to flourish. The paradigms of interconnectedness in the new physics and the new biology in many ways provide an adequate, even though changing and therefore limited, background in which to explore this possibility. Remember that the Freudian thesis is based upon a mechanistic model and, to a lesser extent, so is the Sullivanian model. While recognizing the profound dynamisms of inter-personal behavior, it still is a model that focuses on internal processes. There is no difficulty in noting the symptom picture as the Freudians, Sullivanians, and Shapiro have done. My contention is with the energetic presuppositions of the interpretation of those symptoms.

In terms of the paranoid's symptoms of "ideas of reference" this vantage point is somewhat different from the aforementioned perspectives. It is my belief and experience that there is indeed a shared field of consciousness and that the paranoid is in intimate contact with this at certain times. The achilles heel, however, for the paranoid is that the paranoid constantly experiences the psychological field of others through his own lens, a lens that is hardened by the fear of others, hostility, and the sense of possible ego death. He has almost exclusively identified his reality or existence with his ego's psychophysical existence and therefore believes in only extinction and death beyond this boundary. As a consequence, those thoughts that do naturally cross the boundaries and occur to others within the powerful matrix that the person has established are perceived as hostile. This is partly a result of the fact that they are indeed hostile in their real environment. Anyone who has been around a paranoid ends up usually feeling a combination of ambivalence and anger at them. The paranoid is naturally sensitive to this even though the others may want to deny it for social or family reasons.

In this context Rupert Sheldrake's (1982) interesting hypothesis may be very helpful. Sheldrake hypothesizes that between individual forms that are similar there occurs a certain "morphic resonance." This is similar to the harmonics that occur in music. In this way "information" is transferred from one area that is similar to another area. It is quite possible that a process *similar* to this occurs in the transfer of ideas that the paranoid experiences as "ideas of reference." When this occurs, of course, it is terrifying to the individual because it is another uncanny indication that that ego is vulnerable and may be on the verge of dissolving since it seems to have no impermeable boundary between itself and others. The paranoid process accentuates the datum that "where there is other, there is fear." From a tiny bit of true data the paranoid, who is overideational often by temperament and reinforcement, begins to create numerous self-referent pseudocausal connections and delusions. These delusions are characterized by being highly systematized and always in direct reference back to the body/mind and ego integrity of the person.

PSI AND PARANOIA

Ehrenwald (1948) has documented from clinical practice a number of unusual communications that appear in the paranoid process. These forms of information exchange cannot be accounted for by the social learning models that I have mentioned, nor can it be understood from a purely intrapsychic or even interpersonal perspective. Certainly, the vast majority of the paranoid condition does not involve either direct thought transference or even psi. Let me be absolutely clear about that! I am talking about those significant cases and episodes during the progression of many paranoic situations that do involve hypersensitivity to heteropsychic influences.

Ehrenwald noted that the projection hypothesis of the paranoid delusions advanced by the psychoanalysts appeared to him to be nothing more than the reverse of the telepathy hypothesis, its photographic negative, so to speak. In the case of Dr. Schreber mentioned earlier, in which Freud first formulated the paranoid and homosexual hypothesis, Dr. Ehrenwald points out the influence of psi in that situation. Here the place of psi or telepathic influences in Dr. Schreber's case was taken by "mysterious rays" that seemed to emanate from the sun. The sun itself was taken as a symbolic representation of Dr. Flechsig, who was Dr. Schreber's physician. Dr. Schreber considered Dr. Flechsig to be his torturer. Freud's interpretation of this case was that in actual fact the paranoid Dr. Schreber was tormented by sadistic-aggressive or homosexual tendencies originating from his own unconscious. The patient is seen to be sensitive to what is his own auto-psychic material but not to heteropsychic material. This is only the one-way direction of projection. The intrapsychic model is limited here because of its assumptions about the closed boundaries of energy dynamics, such that anything moving from one place and covering any other must of necessity be an internal psychic process and then therefore narcissistic, not because information and reality are interconnected and interwoven. Freud, always ambivalent and oscillating in this area, did, in his later days, begin to re-entertain the possibility of psi.

Dr. Ehrenwald goes on to give a number of experiences out of his own clinical practice that seem to greatly complicate the traditional perspective on paranoia and psi. Dr. Ehrenwald gives a number of examples of patients who had "ideas of reference" and were either paranoid, borderline, or schizophrenic. In each one of these cases, however, the "ideas of reference" back to the individual in the sense of persecution and harm were operative. In more than a few situations, he found that the paranoid individual indeed was in various ways correctly perceiving Dr. Ehrenwald's own feelings, intentions and thoughts. Technically, this is tuning into the countertransference reactions of Dr. Ehrenwald. Ehrenwald then makes an observation that appears to me to be the functioning of the family unconscious system. In a number of situations, he notes the close similarity in "ideational content" between people in significant relationships over time. These are usually husband and wife relationships. Recall earlier discussions of folie a deux or shared delusions. Ehrenwald surmised that the delusions of the identified patient and the feelings of significant others in the patient's constellation, which usually includes family or family-like members, were derived from essentially "identical sources of the unconscious in which we're always likely to rest upon identical symbols." In other words, from a shared matrix of consciousness, affect and behavior, Dr. Ehrenwald noticed the same process of projection and real, but distorted, information exchange occurring. This is also true in the other related condition of schizophrenia. The ultimate clinical form of this is seen in the patient's process of decompensation or "emotional breakdown." It is called "psychotic insight" when a patient has such an uncanny perception of the therapist's own thought processes. In schizophrenia, the data appeared to be much more "scattered," as opposed to the paranoid condition where there is more thematic material. This is not always the case but is true generally.

There is an excellent book on the market called *An Explosion of Being: An American Family's Journey into the Psychic* (Dillon and Dillon, 1984). This book intricately details the influence of psychic or paranormal communication in a family. It also shows how a family stabilizes around boundaries in a new way in order to deal with this indication of a greater intimacy than many of us may be comfortable with. My suggestion here is that projection is constantly occurring and that at various times we all experience the true parallel thought experience of others. We, in our relationships, are each psychoenergetically enfolded into the innerlandscape of significant others for better or worse, and the affective and informational power of that introjection seems to parallel the inverse square law so often seen in the electrostatic, electromagnetic and gravitational laws that structure the material universe. We project and have a minority representation in the other. This is normal and happens all the time. It is our degree of anxiety and our presumptions about our psychic boundaries as understood by the ego and contemporary society that make this more or less problematical. Also, it is enormously important what comprises the content of these ideas of reference. The difficulty the paranoid has is that, almost without exception, these ideas of reference are usually hostile and confused with their own denied hostile projections. When these ideas of reference are benign or even affectively positive we, of course, do not experience a problem. Then it is called extraordinary insight and empathy!

TRANSIENCE/FEAR AND INSIGHT

The paranoid process has come to be seen in a number of different ways. In each case I have noted that the ego structure of the paranoid is in touch with autistic, pre-egoic, and primitive self-referential processes. Attention has also been brought to the paranoid's actual extraordinary sensitivity and perception in interpersonal relationships. This, of course, is partially learned in the family matrix and partly is an adaptation and accommodation by the intrapsychic system to the demands of the external world. When this occurs in a highly systematized and logical order with the paranoid, the reference is always back to the paranoid's particular and individualized ego. These usually have to do with protection and vulnerability, etc. In extreme cases, issues of physical, psychic and psychological survival are intensely activated that touch upon the world cataclysmic, collapsing experiences of the birth process into this world. Perhaps even lower levels of the triune brain are reached. If this is so, we should be able to find a great degree of autonomic nervous system instability reflecting a deeper limbic system lability, and also perhaps deep, proxamil brain waves on the EEG.

When the perspective of the paranoid can be supported either by science or by the social system in some sort of way, one can either have the mass psychology of fascism, the most intricate of scientific theories, or numerous other manifestations of intricate and elaborate processes. In other words, the paranoid propensity for intricate thought weaving has both a positive and negative aspect. On the one hand, it is a very constructive, systematizing, and analytic intelligence. On the other hand, it is fraught with a powerful predisposition toward certain assumed, and apparently thought to be necessary, positions for security maintenance.

While these above-mentioned situations are true, the ego of the paranoid is also acutely sensitive to information of an unpleasant nature that arrives from "below" and that more luminous information that descends simultaneously from "above." It is my belief, in other words, stemming from clinical practice, that the process of thinking that very often can occur in paranoia is sensitive not only to the person's own denied and repressed intrapsychic frustrations, but is also open to the true insights that go beyond the person and individual personhood. These are in addition to the genuine reflections of the thought processes of others in the shared community.

In stressful situations, the paranoid ego rapidly observes increasing data coming in and a sense of chaotic undivided wholeness, of a fusion of energies rushing into the world. This undivided wholeness of psychic, psychological, and causal relationships is a reality on many levels, but the temporary ego boundaries established by the system are beginning to break down to such an extent that this information creates a sense of dissolution, fear and anxiety. It is swept up in a new storm at sea. The ego first attempts to control this by the security operations that it has already attempted in the past but these, of course, are in the process of failing. The cognitive structures of formal operations with their system of hypothetical-deductive reasoning are enlisted, but not used clearly. Occasionally, as even they break down, hints of fleeting post-formal operations arise but pass quickly because of the opening, yes, but unstable psychic and subtle process. The ego, therein, perceives itself as needing to survive even more and thus becomes more profoundly affected or involved with the survival level. Stress biochemistry sweeps through the system and more primitive mechanisms arise. It may even be that the lower levels of the brain stem, as in the reptilian and limbic mammalian levels of our triune brain, are again activated.

It is at this point that the clinician will very often notice in the productions of the paranoid a number of ideas and associations that are around "survival" themes. In Yoga psychology this is referred to as the first, or root, Muladhara chakra basic structure. You may recall that a basic structure remains after it has emerged consciousness as opposed to a replacement structure. These associations and powerful affective energies around survival brutalize the sense of basic being or ontological security that would normally pervade the psychic system. These feelings, usually repressed, are beginning to break through to consciousness. These are very primitive self-referential processes and primal images. The ego attempts control by contracting upon its own experience even more so, which again, of course, only leads to the fleeting and partial experience of control, then eventually a sense of emotional exhaustion from such a psychic energy construction, and then, finally, to a greater sense of vulnerability. It is difficult to give up because it is partially successful, since it initially does relieve some anxiety and projects blame outward. The paranoid reaches for a *mental grasp* of this always changing scenario and thus fails at the flowing *realization* of the whole process. The upper opens, but so does below. This partial insight of the paranoid into the real, interconnected, and undivided wholeness of reality is an attempt to move toward a higher or more subtle sense of balance between the "inner" and "outer" world. This sense of "balance" is sought after regardless at whatever stage of cognitive, moral, or psychological development.

One of the tendencies the clinician will notice in the productions of the paranoid is a very highly articulate and at times florid display of an integrating conceptual capacity. In many ways the ego, feeling itself to be falling, attempts to reintegrate on higher and lower levels at the same time. It fails in the integration of the arising new and more inclusive consciousness that is open to both higher and lower possibilities. Needless to say, the lower level of integration wins out in most cases. However, in this striving is an attempt by the ego to integrate the dazzling new data coming toward and from within it in a balanced and systematized way, a way that would in other circumstances reflect its unfolding or higher development. We are referring here to the developmental stage of what has been labeled "vision logic" (Wilber, 1981). At this stage, the individual in a healthy context would be expansive and living up to great potentials in creativity and expansion in its world. The cognitive stages of formal operations and systemic and holistic thinking are fully utilized in the understanding of the world process. The clinician witnesses the presence of vision and design in the grandiose delusions of the paranoid. The delusions and fantastic causal connections swirl around a "hero" in this scenario of the paranoid, a besieged hero who often has or knows a great "secret" that others may want and envy him for. Thus, the hero is special and the argument becomes airtight. At this point his automythology is almost unassailable. The emerging potential for world-constructing formal and post-formal thought is therein enlisted to strengthen and gather data for the paranoid stance. The emergent mode of "vision-logic" is distorted by this process. Often all these cognitive and maturational factors occur in a person and family when the 16- to 19-year-old is about to leave home and family to live on his or her own. Here the family therapist regularly sees the first overt signs of a paranoid schizophrenic break with all of the earlier mentioned dynamics.

Piaget, back in Chapter 2, had pointed out how the adolescent with formal operations in cognitive functioning constructed world systems and was at the metaphysical age par excellence, but was still embedded in egocentric perceptions. This has its parallel in the expansive level of vision-logic.

This stage of vision-logic is the stage prior to the full conscious recognition of subtle interconnecting phenomena in the world, yet is involved with it, and a precursor to true transpersonal states. The contracting ego of the paranoid experience is like the swimmer in trouble in the water who reaches for a sense of stability from a life raft but does not quite grasp it. These delusions are an attempt by the ego to explain, and in many ways to swim and survive symbolically in, the world. The paranoid wants to be saved from this. At the same time, it is an attempt to escape all responsibility and blame for the situation and to explain that on the basis of others attempting to hurt one. Others, of course, attempt to hurt them because they have some "special" gift. Since specialness is reinforced by the data that the paranoid receives from the environment, both internal and external, it forms a closed loop or system. It also leads to compensatory self-esteem measures leading inevitably to grandiose ego expansion. This grandiose ego expansion is occurring because unconsciously the ego feels itself to be actually moving in the opposite direction, which is ego deflation and perhaps dissolution. So while observing hostility and deception in the world, he is also searching for a "savior" to save him from the world. Should they meet, then a new process, for better or worse, is loosened into the world.

In essence, the paranoid's particular constellation and mode of defensive maneuvers is, like all other such patterns, a seeking for balance or higher wholes, information processing and harmony or Maat. The paranoid's particular constellation leads him to seek the "hidden motive" and eventually the "ultimate meaning" of their situation. However, any ultimate meaning that the paranoid experiences is referred specifically and egocentrically directly back to them, not the community or others. It is not always applicable to other persons. He again seeks to answer the gnawing question of "who" is the matter with him, not "what" is the matter (Jamal, 1983). This is testimony to the egocentricity of the paranoid as opposed to the transegoic states as outlined earlier. The paranoid wants to mentally understand the innumerable overt and subtle causal relations in the undivided world process and therein fails in the flowing, non-mental realization of the process. As Sankaracarya, the ancient Advaita Vedantic seer and scholar/Yogin observed:

343 The projecting power, through the aid of the veiling power, connects a man with the siren of an egoistic idea, and distracts him through the attributes of that.

Thus seeking balance and transcendence, the paranoid fails. He has an even more tenuous hold on reality than the obsessive-compulsive. But, oh, sometimes what a sense of energy!

Many creative artists are in vital contact with these energetic dynamics and they reflect these tendencies in their work. One can easily see the exquisite sensitivity to interpersonal relationships, yet also the brilliant but floridly egocentric perceptions and primitive, paranoid fears erupt in the great work and private lives of the playwrights A. Strindberg (Meyer, 1985), E. O'Neill, T. Williams, and the poet Delmore Swartz.

> Along with its beauty we find the limits of the illuminated mind: illumined poetry translates itself into a flood of images and revelatory words (because often the vision opens at this stage and also one begins to hear), almost an avalanche of images, luxuriant, often disordered, as though the consciousness was hard put to it to contain the luminous wave and this additional intensity–there is too much of it, it overflows. Enthusiasm changes easily into excitement and, if the rest of the being is not sufficiently purified, any lower part whatever may

> get hold of the light and force which descend to use them for its own ends,–this is a frequent danger. When the lower parts of the being, specially the vital, seize the luminous flood, they harden it, dramatize it, torture it–the power is still there but hardened. . .
>
> Satpren,
> *Sri Aurobindo,*
> *or the Adventure of the Consciousness*, p. 211

In many ways, the mature ego functions like a mature scientific theory. The mature ego observes external and internal phenomena, generates hypotheses about that phenomena, and attempts to deal rationally and in a balanced way with the needs of the system. Like a good scientific theory, it persists in gathering data of increasing complexity and eventually in the gathering of that data will appear material that does not fit with the known facts of that system. The mature scientific theory begins to experiment and confirm or disconfirm data and move onto new insights and efficient functioning where it is appropriate. It lets go and does not frantically cling. The mature ego, like the mature scientific theory, carries within its roots the seeds of its own transcendence. The mature ego that is able to do that achieves balance at each level, while not absolutely identifying with that level, and therein prepares the way for what is beyond it. Structures arise, are functional, then dissipate. The ego that becomes fixated and frightened of its own transience falls into neurosis or, in some cases, psychosis. It is not yet ready to embrace the deeper, boundaryless all and falls into a fearful, self-contracted stance. It is the difference between fear and serenity.

PARANOIA AND THE FEARED LOSS OF POTENCY: A CULTURAL CASE

I have pointed out the paranoid process and how it seems to operate. How might this approach look at the well-known male concern with power, sexual potency, and sperm?

Sullivan (1953) was not the only clinician to recognize that the male paranoid at times became excessively concerned with loss of potency, especially loss of semen and sexual fluids. It is often deeply intertwined with the sense of power in the world. This is implicit in Freud's theories of paranoia and homosexuality. The male phallus is still the preeminent *symbol* of power in our day. I am not talking about "liberated" reality, merely the symbols that most cultures have evolved during the last period of patriarchal hegemony. Feminists have no problem with this position of the male phallus as the modern *symbol* of male power in culture (Greer, 1971).

In the above cases, and in so many others, the paranoid's decompensating system is concerned with losing the virility and power to deal in the world. This may seem nonsensical to with sexually liberated moderns, yet this association and train of thought is echoed in just about every major religious system (with disastrous results, I might add). Beyond primitive animistic beliefs, where the semen is assumed to have magical powers, to those of certain Yogic schools that demand the seeker eliminate or severely limit his sexual behavior, there are excessive concerns with *loss* of semen (Haich, 1975).

There are also, however, some schools, especially those with a Taoic or Tantric lineage, that take a different view toward sexual behavior and the life-current, but also share the same concern with *loss* of semen. Their approach *magnifies* the life-current and seeks to not lose it but use it and other powerful energies for transformation and transcendence. It is a body-positive, highly disciplined and ecstatic path. The benefits of the Tao's way, in particular, have been immeasurably beneficial to Chinese medicine for thousands of years (Chang, 1977).

Thus one can see that the paranoid person with excessive concerns with loss of power and sexual fluids has a whole worldwide cultural/religious backdrop for his delusions. Who of us does not remember the movie *Dr. Strangelove*, with its paranoid, decompensating military general who is obsessed with outside forces trying to steal his "precious bodily fluids?"

My own bias is that the process of conservation of semen in various Yogic and other practices is rooted in biochemical and hormonal processes, and not the result of simply the withholding of semen itself. There is no way that semen can go directly up the spine. Ojas, the assumed essence of semen that is associated with this process, is no doubt an endocrine function that may be related to melanin, the light-interacting molecule that is intimately connected to the pineal gland and other processes associated with both human embryology and evolutionary neurobiology. It is also a responsible agent in the skin pigmentation process.[2]

The conservative religious notion of retaining semen and limiting sexual behavior is brought on by cognitive notions of conservation operative in earlier cognitive modes of humankind. Poor Saint Augustine! He spent many a tormented hour wondering how many thousands of children would not be born because he wasted his ejaculation. Hindu ascetics have a similar worry concerning the loss of sperm (Kripalvananda, 1978). Apparently, no one has told them that semen is continually produced by the system and not a fixed commodity! This is a distorted understanding of the ancient, but *conscious* practice of brahmacharya, wherein the science of subtle energies in the psychic, sexual, and vital life of the organism are regulated and transmuted. In the case of "Urdhvareta," or the process that spontaneously occurs in certain phases of Yogic discipline where the gonads seem to be pulled back up into the body, even then extra or surplus sexual fluids are copiously produced by the body as part of an evolutionary psychospiritual process. The whole body-mind is invigorated, including nerves, endocrines, and the brain. While the *loss* of biochemical fluids may be rooted in the actual loss of vitality in the body, Taoist and Tantric practices also make it quite clear that the sense of body/mind vitality and equanimity can also be increased with a disciplined, joyous approach to the source of energy. The connection between vitality, energy, evolution, and sexuality has been thoroughly explored by contemporary Adepts (Krishna, 1972, Free John, 1978).

Here again, the paranoid partially sees the truth of the relationship between power, sexual fluids, and vitality. Yet given his hostile projections, denial of blame and responsibility for his own hostile

---

2. It is interesting that, historically speaking, as far as we presently know, the first earth cultures with Yogic disciplines of any kind where there is some presumed notion of enlightenment as a goal of evolution (In-light-ment) were dark-skinned peoples in which there was a naturally higher level of melanin in the skin, e.g., Ancient Kemetic/Egyptians and the pre-Aryan Dravidians of India. Perhaps it was just coincidence, but the great process of Yogic discipline has spread to all in "her" family, to all humanity, just as modern science has spread to the rest of the world.

wishes/fears, and the process by which he defends against dissolution as I have outlined, one can see how this area, fear of semen loss and potency, becomes implicated in his delusional system. The "animal" and sexual/aggressive impulses that are denied and projected, along with blame to others, are usually his own unacceptable aspects. With the breakdown of the system and the psychic boundaries to heteropsychic influence, all kinds of ancient and modern explanations for the seeming loss of control and power in the world are enlisted. The excessive concern with semen loss is readily available and an easy one to misinterpret since, like all paranoid explanations, it contains beyond the egocentric distortions, a window on the truth.

CASE HISTORIES

The paranoid process is manifested in the following two cases. Each is somewhat different and highlights various aspects of this clinical syndrome.

Case 1

Brian X. was a 32-year-old white male who presented himself for psychotherapy. He was self-referred to therapy and had a checkered history of on-again, off-again treatment with different therapists.

> He was very concerned with his psychological development and also quite upset about his serious alcohol and illegal drug addictions. These had plagued him since late adolescence. He spoke in a tight, clipped fashion with a sarcastic, but bright, sense of humor. He became invested in therapy after several sessions and said it was time he made some real changes in his untidy life.
>
> He had a child by a former relationship but was "afraid" of marriage. Numerous times he focused on family conflicts with his father, as well as society conflicts and his intense ambivalence about any form of discipline. The drug experiences, he insisted, helped him feel expansive, integrated, intelligent, and

perceptive when he was "high." When he came down, so did his self-esteem. He spoke of his "high" experiences as though they reminded him of a great but lost memory or experience. He was extremely concerned about his loss of vitality and energy, especially in any emotional/sexual committment with women. He had come into therapy partially to learn how to function in a committed relationship.

Apparently he liked his therapist and began to trust the therapist more and more. As exploration of his intrapsychic and interpersonal processes progressed he indicated a growing recognition of his own hostility toward others. He had some strong psychospiritual interests, especially in areas he referred to as "dynamic meditation." The therapist encouraged this area of exploration so that he might better understand his process of extreme self-criticism and increase his spontaneous behavior.

It was at this stage that he began to explore his fantasy life in depth. The dynamics of power, self-esteem, hostility, and paranoid ideation slowly emerged. In his daydreams, which sometimes lasted hours, he saw himself as a representative of his "Aryan ancestors." In particular he saw himself as a Prussian general in the 1870s. Sexual and military control became fused at times as he re-fought legendary battles. He wanted to "get back" at others in his fantasies because in some way they had injured him and thwarted his greatness in the world.

Just as he was progressing in this area he fell back into illegal drug usage. He stopped therapy but let the therapist know, by mail, of his abrupt change. The therapist could not get him to return to treatment. Thus the therapist became another of the many therapists he had seen and rejected. Throughout their brief (four-month) contact he was oriented as to time, place, and person, and evidenced no suicidal ideation, hallucinatory behavior, or overtly delusional material. This is in contrast to the next case of paranoid style.

Next is a somewhat different case in which suspicion spreads overtly to others.

Case 2

Susan X., a young professional, presented herself to a psychotherapist in order to "clarify" a situation she felt had occurred in her life. She was very concerned that her boyfriend, who had just broken off their long relationship, had controlled and influenced her mind by "unknown methods" while she was asleep at night. They had lived together for some time but she strongly denied any anger or depression over the loss of the relationship. The therapist's probes were met with hostility. She said she was not there for therapy, only information. The therapist's area of specialty was hypnosis, and that is why she had contacted this particular clinician.

Her boyfriend had worked in the area of artificial intelligence. The therapist was somewhat apprehensive of all this but decided to listen to her presentation anyway. Apparently, she had awakened from dreamsleep to find him mumbling something in her ear. She could not recall what it was, but felt it was crucial! She wanted hypnosis to uncover this.

Susan X. and the therapist debated the situation and she insisted that it be done since she could pay for it, it was her right, the therapist had the skills, worked for her, etc. She eventually took her demand to the therapist's superior, got him upset and then came back to the therapist. The therapist reluctantly agreed to three sessions of teaching her self-hypnosis.

When it came time for the sessions, she insisted that they be tape recorded for security reasons. The therapist did not resist. The first session was uneventful. During the second session the patient was afraid that the therapist had another hidden tape recorder operating because the radiator was making a clicking noise. The therapist told her that there was a movie camera behind the couch. She was not amused! At other times this humorous approach has cut through the delusion. This time it didn't.

After the third session she became angry that the therapist had not uncovered anything. At this point the therapist saw the quicksand and simply refused to do this anymore unless they could explore the process in psychotherapy also. She refused and left. Later, she came back and demanded to see her clinical records. She would not transfer to another therapist. She quoted the Federal Family Education Rights and Privacy Act, known as the Buckley Act, and stated in writing that her clinical records were not to be seen by anybody!

The therapist suggested to her that she might consider another private therapist. She replied that the only medical problem she had was an undisclosed "ear" disorder and that only a male would insist on therapy for her, since she was obviously OK. The therapist said nothing in response. She then began a series of hostile verbal comments, picked up her things and walked angrily out the door. On her way down the hall she yelled out "Fuck you, bastard." Both were glad their relationship was over.

SUMMARY

From the inception of the chapter, I have tried to give a general portrait of the paranoid style or syndrome. Not all symptoms are present in every situation, but there does emerge a mosaic of patterns that can be effectively differentiated from other clinical syndromes.

Attention was drawn in particular to those aspects of the paranoid process that have to do with the family constellation, often the scapegoat/blame sensitizing that occurs, the use of denial and projection as defensive strategies, and the resultant absence of blame on the part of the system. Also mentioned was the constriction of affect, the use of the constructive capacity of the mind to systematize what appears to be happening to the person, and the general social-cultural context of the person which may *reinforce* the paranoid process. A Jew in Germany in 1936 had his paranoia amplified if he got past the denial stage. A sensitive black in the United States has some degree of socially reinforced and survival appropriate "cultural paranoia."

Also explored at some length were the great contributions of Sullivan and Freud, two clinical researchers who had personal experiences with this process. Eventually I offered another perspective as to the combination of many of these patterns and others in the paranoid process. Much was understood by recognizing the paranoid's reach for transcendence and subsequent fall into auto-psychic and heteropsychic hostility and self-referential misinterpretation of the actual flowing reality of undivided wholeness on the physical, psychological and psychic planes.

The paranoid, in the process of ideation, enjoys and needs the subjective sense of being on the frontier of human knowledge by insight into his or her problem. But since this initially visionary, high ideational energy is pulled back by the "gravity" of fearful egoity, it falls away from conscious absorption in the Absolute. The paranoid does not essentially fulfill his or her specific and unique destiny in our collective and interconnected destiny where each person has a rare role to play in the cosmic dance. The paranoid does not succeed in clearly reflecting its particular aspect of the Real and thereby essentially fulfilling the intuited "Way" in its ultimate, and still personal, sense for him/herself and us. Suzuki (1970) is clear in declaring: "Each one of us must make his own true way, and when we do, that way will express the universal way. This is the mystery." In this sense, the paranoid is the failed Bodhisattva sensing beyond itself in the great shared field of others, yet exchanging compassion for fear, and a cycle of rapid, inflexible half-truths for the seamless current of the life-force.

Finally, this outline was applied to a specific area of heightened paranoid concern in the male of the species in times of crisis, i.e., sex, semen, and the loss of power. It was seen how the partial grasp and egoic misinterpretation of subtle interconnected life-force processes brought about delusions and fear.

The delusions and ideas of reference that the paranoid so intensely feels and experiences are strongly held together by a vigilant ego-consciousness hard won in earlier struggles. These intense states of heightened sense of self form localizations in the field of the person's mind. When held together and kept in some contact with reality, there is paranoia. I want to proceed now to the multiple personality. In the multiple personality these defenses have failed considerably or, in some cases, not developed at all. The areas or sub-fields where the sense of self-localizations arise communicate much less with each other and seemingly discrete states of self-consciousness abide side by side, so to speak. There are even differences of EEG and other psychophysical measures employed by these discrete self-sense fields. We need a new model or schema to grasp this elusive creature. Thus, I want to explore perhaps the most shattering and splintered style of all, the multiple personality. It is into that world of many selves and realities that we now peer.

REFERENCES

Ackerman, N. *The Psychodynamics of Family Life,* Basic Books, New York, 1957.

Chang, J. *The Tao of Love and Sex: The Ancient Chinese Way to Ecstasy,* Dutton Books, New York, 1977.

Dillon, D. and Dillon, B. *An Explosion of Being: An American Family's Journey into the Psychic*, Parker Pub. Co., West Nyack, New York, 1984.

Ehrenwald, J. *Telepathy and Medical Psychology,* W. W. Norton & Co., New York, 1948.

Free John, B. *Love of the Two-Armed Form*, Dawn Horse Press, Middletown, CA, 1978.

Freud, S. *Ego and Id* (1923).

Freud, S. *The Psychopathology of Everyday Life* in the Standard Edition of the Complete Psychological Works of Sigmund Freud, Vol. 6, p. 1-279, 1901.

Greer, G. *The Female Eunuch,* McGraw-Hill, New York, 1971.

Haich, E. *Sexual Energy and Yoga*, Aurora Press, New York, 1975.

Jamal, I. "The Magic of African Medicine," *East-West Journal* 13:7, July 1983, 42-46.

Kripalvananda, Y. S. *Yoga and Celibacy,* Talati Press, Vadodara, Gujarat, India, 1978.

Krishna, G. *The Biological Basis of Religion and Genius*, Harper & Row, New York, 1972.

Menninger, K. *The Vital Balance: The Life Process in Mental Health and Illness*, Viking Press, New York, 1963.

Meyer, M. *Strindberg: A Biography,* Secker and Warburg, London, 1985.

Reich, W. *Character Analysis*, Farrar, Straus, and Giroux, New York, (1949) 1971.

Reich, W. *The Mass Psychology of Fascism*, Farrar, Straus, and Giroux, New York, 1946.

Shapiro, D. *Neurotic Styles*, Basic Books, Inc., New York, 1965.

Sheldrake, R. *A New Science of Life: The Hypothesis of Formative Causation*, J. P. Tarcher, Inc., Los Angeles, 1982.

Sullivan, H. *The Interpersonal Theory of Psychiatry,* W. W. Norton New York, 1953.

Sullivan, H. S. *Schizophrenia as a Human Process*, W. W. Norton, 1962.

Sullivan, H. S. "Schizophrenia, Paranoid States and Related Conditions" in *The*

Study of Abnormal Behavior: Selected Readings by Zax and Strickler, Macmillan Co., New York, 1964.

Suzuki, S. *Zen Mind, Beginner's Mind*, Weatherhill Press, New York, Tokyo, 1970, p. 111.

Wikler, L. "Folie a Family: A Family Therapist's Perspective," *Family Process* 9:3, 1980, 257-268.

Wilber, K. "Ontogenetic Development: Two Fundamental Patterns," *Journal of Transpersonal Psychology* 13:1, 1981, 33-58.

Chapter 6

Multiple Personality: The Wilderness of Mirrors

THE NEXUS OF PANIC

In every corner of my soul there is an altar to a different god.

–Fernando Pessoa

Giving way to the rush and power of the Cromagnon, both her father and brother broke the ancient incest taboo. Repeatedly over the years they forced her through episodes of panic, isolation, and fear, hid her in closets, told her she was crazy. Physical and sexual abuse were almost ritually practiced in her family, while to a more distant outside community they seemed the ideal nuclear unit. Along with famine victims and the holocaust survivors, she is among our ancient mother's most tortured children and progeny.

Margaret X., you see, is unfortunately not an isolated case. I had worked with other similar persons, but this situation was the most dramatic. She had managed to move away from her socially isolated family. She was intelligent and perceptive, though emotionally unstable, and yet by effort and some compassion from others had made it all the way to a professional school. Her degenerating physical disability made her an even more vulnerable person. Despite all this, her intelligence and humor did not fail.

I first met her during one of her emerging suicide situations. As I was to later learn, these calls for help were both genuine and manipulative. Several times her overdose attempts were near misses with the scythe of death. Between periods of seeming emotional balance with only mild depression and then later borderline problems she would "discover" herself rushing home after spending all her money on gifts, garbage, and trivia. Of all the patients in the treatment facility, she was the most difficult. Eventually, many clinicians at the institution became unwilling members of her extended family.

It was late one evening after another emergency suicide manipulation that I first saw her multiple personality. While speaking with her primary personality as Margaret, she complained of feeling as though she was about to lose control. This was her common lament. We were face to face, one of my psychology interns was present, and I was becoming suspicious and angry at all this manipulation. I knew I needed to shift direction. I told her to simply let go and lose control. Her anxiety level increased. I urged her to go on anyway, assuring that some aspect of her would exist even though other aspects may seem to dissolve. Through her tears and fear, which were real and painful, she then revealed to us a startling process. Her eyes went blank, her face contorted, then relaxed. Within a few seconds, both eyes were drawn upward to the spot between the eyebrows. The body shifted, the voice changed and mellowed. Out stepped another persona and a different conversation.

We all talked at some length before yet another persona emerged from a similar sequence of body/mind actions. Eventually three autonomous personas arose and disappeared in her conflicted, painful circus of persons in one body. There was even an extremely young, rudimentary fourth constellation of attributes that we saw as another personality that emerged in later sessions. The major characters, however, were about 6, 12, and 15 years old. All frightened, all in separate "locations" in the system, they were at war with each other with unequal ammunition. Some were aware that others existed, one merely thought she was presently at the age of abuse and had no protection. Her child persona cried repeatedly, "Don't hurt, don't hurt."

Her treatment lasted several years and occurred with a number of different clinicians. While her manipulations decreased, they did not end. Her different personas, however, did all meet each other in treatment and she progressed from a multiple to a more manageable borderline personality disorder.

The above vignette taken from my clinical practice is perhaps the most bizarre and unusual of personality patterns and is what is known in the classical literature as a multiple personality. This is an extremely rare syndrome in comparison to the preponderance of other syndromes. However, the syndrome does occur. It has been popularized in a number of books including *The Five of Me*, (Hawkesworth, 1977) and the classical account of Dr. Cornelia Wilbur's treatment of *Sybil* (Schreiber, 1973) which was eventually made into a movie. The multiple personality as described above tends to be one of the more dramatic personality patterns. It is obviously much more serious than a situation in which we are "not quite ourselves today."

This particular personality syndrome calls into serious question both the intrapsychic or psychodynamic model and also the interpersonal model of personality development. In each case of multiple personality, the psychic system of the organism seems to be possessed of several autonomous and inter- and independent systems or subsystems. These highly personalized subsystems are kept unaware of each other by internalized miniboundaries in an energized matrix rooted in who, us, they, and them. There can be anywhere from three to 13 different personalities in a multiple personality. In other words, there are at least three or more distinct personalities within the organism. Moreover, what is even more startling is that these personalities have dynamics, traits, sometimes EEG brainwave patterns and even dermatologic and allergic responses peculiar to each one of them (*Brain/Mind*, 1983). Almost always these individual personalities do not have full knowledge of each other. Their relative identities are kept separate. A number of different theories have been put forward in an attempt to harness this vortex of separate selves in development. Each major perspective will be put forth before a different paradigm is cast over the path of this elusive creature.

CONTRASTING VIEWS

Europe

The splintered heart who opened this chapter has been known to our kind since the earliest of collective memory. No doubt our ancient mother of primeval lakes under the vast, African sky saw a form of this process among her kind. Most of its history has been her story and even today most victims are female. The later ancients assumed that a form of possession by good or evil spirits caused the problem. It was seen to have an affinity to epilepsy and, in other contexts, to the divine intoxication of poetry and music. While the inherent mystery of the process filtered through all cultures, it was a Europe of science and rational philosophy that sought to tame it in clinical practice. Years before Freud the ability of the mind to manifest several apparently different personalities was well known.

In 1791, a German physician, Eberhardt Gmelin, reported cases of "exchanged personality." Erasmus Darwin in 1810 described the case of a woman "possessed of two minds." The case of Mary Reynolds, a famous multiple personality, was presented by Dr. John Mitchell from the early school of dynamic psychiatry in 1816. In the medical school training of students in 1812 Dr. Benjamin Rush presented several cases at the University of Pennsylvania. It was later between 1880 and 1910 that great interest in this ancient and mysterious process reached its peak. Since then it has declined, only to find renewed energy today. This may be because of a clear connection between physical/sexual abuse and the genesis of this syndrome in the context of our present day awareness of the widespread sexual abuse of children in society. However, not all of the processes of multiple personality functioning were seen as negative or pathogenic.

The United States

William James, always the creative and positively oriented experimenter, saw that a great potential was revealed in this process. The ability of the mind to push away from, or disassociate certain aspects of itself had a definite positive connotation. This process of separating certain parts of the personality from other parts is clinically termed "dissociation." In clinical hypnosis, it is a common practice to teach the patient to dissociate from pain for obvious reasons. In fact, the first great insight into the hysterical personality style involved the capacity to dissociate certain aspects of the body through mental processes such that those aspects of the body were experienced as alien to the basic "I" sense. A very neat trick! James argued quite persuasively, but was ignored by the new hegemony of nineteenth century mechanistic science, that these dissociative states create conditions in the mind "for permanently superior dimensions not normally accessible to waking awareness" to emerge. Out of this whole series of positive and negative reactions to the emerging dynamic of the dissociation process came insights into the workings of primitive psychological splitting, repression and suppression. For the moment I will leave aside the question of who or what is suppressing, splitting, or repressing psychic processes. Suffice it to say here that the ego itself may not be the key since many of these processes began before the rudimentary linguistic ego was operative, as in the splitting seen in borderline personality processes, and also because different psychophysical reactions are seen which imply processes deeper or outside of the ego. The process of dissociation itself, however, has been a watershed to this thirsty clinical field.

Dissociation of ego states with concomitant rigid boundary development between these ego states is one of the most heuristic theories put forward to explain multiple personality development. Gruenwald (1978; 1977), a modern researcher, takes a psychodynamic view and hypothesizes that it is this dissociation of ego states that leads to the syndrome of the multiple personality. In another formulation, Greaves (1980) emphasizes the massive splitting and the narcissistic personality structure as predisposing the condition of later multiple personality development. Some find in the multiple personality (of course) a real borderline diagnosis (Horevitz and Braun, 1984). Lasky (1978) saw the multiple personality as a form of frank psychosis. Suffice it to say there are very few full records in the clinical literature since this is such an exotic syndrome.

As a consequence of these and other diverging viewpoints, there is little real consensus on the development of the multiple personality syndrome. Add to this the new research done on multiple personalities, indicating that each independent or autonomous sub-self within the multiple personality is capable of different brain wave patterns, personality dynamics and other psychophysiological patterns when they are in these different separate self states adds more data to the feeling that a different perspective is needed. One very promising viewpoint is the Sullivanian viewpoint espoused by a number of people, including Lovinger (1983). Finally, there are the viewpoints of a number of researchers who have explored the connection between multiple personalities and the development of usually friendly imaginary companions in childhood. Yet, exactly what little is really known about the history and powerful patterns that affect multiple personality development?

Isolation, Abuse, Me, and Not-Me

One of the most powerful dynamics noted by almost all clinical researchers in this area is the presence of severe sexual and physical trauma in the experience of the childhood of the multiple personality (Lovinger, 1983). It is also noted by these researchers that for prolonged periods in the childhood of the multiple personality there were instances of severe emotional and physical *isolation* often accompanied by physical punishment. This isolation is crucial.

It is of clinical interest that the prolonged isolation and physical abuse of individuals is a technique used in the brainwashing of political prisoners, as exemplified in the Korean War. Contradictory and unpredictable behavior increase one's sense of instability. It has also been noted that very often in child development, during these traumatic episodes, the individual, who later developed a multiple personality, would lose consciousness at the point of the traumatic situation! The psychological bind would often be that the early multiple personality would either have to watch and/or participate in the particular incident or else risk severe danger if they did not. The escape was simply to lose consciousness and attempt to thereby repress or split off the situation, if at all possible, from waking consciousness. This is a kind of hypnotically induced symptom within the family context that gets enfolded and stabilized over time. At the time, the escape is adaptive and ensures survival. These victims appear to come from families that are hypermoralistic despite this socially and culturally repugnant behavior. This further contributes to a splitting on the part of the primitive psychic system during development. Both males and females are known to develop multiple personalities (Hawkesworth, 1977).

It appears that in multiple personalities some of the early defenses that are used are massive splitting and primitive projective mechanisms. The use of the mechanism or process of splitting, it is clear in the histories of these victims, leads during that time to a number of internalized, self-referential processes that could be described in Sullivanian terms as "not-me." In other words, in order to deal with the devastating process of sexual and physical abuse, the very primitive psychic system began to split off and dissociate these experiences in order to maintain its own survival (Saltman and Solomon, 1982). The separate-selves situations had to be developed independently and kept separate from each other through the process of splitting. As a consequence, other alternative personalities or alternative selves were independently developed within the undivided whole of the psychic system. These separate selves, or sub-systems, and planes of experience not communicating with each other yet all in the same "place," so to speak, have a nice parallel or reflection in the mathematical/physicist conception of Hilbert space. This will be addressed again later in this story.

Paradoxically, the use of the defense of splitting is a double-edged blade. On the one hand, there is an affirmation of the defense in the sense that it helps the psychic system achieve some sense of control and survival in an anxiety-fraught, dangerous, and bewildering world. On the other hand, it does not work in the long run and, thus, there is ultimately a failure of the process of denial on the part of the psychic system. However, one thing is clear: the process of developing other selves is kept out of central awareness and therefore perhaps there is no need for the process of projective identification based on fusion by the system. Lovinger (1983) and others (Greaves, 1980) believe that because there is no projective identification based on fusion, the multiple personality actually represents a level of ego organization that is "higher" than the borderline!

The Familial Network

Something needs to be said here about the family network of relationships or family unconscious of the multiple personality. My colleagues and I have noticed that, generally speaking, these individuals arise from family constellations where as children they have been subjected to intense contradictory communications from their significant others. The family has been observed to manifest rigid religious beliefs and to present a united front to the community while it is rifled with internal conflict. This occurs frequently in the sexually abusive family. Of particular interest is the observation that these families are often isolated from the community and therefore quite resistant to outside intervention. Their evil/painful secret must be kept strictly confidential. This secrecy is later taken in or introjected and becomes a prototype for a way of managing the psychic energy field. Things are kept intensely hidden from view. At least one parent or significant other in this shared field of family consciousness is deeply disturbed. Since the "split" occurs before 5 years of age, it occurs in the absence of alternative social and psychological models for the child. Each sub-self must develop a unique way to handle crisis after crisis. This notion of sub-self system fits well with the other data we have on the mind's capacity for diverse functions executed simultaneously.

In family therapy in particular, we can observe the process of the internal family system of each individual member (Schwartz, 1987). The subjective experience of each person, the inner landscape of each individual, is colored and influenced by that person's significant relationships over time. The introjected "objects" of the object-relation school can really be more functionally understood as the enfolded holographic representatives of significant others who share a common psychic and psychological field. Under certain conditions intimate "information" within this shared field of the family is recognized to go trans-temporal and trans-spatial. Just as it does in the material world, energy and also information can go trans-temporal and trans-spatial at certain levels of manifestation. Intersubjectivity emerges, allowing for many unusual forms of communication. This potential for a communion of subjects is implicit in a worldview pervaded by personhood or personalism. This is at its best. When this ability, however, is directed to the primitive psychic and psychological survival of the person, immense capacities for splitting are mobilized and the sub-self systems are kept dynamically separate from each other. This requires structure, intent, and energy. Separate localization or vectors in the overall system are implied in this process. This is, again, why the analogy of Hilbert space is useful.

In a sense, one could say that all the worlds or selves are evolving together, seeking a unity, yet needing to keep the worlds apart for fear of the catastrophe of full realization of what is occurring. The tormentors in this field of family unconscious processes are actively attacking the brutalized personality which must deal with them anyway it can. Therein the multiple personality's sub-selves play out the introjected roles of disturbed parent, violated child, escapist dreamer, sociopathic manipulator, the savior or helper of the child, and all the host of other terrible and bewildering characters of the family inner drama. In fact, it is not uncommon for one of the sub-selves to be similar to a deceased relative of the victim! Here, perhaps, is the partial origin of the notion of "possession" by others so often seen in earlier times.

The consciousness principle has learned to dissociate aspects of itself and perhaps to be absorbed by other realms of phenomena. In a bizarre twist on the medical and somatic aspects of an alien "other" being found in the person's psychic system, one can look at twin studies. In some instances a twin, in embryo, has been known to cannibalize the other embryo, or else the "other" is re-absorbed into the mother's uterine wall by still unknown processes. Some rare people have been surgically operated on only to find bits of hair, teeth, and neuronal growth, the remains of "others," embedded in their own system (Begley et al., 1987)!

Finally, it has been noticed that the multiple style is seen in more than one generation of the family. The family unconscious pattern is deeply rooted in the expectancies, images, and communications of the system over time and persons! Whether or not there is a genetic component is unclear. However, the usefulness of dissociation does become clear, since in a primitive fashion it provides escape and psychic survival for the tormented victim.

MULTIPLE PERSONALITIES VERSUS SCHIZOPHRENIA

Lovinger and others have noted that during development the multiple personality actually lost consciousness or used sleep to escape the terrifying situations he or she had to confront. According to Lovinger and others, a certain necessary and functional amnesia for the alternate selves developed, representing a partial borrowing or introjection of parental attitudes toward the unacceptable behavior. The introjected attitudes of the parent, on the part of the *healthy* aspect of the child, are attempts to identify with the parents, and therein to keep out of awareness certain parts of its own personality that are unacceptable to these parental introjected figures. This assumes, of course, that one of the parents is healthy!

Through development and maturation, the child develops alternative selves that are organized or localized around specific feelings, attitudes, and behaviors to experiences in the environment. It is a matter of localization of repeating patterns in a fluctuating energy field. All these different selves simultaneously exist, yet are kept separate from each other at a certain level of consciousness.

The multiple personality develops separate autonomous systems that are *thematic* and *self-organized* within themselves. They are different, active psychic dimensions of the overall personality style. This is in radical distinction to the schizophrenic, whose personality appears to be more *fragmented* or *shattered* as opposed to split off and thematically developed in alternative ways. I, myself, have witnessed the passage from one subsystem personality to another subsystem personality in the multiple personality patient. During each "transition" the patient would briefly lose consciousness before re-emerging in another personality pattern. This change is not as readily seen in the schizophrenic situation. My observation of this particular situation, and also my reading of the literature, necessitated a re-thinking of the vectors and dynamics of what we understand as unconscious processes and intrapsychic functioning.

THE EMBEDDED AND THE EMERGENT UNCONSCIOUS

The severe sexual and physical trauma experienced by multiple personalities, along with prolonged periods of isolation with concomitant physical abuse, and the early onset of such behavior often before the ego is firmly established, indicates that much of this occurred in the very primitive pre-egoic states. The psychic apparatus uses what splitting and projective mechanisms are available to it during this period to help it put distance between, or split off from, the terrifying reality that it is forced to confront. It seems that at that particular time, as I tried to overview in Chapter 2, that the trauma severely influenced the entire unconscious unfolding process of the individual. At the beginning of development, the unconscious is not only existent as a process, but it is in potentia composed of many elements. The unconscious not only includes the inherited disposition of the individual's collective community, family, and self, it also contains levels of development that have not yet emerged from, through maturation, the individual's Self. In other words, those dimensions of higher development such as vision-logic, subtle, causal and other realms that have not yet emerged are still affected by this traumatic situation. As a consequence of the shattering impact of these experiences, one sees shock waves being sent through the whole system of the person's unconscious. Not only is the subtle energetic level of the individual disturbed, but also the very subtle mental impressions that rarely reach waking consciousness. In Yogic terminology these are often referred to as the Causal level of influence. This Causal level usually does not unfold until the person is maturationally in the mid-thirties or beyond (Wilber, 1981). Even then, it usually emerges through a meditative discipline. However, all these levels exist again in potentia at every period.

PSYCHOLOGICAL SPLITTING, TIME, AND MULTIDIMENSIONALITY

Now in order to understand how a number of simultaneous situations can occur in the same system and yet be separate within that system one has to look for a model in contemporary science that approaches this vector operation. This model is afforded to us by the model from mathematics mentioned previously–Hilbert space. Before that, however, a little introduction to the concept of dimensions and space is necessary.

Eddington (1923) suggested in his classic *Space, Time and Gravitation* that when things were in 3-D, i.e., width, length, and depth, a certain supposed knowledge of things was possible since the observer did not need to immerse him/herself in the subjective/self world of "time." This science, oddly enough, abstracted the observer from the world, made the external physical world real, and the observer's subjective world unreal! This has led, I believe, to the peculiar notion in modern science that we can only trust the reality of the inner world if it can be tested or evaluated by the external world. It is a little like waiting to see yourself in a physical mirror before believing that you actually exist! However, with the transformative $E = mc^2$ and the recognition of space-time or the so-called fourth dimension, we have come to realize that positions are relative and limiting and that not all possible positions of the observer could be known simultaneously. In addition, if there are other intelligent terrestrial beings with other observational views, even more dimensions to reality must be included. Thus we go from 3-D Euclidean space or geometry to the radical geometry of Riemannian which Einstein needed in order to demonstrate $E = mc^2$. The dimensions of reality began to multiply.

In order to deal with other multiple situations beyond we must deal with Hilbert space, which is employed in quantum mechanics, particularly in the many-worlds interpretation of quantum mechanics as put forth by Everett and Wheeler (DeWitt, 1970; 1971). Here many simultaneous, dynamic operations can occur in a system and yet not be in direct communication with each other. It is a helpful tool/model here in this attempt to describe how within the same psychic field there can be so many non-communicative aspects. Science has many working models that fit the "hard data," implicating that both matter, energy, and information can go from one universe to another, or in which matter and energy are potentially lost or gained from another universe (Sewjathan, 1984). Thus we need not fear this notion. This correlation of operations in the intricate field of quantum mechanics with those of our subtle nature may at first seem unsteady, or even worse, a fall into scientism. This is not intended. It is merely an extremely helpful tool. Eddington was aware of this and the limits of science as currently understood. Speaking specifically about Relativity Theory he indicated that

> it is a knowledge of structural form and not knowledge of content. All through the physical world runs that unknown content which must surely be the stuff of our consciousness. Here is a hint of aspects deep within the world of physics, and yet unattainable by the methods of physics. And moreover we have found that where science has progressed the farthest, the mind has but regained from nature that which the mind has put into nature!

Hilbert space, therefore, is a useful conceptual tool. In Hilbert space, a number of simultaneous planes or vectors can exist in the same space without contact with each other. In fact, many cortical processes of the brain, especially when viewed from a holonomic or holographic perspective, are most appropriately modeled in Hilbert space (Pribram, 1991). I use it here primarily as a metaphor and tool created by the mind to reflect upon the many ways the mind has of being enfolded within itself. It is a model discovered or created by the mind, which in its very nature reflects the operation of the mind. I should note, again, that in Hilbert space these vectors are not in communication with each other.

I have hopefully already outlined the survival motivational aspects of being able to keep these traumatic situations separate from each other by splitting. To not do this is to experience overwhelming anxiety, which will disintegrate the psychic system totally. This perspective allows us to understand the diverse brain wave patterns and other psychophysiological measures that have been recorded in different personality substates of the same overall personality. It becomes less and less a matter of objects relating to objects, and more as localizations in fields that enfold, share, and emerge from each other. These capacities have certain parallels to Yogic development at a specific stage of practice.

In the Yogic model of the mind, the Causal level refers to that level of functioning that is associated with the most subtle mental operations. The work of the Yogic meditator at the Causal level is to "reabsorb" the unfolding of thoughts and bring them back to their source, which is not energy, of course, but consciousness itself. In other words, as each potentially separate world unfolds, the Yogic meditator at the level of the Causal mind attempts to reabsorb that world.

> The fine samkaras are to be conquered
> by resolving them into their causal state.
>
> –Vivekananda, *Raja-Yoga*

The multiple personality certainly cannot absorb or control each world but he or she can keep the worlds separate from each other and thus keep the unbearable anxiety from reaching a "critical mass." It is an extreme maneuver on the part of the psyche, deeper and prior to full ego development, and indicates remarkable information processing and survival skills.

The Yogic meditator works with the many potential worlds that are an aspect or subsystem of the real Self. The multiple personality is forced to attempt to do this to survive early on, fails because the structures to do so are not fully operative, and falls into chaos. The night-terror in the adult, which I will discuss shortly, may be a reflection of this struggle to integrate at the Causal level.

The fourth, fifth and sixth sutras in the fourth chapter of Patanjali's *Yoga Sutras* deal specifically with the many worlds of the Causal level (Mishra, 1963; Vivekananda, 1973). These sutras are brief statements of psychological processes witnessed in prolonged, disciplined introspective exploration. They were written perhaps 3,000 years ago. They describe out how a yogic practitioner creates many minds from one mind, how those different minds and activities are controlled by one mind, *and* that the mind which is near being *desireless* approaches "liberation."

> When all obstacles in the course of evolution of prakriti (nature) are removed, a yogin obtains power of forming innumerable mindstuffs, chittam. By power of these innumerable minds he can penetrate simultaneously as many minds as he wishes.
>
> –Patanjali, *Yoga Sutras*

> Though the activities of the created minds are varied, the one original mindstuff is the controller of all.
>
> –Patanjali, *Yoga Sutras*

> The mind of clear light is the foundation of all other minds.
>
> –Geshe Kelsang Gyatso,
> *Clear Light of Bliss*

I simply add here that the Causal mind is characterized by bliss and subtle mental impressions, and is said to be experienced in deep sleep without dreaming. In that state there are no internal or external mental impressions as is recorded in desire-shaded waking and dreaming states. Perception is diffuse and therein difficult to remember. There is the absence of the desire for objects. Eventually the energy or pure light that is the substratum of all objects and worlds arises in consciousness. The Yogin consciously develops and works with this level. The vast majority of us are simply unconscious and indifferent to these many worlds. The multiple personality, it seems, is prematurely forced to deal with them, fails completely, and periodically has these other, unwanted worlds that attempt to deal with a painful reality thrust into waking life.

Thus in the development of the multiple personality one notices a number of things. They have almost always been subjected to extreme and bizarre sexual and/or physical abuse. They often have grown up in families in which such behavior has been hidden but tolerated against the background, paradoxically, of an extremely moralistic code of ethics. These, of course, increase more psychological splitting at an extremely early and vulnerable age. This psychological splitting eventuates in thematic aspects or constellations of ideas, feelings, and patterns localized and stored in different sub-systems around core ideational processes and images. It is much like a holographic or holonomic process. The psychological apparatus of the individual attempts by this process to divest itself of the drives and impulses which it finds to be unacceptable and which seem to generate its abuse and isolation by disowning or splitting off the impulsive or unacceptable behavior into a "not-me"/imaginary companion. In most cases, a child's imaginary companion is merely a good friend and does not imply pathology. In the extreme cases we are focusing on there is the presence of disorder. In these more extreme situations, the child creates a scapegoat and attempts to avoid blame and maintain psychic survival. The "other" personalities are held to be responsible for the child's unacceptable behavior. This, of course, leads to many other splits later on including splits between drives and reason and so on. However, with any system of splitting there are coherent evolved subsystems within the personality. From a certain perspective, all these different personalities are seen to be permutations of the one personality of the individual localized in different fields of experience.

It is reasonable to assume that the high unpredictability of the multiple personality's environment coupled with the early age and the vulnerability to such situations and early ego development probably interfered with the development of the mechanism of denial by the ego (Stolorow and Lachmann, 1980). This seems to be a relatively good working hypothesis. It is unclear, however, whether an ego would have been able to ward off that powerful trauma anyway even if it had been established. Those mechanisms work when there is an "average expectable environment" for that kind of material to arise. The present perspective is somewhat different based upon a new reading of the clinical literature and direct experience.

Instead of the failure of the defense of denial to develop, rather the use of "selective inattention" is emphasized, and the development of alternative views of reality that would allow some sense of stability for the psychic apparatus to occur is the main development. These develop under the impetus of profound psychological trauma. *The mechanisms of attention are frozen in subsystems of the multiple personality.* These systems of frozen attention are necessary in order for the psychic apparatus to distance itself from terrifying anxiety and therein to survive. It is as though the living current is split off into separate oxbow lakes of experience in which each develops its own contours, content, and calibration. At some point the original current is amplified or healed, and the waves of the separate lakes are joined again and the life-force moves toward the ocean of free energy and attention.

Most of this trauma occurs in the prelinguistic phase, perhaps even before the brain's left-hemispheric dominance and thereby in the more unconscious realm of development. It occurs usually in the network of the family unconscious. The unbearable anxiety is warded off into various "not-me" aspects of the personality. That is to say, as "not-me" aspects of the parentally unacceptable personality. However, the "not-me" subsystems may themselves be acceptable to some degree in other situations in society. In each particular situation, the subsystem of the personality very often loses consciousness as he or she goes from one "state" to another. I have witnessed this process. These appear to be splitting or dissociative maneuvers. I emphasize here that in disturbances of deep sleep, called "night-terrors," there is an emergence into awareness of a very primitive level of these "not-me" aspects of the personality. These night-terrors are different from nightmares in that we remember the content of nightmares. In night-terror, we only wake up with a terrifying sense of the uncanny or the unreal invading our psychological and psychic world. This is an indication of how deep and how profound the disturbance is. It happens in the emerging schizophrenic and, occasionally, to the normal person. Historically, it has been observed in cases of supposed "possession" where one person is entering another person's consciousness. Finally, it may be related in certain aspects to the principle and practice of consciousness-transference, or Pho-Wa, in esoteric forms of Tibetan Yoga.

SLEEP AND THE PARASOMNIAS

In the *Mandukya Upanishad,* one of her kind's most ancient texts, the levels of sleep and consciousness are explored. The levels of consciousness are variously, in this psychological text, referred to as the waking state, the dream state, the state of deep dreamless sleep, and the state beyond and enfolding these three, the state of transcendental reality called Turyia. What I am focusing on is the level of deep dreamless sleep which is associated in Yogic literature with the Causal level. Usually this level experienced in deep dreamless sleep is characterized by profound bliss and undifferentiated consciousness. When we wake from it we feel we have had a full, deep, nourishing sleep. It is a state where consciousness is unmodified by shifting mental conditions, and is one with its own current of living energy. On the electroencephalogram (EEG) there is a proliferation of what is termed delta wave spikes in the brain wave pattern. I am pointing out here, in conjunction with Harry Stack-Sullivan's work, that there appears to be a polarity between absolute euphoria and absolute terror. It appears that this dynamic is occurring on the Causal level, the level of deep dreamless sleep, and may be implicated in the process of the multiple personality. In other words, the state of deep dreamless sleep is characterized by a profound peace, a sense of undifferentiated consciousness and bliss. It is an inherently boundaryless condition and therein open to all sorts of influence of a psychological, psychic, and noetic nature. When this level is interrupted it is not interrupted by a nightmare, which has a different EEG profile, but an actual night-terror. Terror is a completely disorganizing kind of experience, much more profound than the nightmare. I have come to believe that *the night-terror is the other side of the night bliss.* Very often when awakening from the night terror one feels that they have had experiences of literally an other-worldly, unearthly kind. Very uncanny.

It is quite possible that deep psychological and behavioral disturbances of sleep, called the parasomnias, represent aspects of the potential for multiple intelligences gone awry. This is again because this state or condition is related to deep sleep, where the usual boundaries are absent. When abruptly awakened from this state, we experience "confusion" and disorientation. Yet there is even more data to suggest this notion.

The parasomnias, e.g., somnambulism, night-terrors, enuresis and encopresis, nocturnal myoclonus (restless legs syndrome), etc., tend to occur in the deep sleep cycle; children, who need time and experience in order to learn to live in the waking state alpha/beta cycle, experience more of the parasomnias than most and also, significantly enough, have more diffuse psychological and psychic boundaries. Such symptoms occur earlier at night when there is more delta brain wave activity; different parasomnias often occur in the same person; all awareness of the state is repressed on awakening. It is as though it were a completely different reality.

When persons experience these states or conditions, they are very difficult to arouse from their "confusion." Indeed, they *actively resist* arousal. It is as though the usual repression function was now operating to keep certain data out of the awareness of the predominate "confusional state" of the sleeper. The person seems to actively prefer a different reality than otherwise. A different localization in the field absorbs the observer's attention. Perhaps attention is even frozen in this subsystem of the psychic process, giving *rise* to many worlds or *opening* to many worlds. One is reminded of the Borges short story "The Garden of Forking Paths" and the innumerable interconnections of a print by Escher. It would be interesting to know what occurs when the "observer," be they deep sleeper or the many-worlds quantum physicist, does not focus or collapse all their attention on discrete observation from this state. When the "collapse of the wave-packet" is avoided, a new or higher state may emerge that interconnects all these worlds.

It is interesting in this light, from a transpersonal point of view, that there are numerous references to uncanny or other-worldly experiences occurring in deep sleep without dreaming. In fact, it is even said that given some meditational procedures the person can enter into the state of deep dreamless sleep with awareness and in a profound way affect not only one's own consciousness, but the consciousness of others. This is said to proceed to states even beyond deep dreamless sleep. I am referring here to the Tibetan doctrine of Trongjug which is related to the previously mentioned Pho-Wa (Evans-Wentz, 1958). Scattered reports also occur of similar phenomena also occurring in certain corrupted forms of voodoo practices (Metraux, 1972; *Time*, 1983). In each case, however, by entering into the profoundest state of human consciousness recognizable by most human beings, that is to say, the state of deep dreamless sleep and undifferentiated consciousness, with its inherent diffuseness of psychic boundaries, certain phenomena involving heteropsychic influence are seen to occur. Certain individuals who have practiced disciplined meditational procedures, such as Pir Vilayat Kahn, Swami Rama at the Menninger Clinic and others, have been able to demonstrate being able to consciously enter into this deepest of all states of normal human consciousness–a state which is characterized by, but not contained in, delta brain wave production. Ordinarily, we are totally unconscious and oblivious at this level. However, Swami Rama and other adepts in meditation have been able to enter into it consciously, as reflected in EEG and other psychophysiological measures, and to bring back information about what was going on in the experimental situation when this occurred. This state is amenable to our conscious influence. During this state meditators report the experience of personality to be immeasurably expanded and diffuse with very permeable boundaries between themselves, other situations, and individuals.

A PRECOCIOUS SUMMARY

This perspective suggests that in most of the very early traumatic and bizarre experiences there arises the early use of primitive splitting mechanisms. These inner world splitting mechanisms are operative before the development of an intact and separative ego. These individual selves are necessarily developed and a great deal of psychic energy is devoted to keeping them separate from each other. The metaphor/tool of the Hilbert space conception is used to show that such phenomena can occur not only in the material and energetic world, but also in the psychological field from which they actually originate. The tool is a mathematical one taken from quantum mechanics. In quantum mechanics, as stated earlier, it is simply used for the analysis of systems of influence that are in *different vibratory states.* In many ways, the multiple personality experiences different independent vibratory states or localizations in the field with each other, yet they are not in direct communication with each other. The events go on concomitantly but are kept separate. The goal of meditation at the Causal level is to create and integrate these selves in order to hasten one's evolutionary progress. The multiple personality, it seems, has been prematurely forced to create, but then does not have the capacity to integrate these various split-off, subselves.

Whether you perceive the multiple personality to be at a higher or lower level of functioning depends a great deal upon your perspective. My own bias in this situation is to perceive the multiple personality at a significantly lower level of overall personality functioning than any discussed so far in this study. It is at an even lower level of personality functioning than the paranoid individual. The simple fact that the autonomous selves appear to be separate does not in any way lessen this. Those independent or autonomous selves that are functioning are indeed relatively independent, but they tend to be rather primitive personalities and not highly integrated, differentiated, and capable of dealing effectively in the world. Also, how do you account for these startling differences in psychophysiological measures, brain wave states and other associations and habits that different selves involved in the multiple personality seem to be able to demonstrate to clinicians and researchers? This can neither be accounted for by the dissociation of ego states nor completely by the development of imaginary companions or "not-me" vectors of experience (Brende, 1984; Putnam, 1984). Because this primitive apparatus of object splitting does seem to occur in the multiple personality at an extremely young age, it indicates that object splitting is certainly not the exclusive domain of the ego. Indeed, this primitive splitting seems to be a more specific form of the more general splitting at a deeper level of mind. In other words, the psychological shock of the multiple personality during the person's traumatic sexual and physical abuse and isolation experience has sent ripple-waves all the way through both the potential embedded and emergent unconscious. As a consequence of this, obviously, profound hypnosis and meditation are the treatments of choice (Gruenwald et al. 1984). These approaches are the only way to reach the mind at such a profoundly deep and intricate level.

Each subsystem of the personality reflects, in a holographic way, each other subsystem and yet is separate from it. An internal harmony of self-images or finer coordination of vibratory intelligence is the goal of therapy. In the final analysis, the various splintered aspects of the mind need to be brought back into contact with each other. This is where the useful analogy to Hilbert space ends.

The multiple personality is, indeed, an unusual phenomenon in human functioning. It also seems to reflect a deeper aspect and capacity of our own psyches which is usually left in the dark. It is the personality syndrome that is the most splintered and, from that perspective, the system that is most out of balance with the person's real Self. This is not to deny the influence of "not-me" experiences, the development of imaginary companions, and the dissociative mechanisms of the ego. The major new emphasis is that the trauma was so devastating, so severe, that it sent ripple-waves through the embedded and potential emergent unconscious of the individual. This, in turn, had a profound and detrimental effect on the person's subsequent ego and self-development. It is a syndrome that goes beyond the ego dissociative mechanisms of classical hysteria and the more conventional splitting of the dual personality. The situation is characterized by overwhelming anxiety and stress, loss of consciousness, psychic energy diverted into the development of alternative realities for the overall personality, all in an attempt to come to terms with a terrifying situation. That situation, of course, is the primordial fear of the *total* annihilation of the known and knowing Self. Defenses arise of necessity, however. The absorption of psychic energies into these avoidance maneuvers on the psychic plane draws energies away from the more transcendental functions of the personality. From this perspective, the multiple personality is the most severely disturbed of all the personality syndromes so far presented. It goes without saying that the multiple personality is dissociated and split off from the *flow* of life-energy. The flow of life-energy is a direct perceptual recognition that life, indeed, is not fragmented but is literally a loving, flowing current–a multidimensional whole. The experience of the multiple personality with the life-force is that the life-force has allowed a profound sense of insecurity to emerge for the person. This personality pattern dealing with the life-force has been fraught with oceanic anxiety and catastrophic danger, given its tormented history. Inevitably, a profound sense of terror, of basic ontological insecurity, has developed in the multiple personality. Its way of defending against this is massive separation, splitting, and fragmentation on a scale extraordinarily difficult for the average person to comprehend. Each separate world gives asylum to the orphans of the injured self.

REFERENCES

Begley, S., Murr, A., Springen, K. and Gordon, J. "All About Twins," *Newsweek*, November 23, 1987, pp. 53-69.

Brain/Mind Bulletin, Issue on Multiple Personality 8:16, October 3, 1983.

Brende, J. O. "The Psychophysiologic Manifestations of Dissociation," *Psychiatric Clinics of North America*, Vol. 7, No. 1, March 1984, pp. 41-50.

DeWitt, B. S. "Quantum-mechanics Debate," *Physics Today*, April 1971.

DeWitt, B. S. "Quantum-mechanics and Reality," *Physics Today*, 23, No. 9 (1970):30.

Eddington, A. *Space, Time and Gravitation*, 1923, p. 185.

Eddington, A. Op. cit.

Evans-Wentz, W. Y. (editor). *Tibetan Yoga and Secret Doctrines*, Oxford University Press, London, New York, (1958) 1978.

Greaves, G. B. "Multiple Personality, 165 Years After Mary Reynolds," *Journal of Nervous and Mental Disease*, 1980, 168(10), 577-596.

Gruenwald, D. et al., Whole issue of journal multiple personality, *International Journal of Clinical and Experimental Hypnosis*, Vol. 32, No. 2, April 1984.

Gruenwald, D. "Multiple Personality and Splitting Phenomena: A Reconceptualization," *Journal of Nervous and Mental Disease*, 1977, 164, 385-393.

Gruenwald, D. "Analogues of Multiple Personality in Psychosis," *Journal of Clinical and Experimental Hypnosis*, 1978, 26(1), 17.

Gyatso, G. K. *Clear Light of Bliss: Mahamundra in Vajrayana Buddhism*, Wisdom Publications, London, England, 1982, p. 76.

Hawkesworth, H. (with T. Schwarz). *The Five of Me*, New York, Pocket Books, 1977.

Horevitz, R. P. and Braun, B. G. "Are Multiple Personalities Borderline?" *Psychiatric Clinics of North America*, Vol. 7, No. 1, March 1984, pp. 69-87.

Lasky, R. "Psychoanalytic Treatment of a Case of Multiple Personality," *Psychoanalytic Review*, 1978, 65(3), 355-380.

Lovinger, S. L. "Multiple Personality: A Theoretical View," *Psychotherapy: Theory, Research and Practice*, Vol. 20, No. 4, Winter 1983.

Metraux, A. *Voodoo in Haiti*, New York, Schocken Books, 1972.

Mishra, R. S. *Yoga Sutras*, Anchor Books/Doubleday, Garden City, NY, 1963, pp. 408-410.

Pribram, K. *Brain and Perception*, New Jersey, Lawrence Erlbaum Associates, 1991.

Putnam, F. W. "The Psychophysiologic Investigation of Multiple Personality Disorder," *Psychiatric Clinics of North America*, Vol. 7, No. 1, March 1984, pp. 31-39.

Saltman, V. and Solomon, R. S. "Incest and the Multiple Personality," *Psychological Reports*, 1982, 50, 1127-1141.

Schreiber, F. R. *Sybil*, Chicago, Henry Regenery, 1973.

Schwartz, R. "Our Multiple Selves," *The Family Networker*, March-April, 1987, p. 25.

Sewjathan, V. *Journal of Mathematics and Mathematical Sciences*, 1984-1985. (Reported in *Brain-Mind Bulletin*, October 22, 1984.)

Stolorow, R. D. and Lachmann, F. M. *Psychoanalysis of Developmental Arrests*, New York: International Universities Press, 1980.

Sullivan, H. S. *The Interpersonal Theory of Psychiatry*, W. W. Norton & Co., New York, 1953.

Time, Medicine Section, "Zombies: Do They Exist?," October 17, 1983, p. 60.

Vivekananda, S. *Raja-Yoga*, New York, Ramakrishna-Vivekananda Center, (1955) 1973.

Wilber, K. "Ontogenetic Development: Two Fundamental Patterns," *Journal of Transpersonal Psychology*, 13:1, 1981, 33-58.

SECTION III. WHERE THREE RIVERS MEET: THE BODY, THERAPY, AND EVOLUTION

We speak of the evolution of Life in matter, the evolution of Mind in Life; but evolution is a word which merely states the phenomenon without explaining it. For there seems to be no reason why Life should evolve out of material elements or Mind out of living form, unless we accept . . . that Life is already involved in Matter and Mind in Life because in essence Matter is a form of veiled Life, Life a form of veiled Consciousness. And then there seems to be little objection to a farther step in the series and the admission that mental consciousness may itself be only a form and a veil of higher states which are beyond Mind. In that case, the unconquerable impulse of man towards God, Light, Bliss, Freedom, Immortality, presents itself in its right place in the chain as simply the imperative impulse by which Nature is seeking to evolve beyond, and appears to be as natural, true and just as the impulse towards Life . . . The animal is a living laboratory in which Nature has, it is said, worked out man. Man himself may well be a thinking and living laboratory in whom and with whose conscious cooperation she wills to work out the superman, the god. Or shall we not say, rather to manifest God?

–S. Aurobindo
The Life Divine

Chapter 7

The Psychosomatic Web

THE ARCH OF EVOLUTION

$$E = mc^2$$

–A. Einstein

$$\lambda = \frac{h}{p}$$

–L. DeBroglie

> . . . conversion symptoms are not simply somatic expressions of affects but very specific representations of thoughts which can be retranslated from their "somatic language" into the original word language.
>
> –O. Fenichel, M.D.
> *The Psychoanalytic Theory of Neurosis*

Perched heroically like an eagle atop the modern city of glass and stone, the assertive character of today has no doubt about our collective near-mastery of nature. After looking out over streets of pressed rock and hearing the ooze and noise from passing radios play against the arresting shrill of taxis, the modern city dweller will then close his windows, turn on the tube and try to ignore most of the stimuli that rivets his senses.

His sense of smell is particularly out of touch. Strange new odors that his ancient progenitor never knew sweep through his system. Perfumes, exotic fruits, even noxious industrial pollutants, have their affect on the sensitive pathways of his nervous system. The pervasive forces by which the various sensory systems stimulate the brain seem to particularly affect the rhinencephalon, or what is called the visceral brain, which in turn strongly influences the cerebral cortex (MacLean, 1949). Indeed it is this smell, or olfactory and visceral brain, located between the inner sense of need or I-sense, and the outer more interpersonal and social world of symbols, that is vitally involved in the development of the deep, somatic anxiety signal. This pathway was alert and responsive for our ancient mother of the lakes and woods. Of this our modern compatriot is largely unconscious, yet still responsive!

Without the slightest provocation the modern cousin quietly realizes he is anxious about something but he does not know what. The lower body somehow knows, however, the visceral brain speaks and acid creeps into his stomach. A pounding-harder heart then alerts him to a shortness of breath while the TV news ups the whole ante with the latest report on blood-letting in a place he once was or merely heard about. He actively suppresses this panic attack. Armed with a college degree and a zigzag history of independent thinking, the modern dweller wonders how evolution has gotten him to this point.

It is clear that evolution continues. Its nature and trajectory seems to be one of those irreversible processes that, once set in motion, bring time into the world and sets up all kinds of increasingly complex structures and situations. Even the hard core materialist says these days that the universe began in an explosion of immense energy and power (Weinberg, 1977). Through innumerable exchanges and spontaneous experiments, au natural, some order far from the usual equilibrium emerged from the apparent chaos of material nature. The materialist may not logically derive from supposed random events "the why," but somehow "the how" of nature moved toward increasing order and away from the expected slow heat death of entropy.

Out of the material vastness, itself a drop in a limitless back ground sea of energy[1] or generalized light, many systems of increasing complexity and novelty emerged on the scene (Jantsch,

---

1. This refers to theoretical physicist David Bohm's calculation of the "zero-point" energy. This is the latent energy of the infinite substructure of matter far beyond the reservoir of the known nuclear energies. If one computes the zero-point energy due to quantum mechanical fluctuations in even one cubic centimeter of space, the order of 10^{38} ergs emerges which is more than the fission of 10 tons of uranium! Thus the unseen universe is a vast, seamless sea of light energy, unmanifest to our scientific instruments. The apparent emptiness is paradoxically full (D. Bohm, *Causality and Chance in Modern Physics*, pp. 163-164).

1980). This eventually became organic life. With more self-regulation, exchanges of energies and fluctuating conditions, eventually the most primitive signs of vegetation appeared. After a thousand million years of cycling, even more complex self-regulating organisms emerged and left the womb of the warm sea from which they spawned.

Crude consciousness, at first transient, then stable, emerged from those animal forms that seemed to increase the negative entropy or trend toward higher organization processes in nature. With mammals, the power to be conscious was stabilized. Out of them and their development, finally, the greater integration and harmony of body-mind processes led to early man. The rest is, of course, the history of ourselves, the five-fingered form.

The ego of modern man seems to feel that the great arch of psychophysical and conscious evolution ends in our era. Yet it is also quite possible that we are but the latest aspects or manifestations on earth of this whole process of evolution. Perhaps we are, as Sri Aurobindo says, a "transitional" man or episode on the evolutionary way to an even more refined manifestation of this vast opening capacity of conscious intelligence to express itself in matter. The present ornament or mental/egoic condition may be a necessary passageway to something greater in evolution and consciousness. Surely we can see that as evolution increases, free intelligence and consciousness become more manifest in the world. Perhaps, as Aurobindo envisioned (Satprem, 1968), matter itself is becoming more receptive to the unfolding, greater consciousness, and that at some point the "mental" way of dealing with the Absolute, mentioned in early chapters of this study, may itself be too limited an expression.

There is much to this view. All of us have seen the increasing self-regulation and complexity of matter reflected in the increasing mental capacity of evolution. The transient dissipative structures lead to structures of increasing complexity, which then allow for a more subtle consciousness to unfold or emerge. There may be a cosmic joke played out in the apparent "magical" ability of "dead matter" to complicate and expand itself by random action. *Or,* there may be some as yet not fully understood process of evolutionary intelligence drawing matter into greater spirals of complexity, subtlety and actualization. The life-force referred to so many times in this book appears to be an *expression* of evolution and its process of innumerable adaptations. Our most intimate association with it appears to be connected to the initially embryonic neuromelanin system and its later unfoldment throughout somatic and nervous system development.

Is it possible that evolution, that grandiloquent wave and still intimate reality, works through and in us individually in a real and tangible way? I feel it does. This life-current around which the ego so often contracts is a luminous, subtle, individual/collective expression of increasing development in matter and consciousness. It is not an abstract idea, but rather is expressed daily, innumerable times in the breathing process, body-mind tension states and other occasions of its overt manifestation. There is a constant pulse, a perpetual contraction and expansion that is the life process. Clinging desperately to this pulsation leads to a focus on contraction, leading to all sorts of psychophysical signs and symptoms. To give is to let go, and paradoxically, to more deeply have. To not give is to freeze, to not let go of the transient and fall into the prior and the transcendental. On the deepest level, it is the failure to forgive and is thus bondage.

From this perspective, stress disorders or initially emotionally/psychologically created disturbances of body-mind integration are the primary source of deep, long-term psychosomatic problems. When one is in balance with the life-current, there is a natural regulation of breath, appetite, and a sense of body-mind equanimity abides. The flow of the evolutionary force is easy, steady, and life-affirming. From this position, one begins to intuit even beyond the body-mind experience of increasing/ascending life energy to the source of its manifestation, which appears to be the Absolute, the transcendental condition itself, beyond the lens of all temporal, matter/energy manifestations.

This chapter will focus on the processes that deflect or distort the natural rise and arch of this evolutionary, teleological, intelligent life-force in us as individuals. These distortions, like those earlier, largely psychological distortions, are also the mirages of light. This light and biolight is rooted in our neural and embryonic inheritance and, perhaps, is the actual urge and pull of evolution. Remember, this physical body is matter and matter is a form of concretized light. Yes, we are moving toward something higher or beyond our present mental, emotional, and noetic expression. Both mind and matter are enfolded and transformed in the process, transformed into more complex, subtle, and harmonious expressions of a more vast and intelligent light source that pervades the known and unknown universe.

This is an evolutionary perspective that sees the process rooted in our blood and genes. Given the structural knowledge offered by the triune brain's levels of development, from the core reptilian to the limbic mammalian, all the way to the spreading neocortex of our common ancient One, it is surely obvious that a directionality is present. This directionality is toward increasing self-conscious intelligence in evolution. From its early weeks in the womb, the embryo has elongated along a spine. Its melanin-sensitive centers have evolved glands whose biochemistry is responsive to light and carbon, carbon being the very basis of life on earth. This cord of nerve is the conduit along which light and intelligence move toward increasing complexity in the brain. This, again, is literally the force of evolution, of which only a fraction is liberated by most of us. This subtle current of light becomes almost infinitely expanded and complex when it interacts with all the other wave-fronts of the neocortex. All the "organs" of the body would appear to have a certain vibrational affinity to each other and are all represented or localized in certain functions of the brain touched by the life-current. In a very real sense, this carbon-based evolutionary life-force that currents through the body-mind and spine, translating light and bioenergy into intelligence is a paradoxically luminous dark force. It reaches back into our deepest memories of blood and race.

THE RITES OF PSYCHE AND SOMA

The Egyptian and earlier Nubian priests were familiar with it as were their later counterparts, the Greek physicians (King, 1982). Long before these, and long before the Aryan invasions of ancient India, there were established elaborate human laboratories in the temples and meadows of the Indus Valley. The peoples of Nubia-Egypt and southern India discussed its operations between each other, and integrated it into the ancient religions. Peoples and cultures all over the earth have known about it. In many hidden and mysterious ways, the mind, thought, and inner breath, or "soul," of a person were felt to deeply affect the body. Indeed, it is only us moderns who believed that the mind and body were ever separate. All the ancient world knew them to be a unity. By the end of the nineteenth century in the West, however, the new scientists were beginning to discover what much of mankind had already known. The brilliant pioneering work of Freud in his early years with hysteria and hypnosis led to a "new" understanding of the relationship between psyche and soma. Out of these startling observations and revelations, Freud discovered the dynamic principles of repression, transformation, and sublimation. This was only another beginning in a process that delights in the forever new.

The whole field has been given various names. Some have chosen to call the negative effect of mind upon the body a "conversion disorder." Others speak of psychosomatic reactions. And still others speak of psychophysiological dysfunctions. For convenience, and out of convention, I will take the traditional word of "psychosomatic." This is obviously somewhat arbitrary, and arguments can be made for any label chosen.

After Freud's pioneering work on the psychodynamics of hysteria, particularly conversion in hysteria, where emotional conflicts are dramatically expressed in physical symptoms, psychoanalysis began to brilliantly extend its tools to other areas of psychosomatic expression. The understanding and operation of symptom-formation as a compromise between conflicted drives was seen over and over in the psychoanalytic hour. Yet, denying a teleological impulse, these new voyagers did not go all the way.

It was Fenichel (1945) who, a number of years after the passing of the great liberator Freud, stated clearly in reference to the psychosomatic process that "conversion symptoms are not simply somatic expression of affects but very specific representations of thoughts which can be retranslated from their 'somatic language' into the original word language." He further went on to indicate that

> the syndromes of conversion symptoms are unique in every individual, and analysis shows where they originate: they are historically determined by repressed experiences in the individual's past. They represent a distorted expression of repressed instinctual demands, the specific type of the distortion being determined by the historical events that create the repression.

This, of course, involves tremendously powerful unconscious processes. We are led to understand from this formulation that it is a psychological necessity that earlier on in the individual's history they turned from reality to the fantasy world, that is to say, they began to replace real sexual "objects" with supposed fantasy representations of those early infantile sexual objects. For us today, however, remember these "objects" are "fields" of psychic energy that interface within and between others.

The hysterics, of course, were supposed to be the most adept people at this particular kind of psychological process. Ferenczi even spoke of "hysterical materialization" of repressed fantasies. This feels like a tacit recognition that mind enfolds and works on matter, that our conscious and unconscious mental energy affects the material body in an intimate play on $E = mc^2$. Coming from the other direction, all matter also has wave-like qualities, $\lambda = \frac{h}{p}$, and these waves are interconnected with other waves in an implicate order. Each aspect of the system reflects and influences each other aspect in sickness and in health. Each density localization in the field has a certain resonatic affinity with the other.

While the classical hysterical disorder is a somewhat rarer bird these days than in the early days of psychoanalysis, the fact remains that the psychosomatic and conversion disorders still continue to predominate in many areas of psychological distress. They predominate either as an active functional aspect of the disorder or as a by-product of it. In early chapters, especially those on the borderline (anorexia nervosa), obsessive/compulsive and paranoid style, I pointed out how often these people are physically very tense in their mode of operation. The constant stress/fear biochemistry produces numerous physical problems (Selye, 1976). There are many events and motivations that lead to the psychosomatic disposition. The major origins or etiologic explanations of this somatization are the following:

1. Somatization or psychosomatic reactions are often a *response or failed solution* to a family systems problem. Many have pointed out how a child's psychosomatic reaction in a family constellation serves to re-focus attention away from a hidden marital problem (Minuchin, Baker, Rosman et al., 1975; Minuchin, Rosman, and Baker, 1978). Family therapy is the treatment of choice and will be explored in the next section.

2. Somatization is often a way of *communicating between family and others* when more direct channels are closed or repressed. The earlier mentioned conversion disorder is a good example. It occurs more often than one might realize (Ford and Folks, 1985). In both numbers 1 and 2 above there is an enormous influence of family roles, images, affect, and ideas communicated in a shared matrix of relationships and feelings. Many wave-fronts are involved. There are other cultural, religious, and sometimes even financial, gains from psychosomatic reactions. Sometimes it is "safer" to have a physical or medical problem than a psychological problem. In each case, however, the system exerts a kind of hypnotic influence on the symptom "carrier" in the system. The family remains perhaps the most powerful of these.

In each case the autonomic nervous system (ANS) is implicated in the body's reactivity to family, environmental, and other stresses. Indeed this labile ANS is sensitive to stress *prior* to the actual disease and/or illness process is overtly manifested. Like the unconscious mind that functions in the dream state, the labile ANS remains generally outside of awareness, yet is tacitly conscious of the process and registers this information subliminally. One suspects this is also registered in the deep core imagery and processes of the brain. These should eventually show up on either EEG brainwave measures or other monitors sensitive to subtle aberrations. In a sense, like dreams perhaps, symptoms unfold out of the ANS process of unconscious activity at a crucial and symbolic time in the person's life cycle.

3. Symptoms are *selectively reinforced by attention* from family, society and others, leading to what are termed secondary gains for

the person. This labile ANS can become a way of life, as can be the internalized family derived images of illness, distortion and so on.

4. A symptom can often be a way of *expressing conflict* when the person has no words or vocabulary to relate the problem. The word for this condition in behavioral medicine is alexithymic.

5. It goes without saying that a reaction to physical injury or accident can be a *somatization of fears and worries*. After a heart attack it is common to become hypochondriacal with obsessive features. These obsessive thoughts may have been only an occasionally unpleasant experience for the person before the physical injury. Now they become more intense, persistent, and annoying to others.

This increase in obsessive hypochondriasis is related to another factor in symptom creation. This is the tendency on the part of many people to habitually entertain negative, panic inducing, catastrophic imagery and thoughts. This, in combination with a labile ANS and a higher response to hypnotic process has been observed by others in the somatization process (Wickramasekera, 1986). When these are combined in a family system they take on literally "massive" proportions. By this I mean that the shared field of family images and these other influences on the matrix lead to an almost *constructive interference or localization of wave-fronts* manifesting as somatic disorder. Remember Ferenczi's (1968) "hysterical materialization" of repressed fantasies! This is a similar process, only carried out in a field of energetically and psychologically shared processes.

6. Finally, it appears that the effect of the breathing process itself is deeply implicated in the somatization or psychosomatic process. The breathing process directly influences every other process in the body-mind. It can be *consciously* directed toward selectively influencing the autonomic nervous system and the limbic system (Rama, Ballentine, Hymes, 1981). The source of many psychosomatic complications seen in the Behavioral Medicine Clinic are directly related to this labile imbalance of breathing and the ANS. Indeed, the first great anxiety is at the dawn of breathing. The most incisive treatment is a clinical intervention at this level (Fried, 1987). The interface between psyche and soma is made abundantly clear in the conscious modulation of the breathing cycle, the only

system in the body that we can be either fully conscious or unconscious of and still have it operate smoothly.

From this brief foray into the rites of psyche and soma it is easy to see the basic pillars of the psychosomatic structure. While environmental, social, organic, and other factors play a role, the decisive role appears to be in those areas where unconscious forces and family influence is most pronounced. Given this remarkable influence of the family and the unconscious on these systems it would be useful to look closer at both of these for some understanding. First let us turn to the unconscious and its most vocal expression, the dream.

DREAMSCAPES AND THE SOMA

Most of us acknowledge the dream messengers of our sleep. Even science knows that the dreams of psychosomatic clients are replete with images of injury to the body. It does not require a doctoral degree to realize that repeated attacks on the body by the unconscious, by way of dreams and catastrophic self-destructive fantasies can influence us toward physical and psychosomatic illness (LaBerge, 1985).

The ancient Chinese science of medicine, long before Freud, had indicated that dreams reflect the processes of the body. The processes of wish-fulfillment and non-conscious interactions were well known and outlined briefly in *The Yellow Emperor's Classic of Internal Medicine* (Veith, 1949). However, it was that group of intrepid explorers in the psychosoma netherland, the psychoanalysts, who have thrown light on this common boundary in the West.

Kardiner (1933) really opened the biological/somatic dimension of dreaming when he focused on the catastrophic dreams of death and destruction in clients with serious somatic disease. He came to believe that dreams were a reflection of the psyche's attempt to libidinize the destructive forces of organic disease. Sabini (1981) has found dreams extremely useful in the diagnosis, prognosis, and attitude toward psychotherapy.

When the separative ego and body-mind is threatened, be it the body or other psychological aspects, this is partially reflected in the dream expression. This was Kardiner's finding. Both Levitan

(1980) and Warnes and Finkelstein (1971) have noted the unusually large number of death and destruction dream contents in their patients with psychosomatic diseases. In addition both Ziegler (1962) and Schneider (1973), have seen how dreams of such content have occurred just before severe heart disease, so there can be little doubt that dreams reflect somatic processes.

A recent clinical study by Smith (1984) indicated that for hospitalized patients with physical illnesses, dreams were indeed *reactive* to biologic functioning. Those men and women with higher incidence of death (men) and separation (women) in their dream content had a much poorer prognosis, *and* vice-versa!

It appears within the range of possibility to assume that since the body obviously affects the mind, that the deeper, unconscious mind affects the body. The body's condition affects the dreamscape and the unconscious. Perhaps then, given the reciprocal and mutual enfoldment of psyche and soma, the dreamscape can profoundly affect the body. Ancient temples and rites of healing from all humankind's cultures testifies to this.

The ancient rites at Delphi involved a long pilgrimage to the sacred sites, washing in purifying waters, cleansing of the body, and finally, the incubation of the healing dream. Whatever the psychosocial context and religious symbols, the fact remains that dreams of a powerful, revelatory nature were seen to have a direct affect on the physical body. With the decline of Greece and its heir Rome, these methods lost power. In their heyday, however, there were thousands of the faithful, the mobilization of all the psychosocial demand characteristics, and the spontaneous opening to transcendental forces we still know precious little about!

Even earlier than this, in the early dynastic period of ancient Kemetic Egypt, dreamwork was practiced for healing the mind and the body. The use of hypnosis and the waking dream were well known over 5000 years ago. These priests were aware of the forces of the dynamic unconscious. They referred to it as Amenta and the primeval waters of Nun (King, 1990). Tehmut-m-hobi and his colleague Khonsu-p-ri-seker, both priests of Thoth, used the dynamic unconscious and hypnotic approach successfully during the reign of Ramses XII of the twentieth dynasty at Thebes. Their client, a royal female, recovered by this method. Much later, hypnosis and dreamwork were separated as treatments. Yet here we can see their common root in dealing with some of the deeper somatic expressions of the body-mind. Both are not only indications that processes of the body affect the mind and are reactive to biologic stress, but that the body may indeed profoundly respond to the unconscious processes of the dream!

The dream is suffused with powerful imagery, symbolic experience, and an extensive matrix on which the themes of our lives, biological, familial, intrapsychic, and cultural, have their play. It is a collage of our particular history against the backdrop of a larger consciousness. Its web of symbols wedded to affect is our idiosyncratic language in which we talk to ourselves on deeper levels of the psyche and soma. Every realm of our existence is connected and represented here. The ancient priests of Africa, India, and later Europe, especially the Druids, skillfully took advantage of this interconnected process of imagery, symbol, affect, and power as they enfolded and reflected each other.

> This connecting function of the dream-formation is reinforced considerably by formation of symbols. When this function takes a hand and condenses masses of experiences, perhaps a whole period of the dreamer's life, into one single image, then all the material which is contained in this synthesis is reconnected with consciousness. Dream-formation thus causes not only a connection of single details, but also of whole "conglomerations" of past experience. But this is not all. Through the constancy and continuity existing in the process of dreaming, there is created a connection with this dream-continuity. Which fact greatly contributes to the preservation of the cohesion and unity of mental life as a whole. (Lowy, 1942)

Notice here how the image in the dream is a "conglomeration" of so many meaningful, powerful, and affectively charged situations in the dreamer's life. The symbol and image in the dream enfolds a great deal of meaning, and this meaning conversely enfolds psyche and soma.

Somatic stimuli are frequently encountered in dreams. This is nothing new. However, it is emphasized here that just as daily stimuli of various kinds, including somatic stimuli, enters into the dream world by way of unconscious channels and pathways, so it is possible for dream imagery to enter the somatic domain by these same pathways. It is only a small step after that to see how conscious or lucid dreaming, with all its access to powerful, idiosyncratic symbols and imagery, may be used to effect and influence the body. Many of the same principles of symbolic dream interpretation will be used to help the person decode or elicit the symbol/affect/somatic "language" of their own body-mind that is unique to them. Just as powerful dream interpretation has the capacity to unleash emotional healing and creative insight in a person's life, the correct "language" of the person's body-mind may allow a person to intelligently interact with their own immune system. This influence is only a matter of time, discipline, intentionality, and insight.

There are good and powerful reasons for this influence and process. Dreams are clearly an aspect of the unconscious mind, and the unconscious mind is present all the time. The waking conscious state, in a very real sense, is the fluctuating foreground of a much more vast and continually present background unconscious. Dreams come from an area that is prior to and enfolds the waking state. Dreams reflect and also have access to powerful affect and to primitive psychological process, and also occasionally reflect creative insight in science, art and life, in addition to transcendental awareness.

The dreamwork also has a great affinity to hypnotic and holographic processes. In all three cases of dreaming, hypnosis, and holographic processes, there is a *blurring* of boundary processes between significant images, situations, and/or persons. In all three cases the image and imagery is primary. In each situation, also, there is ample room for exceedingly powerful identification with strong affective energies and patterns.

When the holographic image is subjected to the correct translation (Fourier transform), it, like the powerful dream interpretation and the appropriate hypnotic image, is capable of releasing enormous healing energies for the individual and the body-mind system. This includes the immune system. When the dream process becomes conscious or lucid, the awareness is greatly expanded. Someday, using biofeedback procedures, the controlled and focused lucid dream stage and the appropriate interpretation of an individual body-mind's language and interactions with its own immune system, we will take a quantum leap in our organism's capacity to heal itself.

In summary then, symptom formation has been viewed as largely the transformation and distortion of energies, drives, and needs, the still-evolving subtle energies of the body-mind that are the trajectory of transcendence. Away from a basic equanimity arises fear, conflict and emotional contraction, a result largely of egoic and unconscious defensive maneuvers against the sense of potential dissolution of the transient ego. Family interactional patterns profoundly influence this process and, indeed, the shared meaning of many family patterns enfolds and informs specific symptom pictures. This dissolution is a misreading of the natural, unfolding process of evolution which consciously and teleologically seeks more receptive material and body-mind systems to more expansively manifest the vaster, intelligent light of evolution. Dreams can also help or hinder this process. *Symptoms are a form of reactive contraction to this unfolding force.* Illness is an alteration in consciousness gone awry from this unfolding, expanding and categorizing life-force as it moves to a higher balance.[2] Equanimity is the body-mind disposition that is expansive and receptive to this force. In addition to the somatic language of the body, there is an even more subtle language involving the finer pulsating energies of the body. How these are dealt with are again largely influenced by the family development in terms of images of health, vitality, or illness.

The emphasis in therapy is on taking charge of the symptom and moving in the direction of a healthy integration and balance of energies or elimination of it. This involves moving away from conflict with the symptom to, at times, paradoxical surrender to it. Surrender does not mean giving up. Rather, it is non-clinging, letting go, a form of forgiveness. By recognizing the symptom to be a modification and a translation of the body-mind, conflict decreases. This is technically achieved in various procedures, such as hypnosis, biofeedback, some limbs of Yoga and other principles of behav-

2. It is an archetype in all cultural myths of the hero that the hero or heroine must go through three distinct stages: the time of preparation which has order and balance; then the period of chaotic forces and potential disintegration; then the emergence into a higher order, understanding and commitment. This archetype too knows the soma.

ioral medicine. I have seen this principle used effectively in private practice and in the Behavioral Medicine Clinic. The subject is taught ease, relaxation, and calm of the body. Gradually he or she is taught to retranslate and redirect the emotional and cognitive characterological attitudes of the body and the way the body handles its energy relationships with itself and others. The conscious sense of energy balance and equanimity is cultivated. Insight almost always accompanies change. Here is an example:

> Ann X. was referred to the Biofeedback-Behavioral Medicine therapist by a physician internist for long-standing IBS or irritable bowel syndrome. Ann was a 24-year-old health professional herself who admitted to new job/professional stress, fears of being incompetent, and constant concerns about losing GI tract and anal sphincter control. This led to more muscle constriction of her GI tract, emergency operations to halt any "gas" escape, which only compounded the process. She watched and attempted to control the whole process with an obsessive zeal to her thinking, but felt trapped and sensed she could never relax.
>
> The clinician explained the anatomy, functions, and natural pulsations of the GI tract, the relationship between autonomic nervous system arousal and smooth muscles of the GI tract, and the need to "let go" repeatedly. Analogies and direct references to the breathing cycle were used.
>
> She was then taught diaphragmatic breathing, alternate nostril breathing, focus of attention at the top of the lip, bottom of the nose and then focused imagery exercises on the target area. The EMG electrodes placements provided direct feedback from the GI tract. She learned the intimate relationship between stress, breathing, and the autonomic nervous system. Surrendering attention into the target area on the extended exhalation phase of the breathing cycle was employed repeatedly. In this way, a sensation of bliss was awakened and directed selectively to regions of the body. Spontaneous trances would also occur. Eventually, in six weeks, her symptoms radically decreased. At this point she brought up related issues, including her family's style of obsessive worry, her fears

of loss of body control with all the social anxieties. Clinician and client also worked extensively on issues of dependency in relationships and some lingering separation problems with her family of origin. As these psychological issues were addressed, her symptoms fell to a low manageable level. She no longer avoided social situations, used obsessive thinking significantly less, and came to a different experience of body balance and control. She cultivated equanimity by way of the breath and the feeling-intuition of a state of balance not controlled rigidly by the ego. Pointing out that the body was always there even when the ego was not proved quite helpful and the clinician used it many times in numerous examples. The clinician also used humor and body imagery at great length. The counter-transference was positive and meshed well with her transference. Eventually, she translated her hourly clinical practice into daily life.

Notice how the insight came along with and after the initial change. Note the institutionalization of body-mind equanimity into daily life and the decrease of obsessive thoughts.

The profound influence of the mind on the body can be effected as said above by Yogas and various principles of behavioral medicine. In these procedures, the autonomic nervous system is almost always affected. The therapist teaches the individual or the system much more effective self-regulation, breath control, and helps a person to observe the body in a progressively more subtle way. The individual gradually begins to see and associate the various emotional situations with the way that he or she handles the body-mind. This is done repeatedly, with humor and compassion throughout treatment. The client is quietly helped to let go of the circus of frozen images and thoughts. Eventually the person's attention becomes subtle enough that they can see very quickly body tensions and contractions associated with various emotional situations. Remember that in Chapter 2, it was pointed out how the ego arises initially from states of bodily tension. It then develops a more systematized matrix of body tensions out of which it stabilizes and develops into a more tension-regulating system. Thus, at the very root of the ego is the awareness of the body's contractions that give rise to boundary formation. To let go, to in a sense forgive, is to lessen the sense of conventional boundaries and relations of all kinds!

It has been suggested that there is a life-current flowing through the body that can be known by direct observation. I have labeled this, along with others, the luminous current or the life-force. It is directly affected by the states of mind, body, and consciousness of the individual. Various pathological manifestations of this can be seen in Reich's (1971) character armor and Lowen's analysis of schizophrenic body types (1971; 1972). Behind each of these assumptions, however, is a direct perception of the life-force as a radiant intelligent current of energy.[3] Reflection upon that current of energy without presuppositions will show that that current of energy is arising in consciousness. The way the person deals with situations arising in consciousness is subtly changed by awareness and observation. Thus, the level of ego contraction and ego stress is brought under control. There are, of course, innumerable ways to see this in a very practical way.

THE FAMILY PSYCHE AND SOMA

The family's influence on health and illness is immense. Whether it be a physical illness or disease process, an emotional or behavioral problem, or that elusive somatizing or psychosomatic disorder, the reactivity of the family matrix is crucial to its outcome on many levels.

There has already been a focus of attention through this study on the recurrent transactional patterns that families establish over years as people live, work, love, and struggle together. The notion of identity itself first arises in this matrix or context. There is even a

---

3. The reader is directed to Chapters 5 and 6 of *The Family Unconscious* for a simple demonstration of the localization of this energy field. It involves the *practice* of balanced alternate nostril breathing and the application of Sushumna at the junction where the Ida and Pingala nadis or the tip end of the governor vessel meridian is situated (Motoyama, 1981). With an investment of perhaps 30 minutes daily for a month this life-current will be empirically and experientially obvious! This is also located specifically in a number of ancient meditational texts.

new and powerful body of research revealing the correlation and covariation of numerous psychophysiological reactions, mostly unconscious, that occur between persons in recurrent significant interpersonal relationships over time (Levenson and Gottman, 1985). These show the psychophysical, emotional, and necessarily mostly unconscious dance between intimates that occurs perpetually. A few clinicians have even noted with curiosity the similarity between hypnotic phenomena, subtle induction behavior, and symptom formation (Simon, 1985; Ritterman, 1983; Wickramasekera, 1986). Family members with a high profile in these areas are at a higher risk, it seems, for symptomatic behavior. Clinical research in the area of family health, illness, and life-span also reveals an inextricable interconnection between family attitudes and influences on physical, psychological somatizing illness processes (Turk and Kerns, 1985). Finally, Kellner (1963) and other family physicians have observed and documented clusters and associations of illnesses in family systems.

In the area of specific clinical theory and intervention a good opening has been forged in a number of areas. Lidz and Rubenstein (1959) long ago looked at the GI tract (gastrointestinal) disorders, specifically the dynamics of ulcerative colitis. Mara Selvini-Palazzoli (1970) has peered into the family dynamics implicated in anorexia nervosa. Minuchin et al. (1975; 1978) has really delved deeply into the family processes surrounding such diverse symptoms as diabetes, asthma, and anorexia nervosa. Many of his interventions are foundational today in clinical practice. Nothing has yet matched Meissner's (1966) early summary of family processes and psychosomatic reactivity which covered much ground, e.g., ulcers, colitis, arthritis, diabetes, even cancer and leukemia. However, it was largely speculative and needed the later specific clinical interventions of Minuchin and others. All these insights have arisen in the family therapy context. Here we are attempting to extend the dynamics of psychosomatic processes into the notion of "field" interactions. Despite the obvious advance in terms of boundary notions, hormonal influences, and symbol genesis, the "field" still is too often limited to the intrapsychic field of the individual. At this junction it would be helpful to take this all one step further toward a new direction and synthesis.

It seems relatively modest to suggest from all of the above that some systems-wide influence powerfully affects and sometimes informs illness dynamics in a family field or matrix. This overarching field or "wave-front" over the "discrete" individuals of the intimate group is termed the Family Unconscious. It is a matrix of shared imagery, ideation, and affect developed over time and enfolded in a holographic way into each individual member of the matrix. It is both a psychological and an energetic field capable of influence beyond the usual understanding of the constraints of space and time. Many other aspects of nature already manifest these dynamic operations.

We already know for instance that resonators operating in what is termed "phase coherence" are more difficult to break out of entrainment and, indeed, seek to maintain that entrainment over disruptive behavior. Family members certainly have a "resonate affinity" to each other that strangers and casual friends do not. Whenever there is an initial unity in a process and then a subsequent break-up into "separate pieces," these separate pieces will retain some degree of coherence or vibratory interaction with each other, even over great distances. These facets are born out in principle by the findings of Bell's theorem, by the logic embedded in the inherent indivisibility and interconnectedness of the quantum field, and by the dynamics of the implicate order where each aspect enfolds and reflects each other aspect. An intelligent "field" overarches the seemingly separate processes.

This has a direct clinical relevance to family illness processes. In the case of symptoms, somatic, psychosomatic, and emotional, which are transmitted and manifest from generation to generation, this overarching wave behavior just mentioned is seen. Bowen and others refer to this as the "multigenerational transmission of symptomatology." Here all the principles outlined are implicated. The multigenerational symptom acts much as an overarching wave or envelope over the individual or "discrete" behaviors of the individuals who maintain this resonate affinity with each other. The allusion to the Copenhagen interpretation of quantum mechanics is intentional but only heuristic. For in addition to a somewhat "external" overarching field, there also appears to be a more "internal" or implicate field that enfolds the apparently discrete individuals in the system.

There are many other models of processes in science that could be enlisted to make the point. Sheldrake's morphic resonance, where information about the form of events and species is communicated over spatial and temporal boundaries, is another example. It arises from biology and music. Biomagnetism and biomagnetic coupling is still another example. The point is that our psychic and somatic processes are also embedded in nature and reflect similar laws of operation. In each situation, what we might call deep family memories, ideas, and patterns, "family samscaras" if you will, are shared and *enfolded* by each member of the family system. Each member has a certain "evocative pull" on each other member.

In a very real sense, the family has and evolves a "body" of shared imagery, roles, affect, and ideation in a common matrix, almost a shared matrix or "homoculus of images" and feelings that influence behavior. This shared body of images, beliefs, dispositions and even mannerisms is unevenly developed over time and experience with some areas used more often in collective family development and thus reciprocally exercising more influence on individual behavior and perception. Where there is a constant, unbalanced excess or focus on a shared image and meaning in this system, a symptom arises. In the case of a specific individual psychosomatic illness, the symptom is really a contraction of the life-force around a shared dysfunctional family unconscious image.[4] A localization or materialization occurs through this focus and contraction that can affect the "denser" forms of energy we call matter. These symptoms will then tend to unfold out of the matrix at significant, symbolic, and often the same crucial periods in the life-cycle of the individuals in the family (see Chart 7.1).

An extreme and rare example of this may be the spontaneous psi energetic PK, or so-called poltergeist phenomena, observed in fami-

---

4. Think of the affectively charged image as a metaphor that is an ordering principle operating in the world much as the Cartian grid coordinates are seen as complex ordering principles embedded in nature. The metaphor, however, is closer to our everyday literal reality of images and details but is better described by the complex mathematics of fractals (B. B. Mandelbrot) than the linear functional systems of Newton and Descartes.

lies with a disturbed and angry adolescent. Objects symbolic to the family and its angry, repressed adolescent are inexplicably moved or broken (Rogo, 1986). A more common example, however, is the symptom that occurs to a family member at a certain age that also occurred to the parent at a similar age. Numerous times upon questioning a patient in a behavioral medicine intake session the clinician can notice the striking similarity of family symptoms at specific development periods in the family life-cycle.

Case 1

Edward X. is a 23-year-old second-year graduate student who was referred to the behavioral medicine clinic for recent "stress-related" problems. The patient was of average frame, intelligent, and had a moderate diet. His problems were seen to be "panic attacks," often occurring with sleep onset, mild insomnia, prolonged free-floating anxiety, a morbid preoccupation with having a heart attack and a sense of directionlessness in his academic career. He often felt helpless to influence events in his life. This information was elicited on intake.

Upon later probing in biofeedback sessions, it emerged that his father, a physician who he very much admired and identified with, also transiently felt "lost at sea" in his second year at medical school. The father reportedly also experienced "panic attacks" during this same year. Indeed, his father was the first to "diagnose" the problem. The sister of the patient is reported to have had GI tract problems recently in her professional career. The mother, interestingly enough, was described as "laid back" and relaxed.

The patient responded well to biofeedback/behavioral medicine intervention along with some psychotherapy.

Please note the following:

a. Similar family *era of differentiation* for patient and his father;
b. *Identification* of patient with father on several levels;
c. *Similarity of symptoms* between father and son:

   i. goallessness and helplessness
   ii. "panic attacks"

d. Labile ANS; shared family imagery of dis-ease process; *blurred boundary* of mutual identification as in both hypnotic phenomena and holographic imagery.

This process is usually an unconscious process. However, many clinicians have witnessed how a patient may consciously dread a certain upcoming date or year in his or her life because the individual remembers vividly how the same year in the life of a significant family member was catastrophic. The family member may have committed suicide, been psychiatrically hospitalized, or diagnosed with a painful and terminal disease. The person then selectively attends to the psychic, psychological, and somatic stimuli that is identified with the unfortunate relative. The patient may even reinforce this behavior and perception and also subtly manipulate those around him or her to acknowledge the symptom process. Again, this works unconsciously in the case of a parent who executes a projective identification with the offspring symptom barrier.

The "meaning" of the symptom is *implicit* and *unconscious* in the shared field which then informs the psyche and soma. Boundaries are blurred and it is literally somewhat hypnotic. The family member and the large Tavistock group member can both experience the subtle hypnotic induction of the group mind or process. Many a family therapist will testify to the hypnotic way a family can sometimes "take in" the therapist such that the family's fears, defenses, and dynamics are keenly felt by the therapist by way of the therapist's countertransference reaction. This includes the induction of somatic symptoms!

The soma, or body, bears a certain meaning or significance to the person and family, and the meaning of this process is enfolded and implicitly shared by all members through mutual enfoldment (see Chart 7.1). In each case, the boundary between mind and body, and between members of the system, are blurred at a certain level. It is meaning that integrates psyche, soma, and extended environment.

The notion that information and meaning are contained in the "field" around and through an "object" is not new. Bohm (1987) has pointed out that Bohr, himself, and others in quantum mechanics have demonstrated that the quantum field around an object was both indivisible from the object and contained information about

CHART 7.1. Family Unconscious "Field" (Holographic).

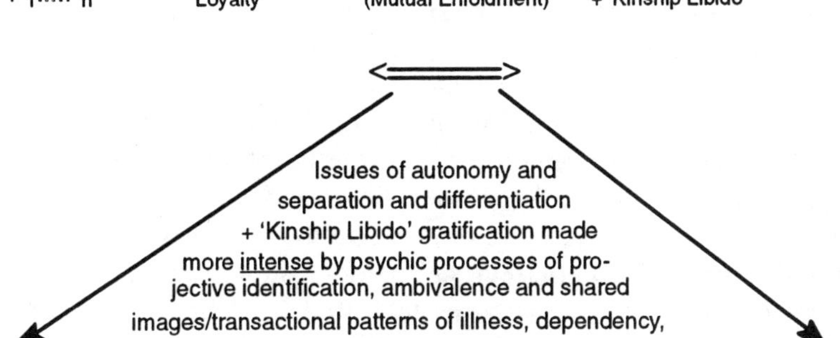

Psychological Identification
(Conscious and Unconscious)

I. Personality and Ego style

II. Anxiety Management
(Psychological boundaries)

III. Resistance Styles

IV. Perceptions of body and values of bodily functions

V. Epigenetic Life stage when symptoms occur.

a) Times to be as others were at this time in life (e.g. 2nd year in college, birth of 1st child, etc.)

b) New family crisis and emergent needed new structures to cope

c) Losses, fears, guilt and conflicts.

Somatic Identification
(Unconscious & Autonomic Nervous System

I. Anxiety of psyche ⟹ Anxiety in body. (Dissociation; conversion; Labile ANS)

II. Behavior and habits ⟹ symptom expression in body, then reinforced by family system.

III. Perceptions of Reality

Values, Attitudes, Disposition } Bodily fluids and functions

Catastrophyzing images and memories. Fatalism/Suffering

IV. Epigenetic Life State when symptoms occur.

a) Psychosomatic Symptom unfolds in similar or identical organ system in body.

b) Alcoholism, suicide

the object. Again Bell's theorem, indicates a non-local "field" "reconnecting" objects that have an affinity to each other. The information and meaning of a field are shared by all regions of the field. This, of course, requires a blurring of the notion of discrete energetic boundaries at a certain point between relations in that field. This is where the influence of hypnosis and hypnotic phenomena, with its *blurred boundaries,* and the holographic image, with its *blurred boundaries,* have their impact on the process. The boundary and wave-fronts are blurred, but the affect is not blunted! We will return to strong affect and emotion in a moment when we discuss the intense ambivalence suggested by Murray Bowen. In each case, however, the information and meaning are enfolded in every region of the shared field.

What does this look like, then, in family symptom formation? It appears that the meaning of the symptom, whatever it is in reference to the family system and its members, *enfolds* both the discrete "objects" or individuals of the family system and its members, i.e., it *enfolds* both the discrete "objects" or individuals of the system and the energetic aspects of their relationship. Given the blurred hypnotic boundary process between significant others, the affinity to blurred holographic imagery and wave-front phenomena, and the mutually shared identification processes, each of which is enfolded in each region of the shared matrix, it becomes necessary to see both matter-energy and consciousness potentially exhibit trans-temporal and trans-spatial phenomena. Indeed not only *what* is the matter with me, but also *who* is the matter with me!

Said another way, shared imagery implies or implicates and enfolds shared meaning. It is meaning that structures both matter and mind. In the family unconscious shared field of affect, memory and imagery, the shared nuances and meanings of the field give rise to the processes and relations of both psyche and soma. The different, complementary and differentiating roles in the family matrix in time and over development are rich with shared meaning, dependency, need, and behavior. Sometimes we act in the roles we play and sometimes the roles act in us.

It could be argued that the above accounts for the process and structural dynamics of somatic symptom expression in families, but what about affect or strong emotions? Well, Murray Bowen (1960) has drawn attention to how "intense" relationships in the family, especially *ambivalently* intense relationships, are relationships "in which the thoughts of both, whether positive or negative, are largely invested in each other." He points out clinically how often in the family matrix the specific worries, anxieties, etc., of the mothering one eventually manifest in the symptoms of the identified patient. These symptoms are even often those the mothering one fought against. This *externalization* of the mothering one's own fears, anxieties, and inadequacies becomes enfolded in the inner landscape of the identified patient.

> Thus, a situation that begins as a feeling in the mother, becomes a reality in the child . . . The "projection" occurs also on the level of physical illness. This is a mechanism in which the soma of one person reciprocates with the psyche of another person. (Bowen, 1960)

Notice how this process of projection, ambivalence, and identification are unfolded in a family crisis situation (Case 2) and in a non-crisis family matrix (Case 3).

Case 2

> Ann X. was a 38-year-old mother of four daughters who presented to a Behavioral Medicine clinician for polysymptomatic problems. She was constantly anxious, experienced the "shakes," diarrhea and irritable bowel syndrome, and also mild tight chest pain and tachycardia. There were numerous family therapy issues of anger and control, especially the impulse/behavior control of her four daughters. Both family therapy and behavioral medicine intervention were used in the reduction of stress and anxiety. The interesting fact, however, is that the adolescent daughter that she and her second husband had the most difficulty with was also the only one with symptoms like her mother! This 16-year-old identified patient (by the family and herself), also had GI tract problems, and occasionally, the shakes. These two had been very close until the daughter's adolescence. Fortunately, therapy was successful with this family.

Case 3

> Debbie and Eddie X. were both seen by a Behavioral Medicine clinician for different stress/anxiety problems. Debbie experienced anxiety attacks and irritable bowel symptoms. The EMG, psychotherapy, and other procedures were used successfully with her, though she did experience a brief relapse at the end of treatment. She then quickly recovered when she practiced the procedures at home again. Her older brother Eddie appeared to the clinic with stress headaches, excessive anxiety levels, and neck pain. He too responded well and demonstrated considerable insight between his symptoms and interpersonal relations. Both described a family matrix of conflict over certain issues, and common images of family and parental power interactions. Both tended to be somewhat obsessive in their psychological field. Family therapy was not done directly.

With the individuals in these cases, one sees how anxiety is experienced as a threat to the system and must be managed. The individuals may seek to decrease anxiety by *identification* with how other family members have managed their own anxiety. The process is "taken in" so to speak, like a propagating wave and hopefully dissipated in some region of enfolded inner space. The anxiety or symptom can also be repressed and *projected* away from the system towards another. Optimally, the anxiety is integrated by insight and bodily-somatic acceptance and release.

In the above cases of somatic symptoms in a family context, the influence of the Family Unconscious dynamic field is operative. Peper (1985) has used the family system to treat asthma rather successfully, drawing on the subtle underlying matrix of family consciousness to work with biofeedback procedures. Minuchin, as mentioned earlier, did some pioneering work with families and psychosomatic problems, and ever since his work in *The Family Kaleidoscope* (1984) has come to see the "common image" in families more and more. Also, recently, Barber and Wilson (1985) have found a large number of correlations between imagery, psi, psychosomatic symptoms and family dynamics in their exhaustive study of the fantasy-prone personality. These are all the different influences that boundary flexibility and family processes have on symptom formation.

So, really, what can be summarized about the implicate and interconnected dynamics of family-influenced psychosomatic processes? First of all, a symptom in the body-mind field has a meaning to both the psyche and the soma. Indeed, like certain other "fields" in natural science, the meaning and information of the field cannot really be separated from the "object" in the field. In this case, the meaning of a symptom enfolds both matter and psyche as they interact with and infuse each other in the overarching Family Unconscious field. The overarching field acts as an envelope or wave-front over the separate individuals of the shared field.

Second, there is abundant research in psychophysiology to suggest that people or psyches influence each other in recurrent ways that are measurable by way of psychophysiological monitoring devices, e.g., galuanic skin response or GSR, electromyogram or EMG, thermoregulation measures or TR, and perhaps, electroencelographic brain wave monitoring or EEG. Interpersonal behavior can elicit a certain signature pattern on biophysical reactivity on the part of the organism.

Third, it would appear that through selective use by members of the system over time, mutual experiencing and the above recurrent transactional patterns that simultaneously manifest biophysical patterns, certain images and patterns are amplified and identified with by members of the system. This occurs down even to the level of similarity of symptoms, organ systems, and periods of occurrence in the life cycle. This body of shared images, associations, dispositions and meanings is almost like a shared homoculus, differentially reflecting the idiosyncratic patterns of the specific family matrix. These patterns are mutually enfolded into each member of the system by certain shared meanings. These shared meanings enfold both psyche and soma.

Fourth, one must consider how hypnotic processes and hypnotic inductions require a psyche responsive to the capacity to *blur boundary* notions yet retain *affective intensity.* Powerful empathic identification with another or intense ambivalence provide the energy for this process. Here the blurred boundary processes of hypnotic responsivity and the blurred boundary processes of holographic wave-front interactions can be seen to have a striking affinity to the psychic process. A labile ANS provides a certain openness for the system in this regard. It keeps certain processes vague or blurred and allows room for a great deal of reactivity. What is necessary at this juncture is to realize that these labile wave-fronts of all kinds have the capacity to go both trans-temporal and trans-spatial under certain conditions.

Finally, when these processes are active in the life course of an individual and family as they literally move through life, psychosomatic reactivity is initiated and unfolds at crucial stages and by definitive events that have a shared meaning for people. The case of the physician father and graduate school son in their second year, confronted by goallessness, panic attacks, and helplessness is an example. The situation of the once very close mother and daughter, who both later develop nearly identical symptoms in a matrix suffused with intense ambivalence, projective identifications, and shared body-illness imagery, is another example. The individual ego contracts the life-force around a specific, shared dysfunctional Family Unconscious image. In each case the enfolding meaning of the symptom is psychically operationalized by the processes of projective identification and loyalty motivations (see Chart 7.1). Loyalty is another fact of deep and mutual identification. Indeed, in so many cases having a symptom similar to that of someone loved or felt about intensely ambivalently is a form of loyalty to that person or system. "Oh yes, many people in our family get. . . ."

But we may well ask if the enfolding meaning of something can effect both psyche and soma in the family and individual by way of a labile ANS, hypnotic and holographic processes, and the ego's own clinging at crucial times in the life-cycle, then it must be possible to observe this process as it unfolds in our own individual system. There must be some way to look into our own depths and see the process emerging from the realm of vast unconscious processes. If so, then where and how would we look?

A WORKING MODEL THAT WORKS

In order to seriously look at the operation we have been outlining, it will be necessary to become a little more technical than usual.

If you are not that interested in this brief section, then by all means skip it and the next four sections and go to the final section. However, since much is suggested by modern research on the actual process of healing and its relationship to energy, attention, bio-energy and imagery, this short section may throw some light on what seems to actually occur. We will move level by level into the recesses of the brain.

First of all take a look at an outline of the human nervous system on Chart 7.2. While this is generally accepted medically and neurologically, there is a great deal about the brain and nervous system that is either still unknown or at least controversial.

Notice that the brain and spinal column/cord are not separated and that, indeed, the spinal cord is itself brain matter! All the nerves of the body are rooted here, e.g., cranial (12), cervical (7), dorsal (12) etc. (Netter, 1972; Gatz, 1973). The pulse and "flow" of evolution is upward along this column and cord, as previously indicated by the triune brain neuroanatomy/physiology research of J. D. MacLean. In fact, the deeper roots of attention begin way back in the basal ganglia and limbic formation of the forebrain (Pribram and MacLean, 1953) and only later do the frontal and parietal areas influence any control on this force of attention (Pribram and McGuinness, 1975). Your attention is drawn toward the gray matter in both brain and spinal cord which is suffused with the *light sensitive* melanin and neuromelanin mentioned in earlier chapters. Carbon is the basis of the life-cycle on our planet. It would appear that there is a subtle life and neuromelanin-associated light-current here along the spine that domes and innumerably interconnects in the vast neuro-cellular ocean of the brain. Who knows what the effect of this light/energy sensitive melanin process is when it reaches all the wave-form potentials of the awakened brain!

While the functions of the left hemisphere are better known to us, and in our technologically intoxicated culture are more highly valued than those of the right hemisphere, it is also clear that the right hemisphere is rich and multi-faceted. The right-hemisphere, in general, is more highly associated with imagery, novelty, or creativity and emotionality. It also has many neural connections to the limbic system, the fountainhead of our affect and perhaps our collective imagery.

CHART 7.2

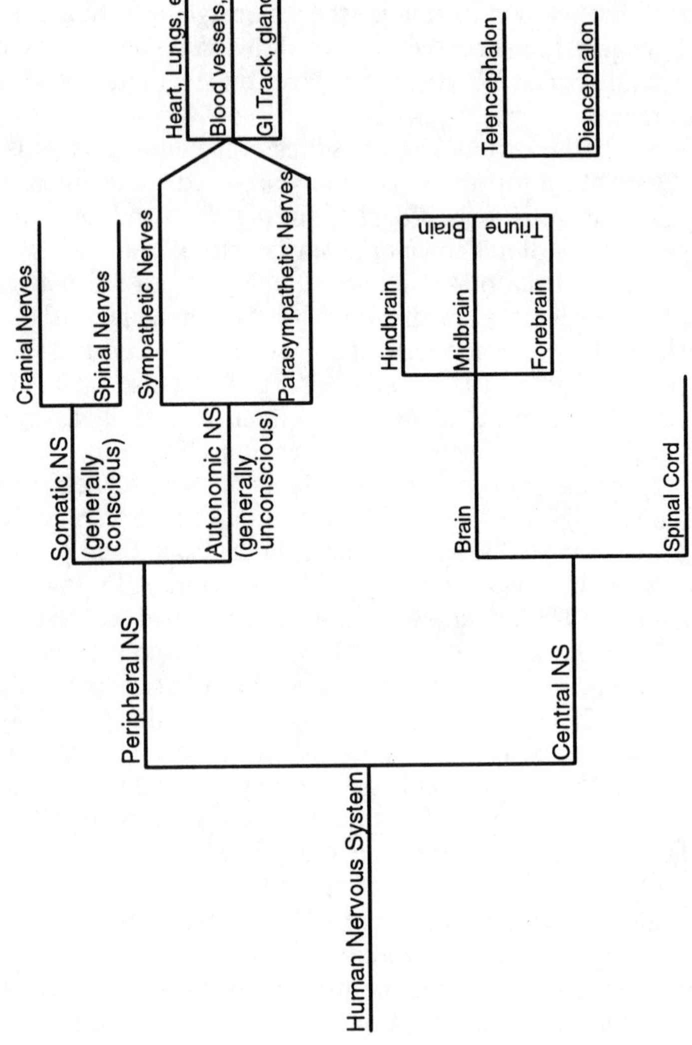
Human Nervous System
Peripheral NS
Central NS
Somatic NS
(generally
conscious)
Autonomic NS
(generally
unconscious)
Cranial Nerves
Spinal Nerves
Sympathetic Nerves
Parasympathetic Nerves
Heart, Lungs, etc.
Blood vessels, etc.
GI Track, glands
Brain
Spinal Cord
Hindbrain
Midbrain
Forebrain
Triune
Brain
Telencephalon
Diencephalon

In primates it is the cortex of the brain that is most developed. In the higher primates and man it is the neocortex that reaches the crown of development. Yet, despite all this, there is a vibrant universe of the brain that we still know embarrassingly little about. We usually think of many parts of the cortex as composed of different receiving areas (sensory cortex) which operate to transmit information or receptor events to the adjacent areas of "association" in the cortex. In these areas of association in the cortex, the various neural events are expanded, elaborated, and "associated" with many other neural events and wave-fronts before they are then "transmitted" to the motor areas of the cortex. These motor areas have been thought to function as the primary effector mechanisms of all cerebral activity. For nearly a century this view with increasing refinements has been the central theory of the brain's function. This neuroanatomical model, regardless of how widely accepted, is still inadequate to explain some of the following mysteries:

1. Memory does not appear to be located in any one place as you might expect, but instead seems to be organized in several locations that overlap and interconnect with each other. Thus the loss of a memory is more accounted for by the size loss of brain material rather than specific brain area.
2. Because of this, and other factors, a specific capacity that may have been damaged or lost through misfortune, etc., can sometimes be recovered. This is apparently not due to neural regeneration, but to some other non-local field effect.
3. In terms of information storage, the generally accepted neuroanatomical model of the brain would require each bit of information to be processed by 3×10^{10} nerve impulses per record (van Heerden, 1968). This is way beyond any neural capacity we can handle.
4. In the area of psi or paranormal processes, which appear to require non-local processes of information "transfer," the present model is woefully inadequate in energetic terms.

The list could go on and on. Yet these do appear to be some of the processes that can potentially be accounted for by an expanded model of brain and neocortex functioning if we are willing to entertain the possibility. To make this possibility more *clinically rele-*

vant, we need to embed it in the actual situation a clinician faces. For that reason, the clinical hour of biofeedback opens the next area of this section. After this, we will return for a deeper look at this newer view of the brain–neocortex and its operation embedded in treatment.

The Clinical Hour

In actual treatment, the client is first assessed for other psychological and medical complications. Styles of resistance are taken into account and a vocabulary that the client will "hear" is used to present the treatment plan. The therapist must make a professional and intuitive "connection" with the client in order for the full benefit of treatment to occur. All the skills of a well-trained psychotherapist including an awareness of transference and counter-transference dynamics are enlisted in order to engage the usual dynamic processes of therapy.

When this has been done, and a formal treatment plan outlined, the next stage of intervention begins. The client learns to *relax the body and focus the mind and attention on the target area.* The person then slowly *breathes diaphragmatically,* which increases relaxation more. It also moves the lungs rhythmically and begins to affect the autonomic nervous system by way of the tenth cranial nerve, the vagus, or so called wandering nerve. At certain points the *exhalation* phase of the breathing cycle is amplified and the clinician may choose to coordinate his or her breathing with the client's. All sorts of images, mostly personal and familial, arise. If you have seen or experienced the behavioral treatment of systematic desensitization, you know that the client does not merely relax in the face of formerly anxiety-inducing stimuli. They actively re-learn images, responses, and associations to these stimuli in addition to psychophysical relaxation. Excessive electrical activities of the cerebral cortex are decreased. Classical psychodynamic processes are readily observed here, from primary process to secondary elaboration with the somatic expressions of this available for interpretation and reflection. All the defenses become obvious. Some of this occurs in the initial stages of biofeedback and clinical hypnosis. The conscious and unconscious mind is accessed in this method.

I and others have the distinct impression that these ceaseless modifications of images, ego tensions and feelings, those perpetual subtle, somatic, and largely unconscious oscillations become, and are intimately involved in, these psychosomatic transformations. A certain vibratory operation appears to occur. These oscillations, or subtle vibratory effects, are quietly but intensely fused and correlated with the image of that somatic area in the mind of the client. The autonomic nervous system, by way of the breath, and specific focused mental/imagery attention are synchronized in a way not totally understood by contemporary science. Heat is almost always produced.

Clinicians have known for some time that external stimuli deeply influence internal bodily and somatic processes. We each know from direct experience that strong sexual or aversive imagery itself can stimulate powerful psychophysiological processes. Even the *intentionality* and *potential action* of some event can increase muscle tension, as measured by biofeedback EMG, GSR or thermoregulation monitors. Beyond that, Barber (1978) has shown how intense images can lead to measurable changes in blood glucose levels, GI tract activity, and even skin blister formation. Finally, even into the immune system, which we will look at later, the effect of powerful imagery can be seen. Hall (1982-83) and others have shown that imagery can and does have a powerful influence on immune system reactivity, especially on white blood cell functions. Thus, the careful and systematic use of intense, focused imagery, bodily-somatic processes, and respiration or bio-energy management can lead to therapeutic results. This is largely because imagery, more connected to the right hemisphere than the left, can be trained and intensified by attention and appropriate harnessing of the autonomic nervous system. The right hemisphere, while generally not a locus of speech functions and the more logical forms of mental organization associated with speech, is nonetheless more *directly implicated* in perceptual processes and proprioceptive feedback with the sensory body itself on many levels and the external environment. An image can and does deeply interact with the soma.

The holographic or holonomic analogy is quite useful here. The image of the soma or body is reflected in the mind. Along with this holographic analogy is focused attention controlled by the breath.

The new behavior or image is the one gently created by the mind directed to a clinical goal. There is no reason to draw the line at the somatic level; the biochemical and immune system may also be implicated. This is partially where psychoimmunology is taking us.

A Deeper Look: The Sensory Motor Cortex

Let us return now to a closer look into the levels and operations of the brain from surface "lens" to the deeper "projection" areas as they relate to our feelings and images of the body.

It is a curious fact that the whole of the human sensory and motor organization is precisely mapped and projected out along the cortex that forms the banks of a fold called the central sulcus. This fold, located about mid-way across the hemispheres, is neuronally connected and "associated" with many other areas of the brain, especially its adjacent areas, the postcentral area, and the posterior part of the frontal gyrus or fold. Both are profoundly implicated in the operation of the human action or motor systems. The precentral cortex or motor area includes both the precentral gyrus and the posterior part of the frontal gyrus. See Figures 7.1, 7.2, and 7.3.

Electrical stimulation of this area causes contraction of the voluntary muscles of the body. Also, if cells are removed from this motor area, paralysis occurs in the voluntary muscles, especially on the opposite side of the body. In the frontal area, which is the site of the drastic lobotomy operation, stimulation leads to autonomic nervous system effects on circulation, respiration, papillary reaction and many other areas of visceral involvement.

The postcentral area, right behind the precentral gyrus, is the sensory or conscious somesthetic area. It receives both exteroceptive and proprioceptive afferent fibers from the spinal cord and the brain stem relayed through the thalamus (see Figures 7.4 and 7.5). Here, also, the different areas of the body are projected and represented in a detailed sequence, like they are on the surface or "lens" of the precentral gyrus.

Electrophysiological experiments show that these somatic afferents are extended on both sides of the central fissure in all primates. The afferents reaching the precentral motor areas and the postneutral sensory areas originate in both the surface of the skin and in muscle nerves (Malis, Pribram, and Kruger, 1953). Yet it is not

FIGURE 7.1. Lateral surface of left cerebral hemisphere, viewed from the side.

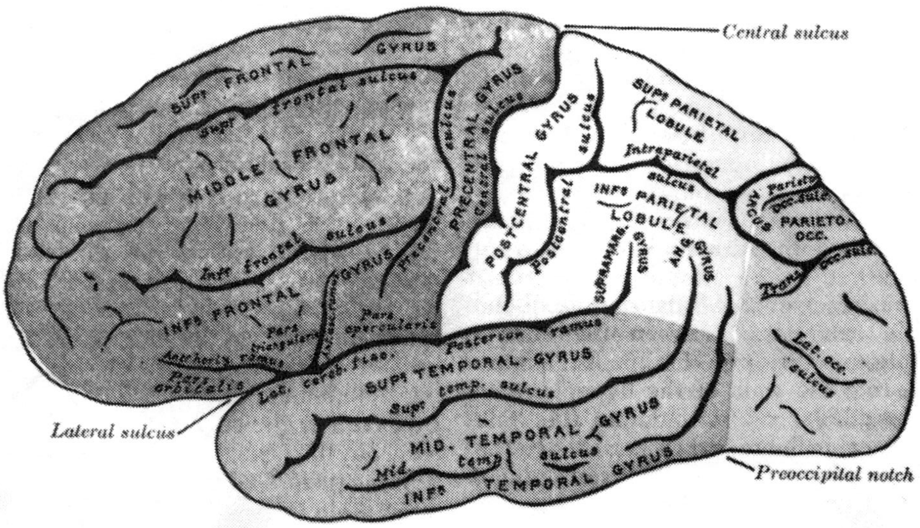

FIGURE 7.2. Cross-section of the brain revealing the motor cortex and indicating the areas of the body as mapped along the precentral gyrus. This is the motor homunculus–the symbolic man lying within the brain mattter.

1. Toes
2. Ankle
3. Knee
4. Hip
5. Trunk
6. Shoulder
7. Elbow
8. Wrist
9. Hand
10. Little finger
11. Ring finger
12. Middle finger
13. Index finger
14. Thumb
15. Neck
16. Brow
17. Eyelid and eyeball
18. Face
19. Lips
20. Jaw
21. Tongue
22. Swallowing

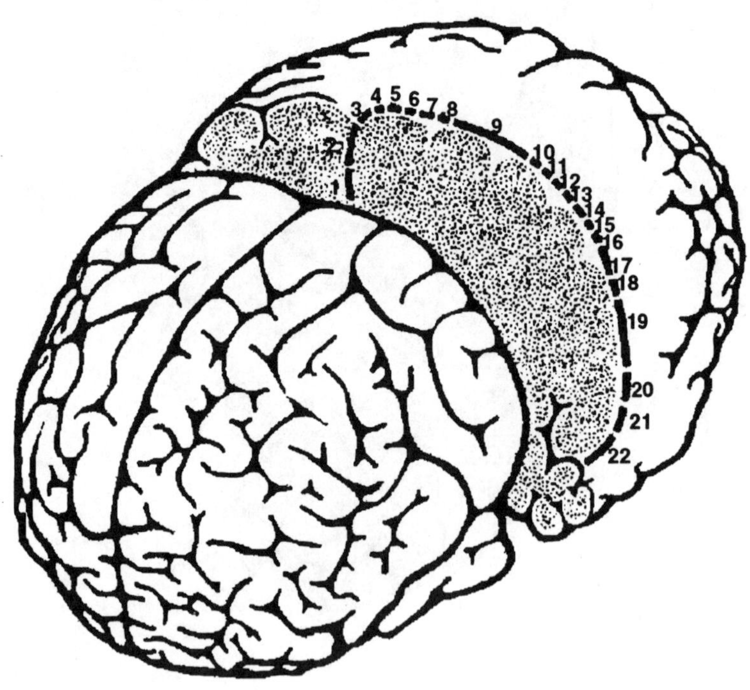

FIGURE 7.3. Somatic sensation. Cross-section of the left hemisphere along the plane of the postcentral gyrus. The afferent pathway for discriminative somatic sensation is indicated by the unbroken lines coming up, through the medial lemniscus, to the postcentral gyrus.

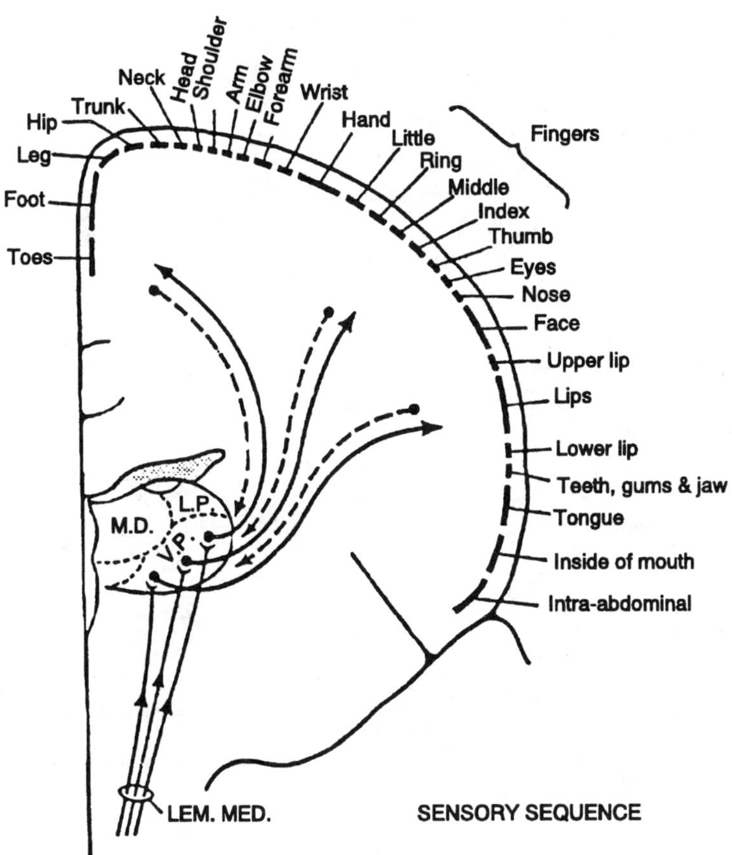

simply a matter of afferents reaching postcentral and efferents leaving the precentral cortex, etc. There is a great deal of overlap of input-output information, of these afferent and efferent "lines." This is not confined to the somatic areas where the sensations of the body configuration are projected. The other senses of vision, gesta-

FIGURE 7.4. Cerebellar circuits. The spinocerebellar and cortico-ponto-cerebellar pathways to the cerebellum are represented by thin fibers. Thicker fibers show efferent paths from the denate nucleus to the spinal cord and to the precentral gyrus. The pyramidal tract is shown as a dotted line.

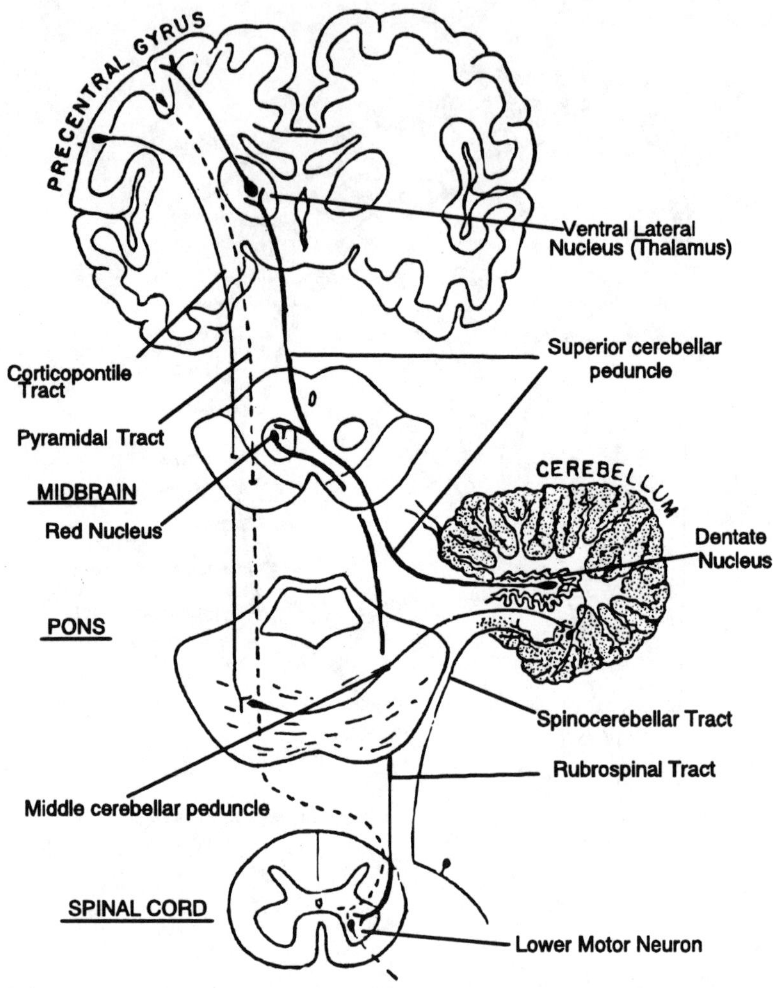

FIGURE 7.5. Proprioception-Stereognosis.

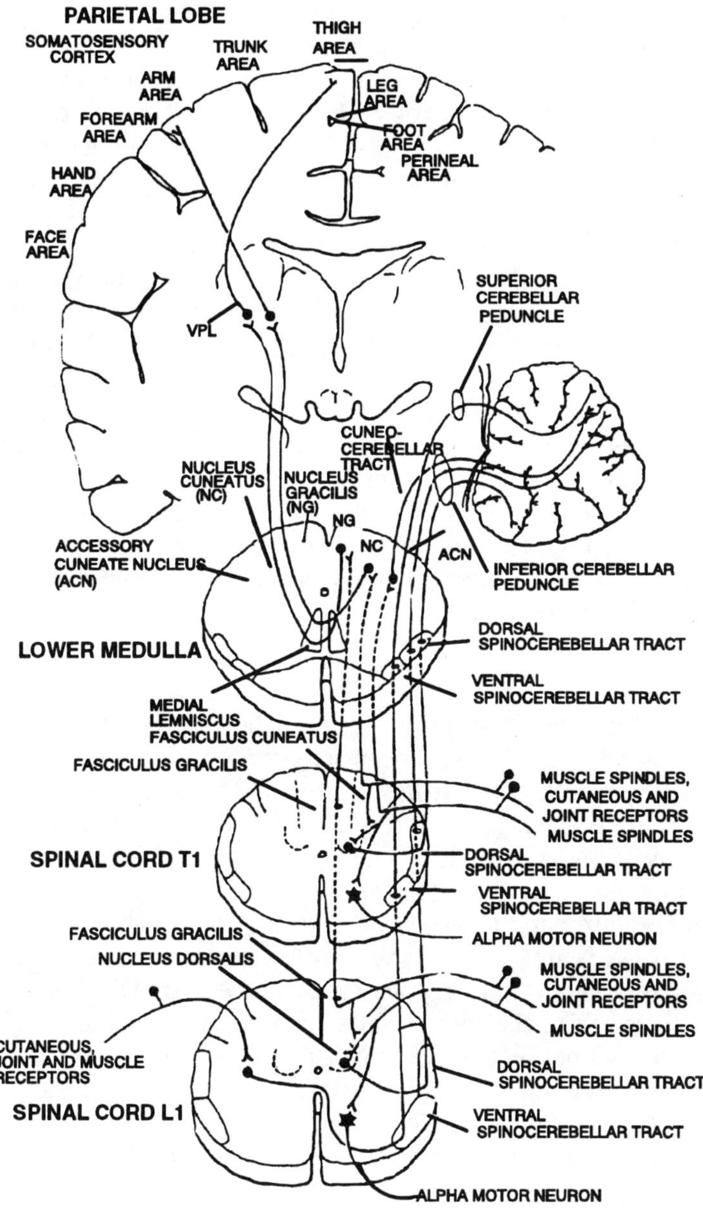

tion, and other functions seem to reflect an overlap of afferents and efferents.

Thus, the whole body, especially the areas under voluntary control, are located along a certain somatopsychic route that is enervated by both the autonomic and the central nervous system. The areas that are the most developed in terms of their representative size in brain tissue, e.g., hands, fingers, lips, nose and internal throat/tongue area correspond to those areas the ancient one and her progeny have developed beyond the other animals in the coursework of evolution. See Figures 7.6 and 7.7.

Therein we see that along this surface or lens, especially of the precentral gyrus, a representation of the human body amenable to conscious interaction is found. A motor homunculus or "little man" is embedded and projected in a neuronal map or hologram of the physical body. It exists primarily as a neuronal abstraction of the physical body that operates in the realm of the neurotransmission and flow of electrical and bioenergy throughout the central and autonomic nervous system. It interfaces with all other energy systems of the body, creating numerous *interference patterns* that communicate with each other. It has great affinity to the holographic process.

Coda

The actual fine detailing of behavior falls to the cerebral motor cortex. It is located in the precentral gyrus of the hemisphere right behind the frontal lobe. It has important connections to the basal ganglia and the cerebellum. The receptive fields of nearby cortical units covers a wide sample of muscles (Phillips, 1965) but are not as once thought to have a point-to-point correspondence like a keyboard (Woolsey and Chang, 1948). Rather, a projective and implicate process is involved. Many muscles are coordinated in a very subtle, smooth fashion if you stimulate the area with electrodes. Thus, it is really the more subtle movement or action itself, not gross muscles per se, that are represented in this most sensitive area. The role of directing action itself, and thus achievement and higher order *intentionality*, is implicated here.

The real data or stimulation from the external environment to this sensory motor cortex comes by way of the dorsal thalamus, *not* by the sensory areas adjacent to it, such as the somatosensory cortex. The thalamus is a relay station for incoming information from the body.

The original input from the external environment issues not only from those nerve fibers that innervate the muscles of action, but also from those that connect with the skin. This is one reason why biofeedback can be so effective and why imagery can effect a subtle change in the system. Taub (1977) has demonstrated the surprising

FIGURE 7.6. Sensory homunculus showing representation in the sensory cortex (after Penfield and Rasmussen, *Cerebral Cortex of Man*, The Macmillan Co.).

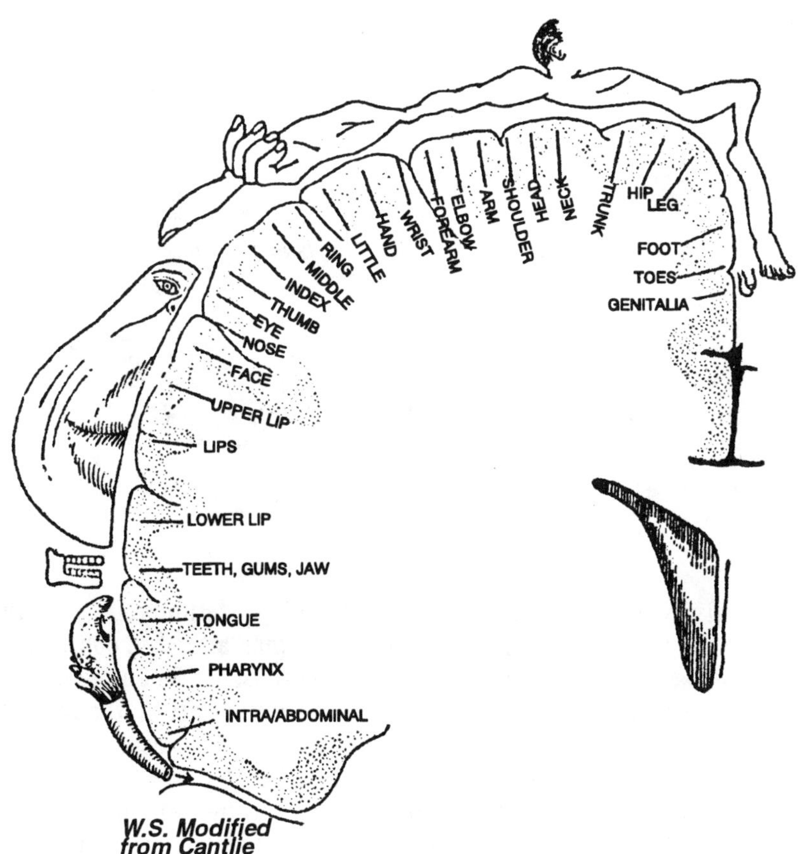

FIGURE 7.7. Motor homunculus illustrating motor representation in area 4 (anterior central gyrus). (After Penfield and Rasmussen *Cerebral Cortex of Man*, The Macmillan Co.).

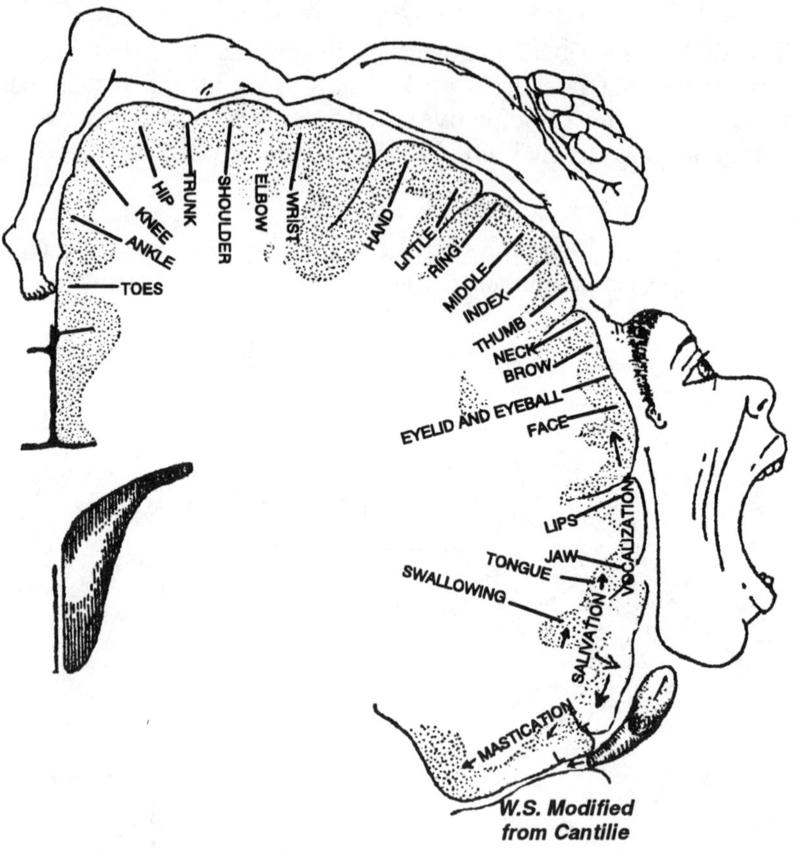

responsivity of skin tissue sensitivity to such procedures. Basmajian (1979) has repeatedly demonstrated that human attention can selectively isolate and fire single motor units of muscle. When the directive is given to "quiet" the system, it usually issues from the frontal and prefrontal lobes of the brain. The frontal lobes, especially the medial and basal portions, are connected by well-developed bundles of ascending and descending fibers to the reticular formation at the base of the triune brain mentioned in Chapter 1 in connection to the superimposition of the limbic system by the later cortex and neocortex of evolutionary development from reptile to mammal to man. These regions of the neocortex receive extremely strong impulses from the lower reticular system, but can also consciously influence this system! This is one of the pathways the Yogin and the healing process use, and why an image, in deep relaxation and a focused autonomic nervous system, can be so powerful. There are many other clinical examples.

Movement or action and effect therefore occur by way of their transformation into an imaging process in the motor cortex which contains input and output for achievement of actions. Neuromelanin configurations have also been found to be parallel, at times, to the motor area of the cortex. Bernstein (1967) in the former U.S.S.R. and Pribram (1977) in the U.S.A. show that such movements generate a temporal holographic process in the brain as representations of the properties of perception and the environment. These are encoded in the brain.

Experiments also show that neurons respond to the *intentionality* of the agent (Evarts, 1967) and not solely to the *force* needed to move the muscle or organ system. These occur actually before the movement itself! Therein, again, an image and intentionality is created and present which guides the actions of the body-mind through various sequences. In a very real sense, Pribram and others suggest that this motor cortex is a "sensory cortex for action." The localized action of muscles and organ systems is directed by a more non-local field of enfolded, higher order action/intentionality or intelligence. In other words, a sort of top down model of cognitive influence at times.

All of this is not to say that the *exact* physiological determinants of motor behavior are specifically localized in the precentral gyrus. No. Each area of the total brain has some influence, some contribution to make. Rather, it is stressed that the specific motor and sensory area of the body-mind is more easily and directly influenced by these areas outlined here when imagery and technique are skillfully applied.

When the clinical intervention is executed, there is some sensory withdrawal with the technique of focusing sequentially on the precentral gyrus map or body outline. The body-mind is slightly defocused. It has a certain affinity to the Yogic sensory withdrawal procedure called pratahyara. As in a classical hologram, the new target image can be unfolded from the defocused and higher enfolded order. The *new image* and *meaning* must be symbolically and somatically egosyntonic indigenous to the person, otherwise it will not be effective. Just as the correct code or interpretation will unlock the real meaning and affect of a dream to the dreamer, so will the correct and incisive imagery of the body-mind release the idiosyncratic and appropriate powerful forces of the body. This appears to be one way in which the healing capacity of the system is enhanced.

Integrating what we said earlier in terms of just the behavioral phenomenology or mechanics of treatment, and the inference we can take from these holonomonic processes, the following scenario arises: The patient begins to relax after a treatment plan has been devised and agreed upon. The appropriate imagery drawn from their specific life context is employed that *both* induces relaxation and corresponds to the specific location of symptomatology. By focusing attention through the "lens" of the somatopsychic area of the precentral gyrus and related areas in the brain, the target area and system is activated. The breathing process, which can be both voluntary or involuntary, is engaged along with the continued focus or "laser" of attention. The new image of healing, in a top down cognitive fashion, is gradually unfolded and brought to bear on the symptom. Breathing diaphragmatically both stimulates the lungs and thus the vagus nerve and therein the autonomic nervous system (Rama et al., 1979). The associated areas of the precentral gyrus, and therein the central nervous system, are also stimulated and given a new image and vibrational matrix to engage. The healing process thus occurs. The subtle, and also the somatic, energies of the body are also enlisted since not only the conscious, but also the vast resources of the unconscious, mind are opened.

ANCIENT HORIZONS: THE FUTURE OF HEALING

A working model of the brain and its sensorimotor functioning has been presented in some detail as it appears to apply to the process of imagery, biofeedback, and behavioral medicine. The model was embedded in the actual treatment situation such that it does not appear to have been abstracted from working reality and thereby, hopefully, avoids too large a disparity between theory and technical description. In particular, a holographic and holonomic perspective was advanced, which is believed to account for more anomalous information that arises in both research and clinical practice.

This holonomic paradigm has implicated in it the notion of the brain, body, mind, and consciousness as a vibrating, information- and light-processing organism. This vibratory, frequency model, in which the image and intelligence are interconnected on innumerable levels has the capacity to coordinate and direct energy by way of pattern recognition, oscillation, and holonomy. On a more subtle level in the body-mind, how might this look? How would mind, attention, and biochemistry be involved in the most subtle form of self-healing, the immune system process?

Psychoimmunology is the study of the mind and brain's influence on hormonal and immune system functions. In recent years psychoimmunology has revealed the vast and subtle influence of mind-body interactions on disease and health. Ader (1981), then Locke and Hornig-Rohan (1983) have compiled and presented in some detail the interaction of mind, environment, and immune system. At present there seems to be a general agreement that the immune system is an interactive, self-regulating network of cells that respond differentially to "perceived" dangers to the organism (Cunningham, 1978; 1981). This form of specific response capacity to a specific "invader" implies both creativity and pattern recognition. It may also have the capacity to interact with consciousness. Some emotional patterns that increase stress will decrease immune system capacity and conversely, some psychoemotional patterns may amplify immune system powers (Stone, 1987). The initial pathway of this influence is generally agreed upon (Jerne, 1973). What is not so clear is the exact function of the now proliferating body of new cells of the immune system that are being recognized as research unfolds. Specifically, we know the origin and function of white blood cells, but as we "see" more, it becomes more complex. After the discovery of the initial lymphocyte "T" cell, which is derived from the thymus and is the basis for cell-mediated immunity, later researchers discovered many different varieties of T-cell: T-helper, T-suppressor, T-killer, etc. The presently called "B" cell is a lymphocyte involved in defending the body against bacteria and other toxic substances. Unlike the "T" cell, which is the basis for cell-mediated immunity, the "B" cell is an agent of humoral immunity. Both B and T are lymphocytes and are different branches of the immune system. The more one looks at the interconnected web of cells and agents, the more the whole process parallels the proliferation of elementary particles in quantum-field theory.[5]

In passing we should note that melanin–which travels through the system by way of leukocytes and mast cells and is also generally present in the autonomic nervous system and many organs of the body, including the perineural cells, diffuse neuroendocrine loci, heart, lungs, and bloodstream–may in all likelihood be a molecular "homeostatic regulator." In that role it can direct such stabilization and re-stabilization processes as tissue repair and regeneration, autonomic balancing operations and immunological responses.

You may well ask what all this has to do with emotional and psychological healing. Well, a number of clinicians and researchers are finding a strong relationship between the immune system competence and other psychological social and interpersonal relationships (Kiecolt-Glaser and Glaser, 1986; Kiecolt-Glaser et al., 1984). They also repeatedly point out the relationship between our intrapsychic motivations, imagery, and the immune system in the production of white blood cells (Schneider, Smith, and Whitaker, 1983). As research continues, more and more will become clearer to us as to how we can affect the immune system by way of focused attention, imagery, and a powerful use of the body-mind's focus. Psychoimmunology is strongly indicating that influence over certain somatic functions can powerfully influence other functions and areas of the body-mind. Indeed, as suggested in earlier sections of this chapter, there appears to be an enfolded order of matter, energy,

---

5. The notion that the "inner" dynamics of our bodies reflect certain "outer" dynamics of the universe is an old idea. Yet if we are indeed embedded in the same universe there must be some degree of co-variation or communication between and within systems. Remember the Dogon tribes' "divination" of the body and the accurate orbit of the dark companion star of Sirius.

soma, and intelligence in the body-mind where each area can influence each other area.

The immune system is itself interrelated to all other systems of the body-mind. The immune system is implicated in emotionality, cognition, motivation, and behavior. Therefore it is also deeply involved in imagery. Imagery, as we all know from direct experience, is interrelated, and perhaps we could say "enfolded" in affect, motivation, fear, and numerous images, especially unconscious family images and memories. Imagery of an intense and novel kind is more highly associated with right hemispheric activity with its denser connections with bodily and inner somatic perceptions of the body. From here, there is no problem seeing that imagery is enfolded in the immune system and can be amplified and focused for therapeutic gain. Indeed, the history of healing is full of such discoveries and methodologies, often many have been lost to time.

Actually, the immune system, unlike the central nervous system (CNS) and brain, or the circulatory system and the heart, or even the respiratory system and the lungs, has no known center per se. Indeed, it is implicated or enfolded and interconnected with every other system of the body.

However, we do know that the CNS, the one most directly connected to the brain and ordinary consciousness, has innumerable interconnections to all other organs of the body *and* the organs known to be intimately related to the immune system network, e.g., thymus gland, spleen, lymph nodes, and bone marrow. By intense, focused imagery, affect and CNS activity with the immune system, the body-mind manages to heal itself. The actual "how" of imagery, affect, and intentionality influence on/in the body will never be really clear to us until we drop the dichotomy of mind vs. body and actually perceive that, in some degree, *all* of this is that. Perhaps it would be better to say that the relationship of mind to body arises in consciousness itself. In other words, we need to recognize that we are ultimately a localization of an all-pervasive process, not a series of discrete entities or objects with an absolute boundary. In this way, we can see, feel, and identify with the imagery of events, recognizing ourselves in various modes and perspectives. The oxygen outside the body would appear not to be us; by the next inhalation it is an intimate realty of our brain and consciousness. Even for clinical reasons, we can and may need to expand our sense of boundary, to see ourselves to some degree in everything, because even inert matter is a form of all-pervasive light, and living matter has already begun the arch toward consciousness.

Curiously enough, even from antiquity other areas of the body have been known to reflect all other parts of the body in some mysteriously interconnected way. From the sole of the foot, various body organs can be manipulated, from the ear, numerous body zones can be stimulated. Both the hand and the pupil of the eye are held to be reflections of the body-mind and all its parts. Embedded in these largely not understood but yet empirically practiced and ancient methodologies are insights into the workings of the human body as yet unimaginable to present day science. There may be numerous micro-holographic systems of the body with interconnected energy or meridian lines that will be the domain of some future science. Undoubtedly they are ecologically connected to the energies of the earth. In time they will unfold. Until then we can certainly take advantage of their phenomenological and psychophysical effects, as we shall do in the methodology section of this study.

As mentioned earlier, the holonomic or holographic model of energy transformation, already in use in contemporary physics and neurology, does not fully localize its operations in one area. The energy dynamics can extend beyond the local body in a non-local way.

Other research has shown that the life-force can extend beyond the local body, that it is attractive in nature, and can be focused. It also interacts with the other known "forces" in nature. It may always be connected with our most adventurous understanding of light. It feels very much as though we are in the position with respect to the dynamics of this life-force today, as we were 200 years ago with the electromagnetic force. For countless centuries, sparks were observed, but it took experimentation in numerous forms to harness this force. Today, we turn on a light switch and there it is! To my knowledge, we have not invented or increased the electromagnetic force in nature, only finally recognized it, harnessed it, and forgotten how mysterious and non-scientific it was once thought to be.

One day, when our sophistication in science helps us better understand the interaction of the known forces of nature with our less well-known inner nature, we will grasp the non-local dynamics that operate in some of the more unusual or latent aspects of our bodymind. Various individuals from time to time have demonstrated to us what is possible if we only knew its mode of operation. Sometimes it is a matter of someone else showing us that it can actually be done at all! Then we see, believe, and do it ourselves. After long periods of trying to run the four-minute mile, it was done. Now it is done by many on a regular basis. Pain control by meditation or deep hypnosis is another example. Even that rare, exotic ritual of firewalking, once thought to be impossible, or at least a trick, is now done in groups all over the U.S.A. Yes, perhaps it is a passing fad, but the fact remains that the average human body, with intense training, is capable of walking on 1200° F coals without burning the body! This is theoretically impossible by the reasoning of all our contemporary science, but still, we can do it. The feats of Yogis are another whole domain in which data abounds of how the bodymind, with disciple and insight, can be profoundly affected in ways that the usual scientific models say are impossible (Benson and Proctor, 1987). There appears no limit to the effect of psyche on soma, be it in the creation of psychosomatic disease, or these other unusual abilities.

Finally, from era to era, certain gifted individuals arise who radically alter or at least challenge our prevailing concepts on the limits or reach of the mind itself. These people afford us fleeting glimpses of mind extended in nature beyond all discernable boundaries. A better understanding of non-local dynamics will greatly expand our understanding of how psychics, of all degrees of evolution, execute their operations. How the process of remote viewing and other psi processes occurs is still a mystery, but is an experimentally validated and replicated mystery! These are laboratory studies by "solid" experimental physicists and psychologists (Targ and Puthoff, 1976; 1977; Targ and Harary, 1984; Hasted, 1981). The literature is also replete with other experiments, data, and clinical research from numerous others (Wolman, 1977; Jahn, 1982). The scientific data is overwhelming at this point; the resistance comes from mechanistic, reductionistic, atomistic models of ourselves, the psyche, and what is thought to constitute the material universe.

These intrepid explorers, encountering professional prejudice and, until recently, a history of only spotty results, continue to push back the orthodoxy of purely materialistic science. A new integration dawns slowly.

Perhaps, indeed, we are all aspects of a vast body, each of us a particular area, section, image, or wave-front. This vast holonomic body[6] is conducive to transformations of energy and the life-force as yet unimaginable. To view something from afar means some new or latent mode of perception is operative in us. The human of the future may exercise these perceptional modes in a tangible way.

As the literal light of greater and more inclusive intelligence descends and takes root in human consciousness, more and more such phenomena will arise. Some will be psychic, some will be much more. It is the coursework of evolution to unfold these now latent modes of perception. Already, we see that this new mode "will not set truth against truth to see which will stand and survive, but [will] complete truth by truth in the light of the one truth of which all are the aspects" (Aurobindo, 1955). Such is the case in "bootstrap" theories in scientific thinking already, especially in particle physics. In a holonomic sense we see with Aurobindo (1955) that

6. There are numerous references to this shared or holonomic body in the collective mythology and psychospiritual methodology of many peoples. The Iroquois believe in a shared, tribal body in which the memories, affects, and meanings of the tribe are enfolded in each member. Also in the intuition and practice of so-called "divination" in sorcery and other religious practices, the body of the individual (microcosm) is said to reflect the body of the greater universe (macrocosm). Most of this is unsubstantiated or even simply false. However, there are documented cases of so-called "primitive peoples" and divination where detailed predictions are later found to be scientifically accurate. What comes to mind are the Dogon people of West Africa who trace their lineage back to predynastic Egypt. The methodology of their ancient ancestors describes and precisely locates the inner workings and physiology of the human body and correlates it with the stellar operations of the recently "discovered," distant, and invisible dark companion stars of Sirius in its orbit! They also knew of the different density of these stars and the years of their special orbits long before the telescope and computers of contemporary science (Griaule and Dieterlen, 1986).

> nothing to the supramental sense is really finite: it is founded on a feeling of all in each and each in all . . . all particular sense knowledge and sensation is a wave or movement or spray or drop that is yet a concentration of the whole ocean and inseparable from the ocean . . . the material object becomes to this sight something different from what we now see, not a separate object on the background or in the environment of the rest of nature but an indivisible part and even in a subtle way an expression of the unity of all that we see.

Experimentation is necessary in order to break through to this new dimension. Much of this will appear "flaky" at first, but then again, how many models of the airplane were around until the Wright brothers at Kitty Hawk? Now we look to the planets and send messages beyond our local solar system. Those explorers who go to the great sea, the vast, perhaps holonomic body we all participate in and through, bring back knowledge that extends and deepens our perception. Who knows what the non-local dynamics are behind distant healing or even that perennial intuition, prayer. All we do know now is that this psychosomatic web, this complex constellation of matter, energy, intelligence and life-force we call ourselves, is more open to inquiry, more navigatable than we have thought. It is another transformation in evolution, an evolution that promises a body even more mysterious in the future. Let us therefore not keep assuming the world is flat, let us forgive and transcend the notion that the body is linear and totally localized. Indeed, it may be a great sea, a vast holonomic ocean of energy and intelligence that, if we sail it openly, intuitively, will bring us back to the shore of that ancient one, and to that luminous mystery, ourselves.

REFERENCES

Ackerman, N. *The Psychodynamics of Family Life: Diagnosis and Treatment of Family Relationships*, Basic Books, New York, 1958.

Ader, R. (ed.). *Psychoneuroimmunology*, Academic Press, New York, 1981.

Aurobindo, S. *The Synthesis of Yoga*, All India Press-Aurobindo Ashran, Pondicherry, India, 1955.

Barber, T. X. "Hypnosis, Suggestions and Psychosomatic Phenomena: A new look from the standpoint of recent experimental studies." *The American Journal of Clinical Hypnosis*, 21:13-27, 1978.

Barber, T. X. and Wilson, S. "The Fantasy-prone Personality: Implications for Understanding Imagery, Hypnosis and Psi." (Unpublished paper) 1985.

Basmajian, J.V. "Control and training of individual motor units", in *Mind/Body Integration*, eds. E. Peper, S. Ancoli and M. Quinn, Pienum Press, New York, Chapter 31, pp. 371-376, 1979.

Benson, H. and Proctor, W. *Your Maximum Mind.* Random House, Inc., New York, 1987.

Bernstein, N. *The Co-ordination and Regulation of Movements.* Pergamon Press, New York, 1967.

Bohm, D. *Causality and Chance in Modern Physics*, Philadelphia, University of Pennsylvania Press, 1957.

Bohm, D. *Unfolding Meaning*, Ark Paperbacks, London and New York, 1987.

Bowen, M. "A Family Concept of Schizophrenia," in D.D. Jackson, ed., *Etiology of Schizophrenia*, Basic Books, New York, 1960.

Cunningham, A. J. "Gestalt Immunology: A less reductionist approach to the subject," in G. I. Bell, A. S. Perelson and G. H. Pimbley (eds.), *Theoretical Immunology*, Marcel Dekker, New York, 1978.

Cunningham, A. J. "Some similarities in the way the immune system and nervous system work," In *The Immune System*, vol. 1, Basel, Switzerland: Kargen, 1981.

Dossey, L. *Space, Time and Medicine*, Shambhala Press, Boulder & London, 1982.

Evarts, E.V. "Representation of movements and muscles by pyramidal tract neurons of the precentral motor cortex." In Yahr, M. D. and Purpura, D. P. (Eds.) *Neurophysiological Basis of Normal and Abnormal Motor Activities.* Raven Press, Hewlett, NY, 1967, p. 215-254.

Fenichel, O. *The Psychoanalytic Theory of Neurosis*, W. W. Norton & Co., Inc., New York, 1945.

Ferenczi, S. *Thalassa: A Theory of Genitality*, W. W. Norton, New York, (1938) 1968.

Ford, C. V. and Folks, D. G. "Conversion disorders: An overview," *Psychosomatics*, 26:371-383, 1985.

Fried, R. *The Hyperventilation Syndrome: Research and Clinical Treatment*, Johns Hopkins University Press, Baltimore and London, 1987.

Gatz, A. J. *Clinical Neuroanatomy and Neurophysiology*, Philadelphia, F. A. Davis Co., 1973.

Griaule, M. and Dieterlen, G. *The Pale Fox*, (trans. by S.C. Infantino), Continuum Foundation, Chino Valley, AZ. (USA), 1986.

Hall, H.R. "Hypnosis and the Immune System: A review with implications for cancer and the psychology of healing," *American Journal of Clinical Hypnosis*, 25:92-103, 1982-1983.

Hasted, J. *The Metal-Benders*, Routledge and Kegan Paul, Boston, London and Henley, 1981.

Jahn, R. "The Persistent Paradox of Psychic Phenomena: An Engineering Perspective." *Proceedings of the IEEE*, Vol. 70, No. 2, February, 1982.

Jantsch, E. *The Self-Organizing Universe: Scientific and Human Implications of the Emerging Paradigm of Evolution*, Pergamon Press, Oxford/New York/Toronto, 1980.

Jerne, N.K. "The Immune System," *Scientific American*, 1973.

Kardiner, A. "The Bioanalysis of the Epileptic Reaction," *Psychoanalytic Quarterly*, 1:375-483, (1933).

Kellner, R. *Family Ill Health–An Investigation in General Practice*, Thomas, New York, 1963.

Kiecolt-Glaser, J. K., Garner, W., Speicher, C. E., et al. "Psychosocial modifiers of immunocompetence in medical students," *Psychosomatic Medicine*, 46, 1984, pp. 7-14.

Kiecolt-Glaser, J. K. and Glaser, R. "Psychological influences on immunity," *Psychosomatics*, Vol. 27, 1986 (September), 621-624.

King, R. D. "Black Dot. The Black Seed: The Archetype of Humanity, Part II," *URAEUS: The Journal of Unconscious Life* (1302 W. Martin Luther King Blvd., Los Angeles, CA, 1982.

King, R. D. *African Origin of Biological Psychiatry*, Seymore Smith, Germantown, TN, 1990.

LaBerge, S. *Lucid Dreaming: The Power of Being Awake and Aware in Your Dreams*, J. P. Tarcher, Inc. Los Angeles, CA, 1985.

Levenson, R. W. and Gottman, J. M. "Physiological and affective predictors of change in relationship satisfaction," *Journal of Personality and Social Psychology*, V. 49, No. 1, 1985, p. 85-94.

Levitan, H. "Traumatic Events in the Dreams of Psychosomatic Patients." cit. (1980).

Lidz, T. and Rubenstein, R. "Psychology of gastrointestinal disorders," in S. Arieti (Ed.), *American Handbook of Psychiatry*, Vol. 1, Basic Books, New York, 1959.

Locke, S.E. and Hornig-Rohan, M. Mind and Immunity. *Behavioral Immunology. An Annotated Bibliography*, 1976-82. New York: Institute for the Advancement of Health, 1983.

Lowen, A. *Depression and the Body*, Penguin Books, Baltimore, MD, 1972.

Lowen, A. *Language of the Body*, New York, Macmillan, 1971.

Lowy, S. *Foundation of Dream Interpretation*, London, Kegan Paul, Trench, Trubner, 1942.

MacLean, P. D. "Psychosomatic disease and the visceral brain," *Psychosomatic Medicine* 11:338, 1949.

Malis, L. I., Pribram, K. H. and Kruger, L. "Action potentials in 'motor' cortex evoked by peripheral nerve stimulation." *Journal of Neurophysiology*, 16:161-167, 1953.

Meissner, W.W. "Family dynamics and psychosomatic processes," *Family Process*, 5:142-161, 1966.

Minuchin, S. *The Family Kaleidoscope*, 1984.

Minuchin, S., Baker, L., Rosman, B. L., Liebman, R., Milman, L., and Todd, T. "A Conceptual Model for Psychosomatic Illness in Children: Family Organization and Family Therapy," *Archives of General Psychiatry*, 32:1031-1038, 1975.

Minuchin, S., Rosman, B. L., and Baker, L. *Psychosomatic Families*, Harvard University Press, Cambridge, MA, 1978, p. 23-50.

Motoyama, H. *Theories of the Chakras: Bridge to Higher Consciousness*, Quest Books, Wheaton, IL, 1981.

Netter, F. H. *The CIBA Collection of Medical Illustrations, Vol. 1 Nervous System*, 556 Morris Ave., Summit, NJ, 1972.

Penfield, W. and Rasmussen, T. *The Cerebral Cortex of Man: A Clinical Study of Localization of Function*, Macmillan Co., New York, 1950.

Peper, E. "The Treatment of Asthma: Combining Biofeedback, Family Therapy, and Self-Regulation." Paper and video tape presented to the 16th annual Biofeedback Society of America meeting, New Orleans, April 1985.

Phillips, C.G. "Changing concepts of the precentral motor area," in Eccles, J.C. (ed.) *Brain and Conscious Experience*, Springer-Verlag, New York, 1965, pp. 389-421.

Pribram, K. H. and MacLean, P. D. "Neurongraphic analysis of medial and basal cerebral cortex. II Monkey." *Journal of Neurophysiology*, 16:324-340, 1953.

Pribram, K. H. *Languages of The Brain*, Brandon House, Inc., New York, NY (1971), 1977.

Pribram, K. H., and McGuinness, D. "Arousal, activation and effort in the control of attention," *Psychological Review*, 82(2):116-149, 1975.

Rama, S., Ballentine, R. and Hymes, A. *The Science of Breath*, Himalayan Press, Honesdale, PA, 1981.

Rama, S., Ballentine, A., and Hymes, A. *Science of Breath*, Himalayan Press, Honesdale, PA, 1979.

Reich, W. *Character Analysis*, Farrar, Straus and Giroux, New York, (1949) 1971.

Ritterman, M. *Using Hypnosis in Family Therapy*, San Francisco; Jossey-Bass, Inc. 1983.

Rogo, D.S. *Mind Over Matter: The Case for Psychokinesis*, The Aquarian Press, Wellingborough, Northamptonshire, England, 1986.

Sabini, M. "Dreams As An Aid in Determining Diagnosis, Prognosis and Attitude Toward Treatment." *Psychotherapy/Psychosomatic*, 36:24-36 (1981).

Satprem, *Sri Aurobindo, or the Adventure of Consciousness*, Harper and Row, New York, 1968.

Schneider, D. "Conversion of Massive Anxiety Into Heart Attack," *American Journal of Psychotherapy*, 27:360-378 (1973).

Schneider, J., Smith, C. W. and Whitaker, S. "The relationship of mental imagery to white blood cell (Neutrophil) function: Experimental studies of normal subjects." Uncirculated mimeograph. Michigan State University, College of Medicine, East Lansing, MI, 1983.

Selvini-Palazzoli, M. "The families of patients with anorexia nervosa," in: E. J. Anthony, and C. Koupernick (Eds.), *The Child in His Family*, Wiley, 1970.

Selye, H. *The Stress of Life* (Revised Edition), McGraw-Hill Books, New York, 1976.

Simon, R. "Deeper, Deeper, Deeper: The Family's Hypnotic Pull," *Family Therapy Networker*, Vol. 9, #2, 1985.

Smith, R. C. "A Possible Biologic Role of Dreaming." *Psychotherapy/Psychosomatic*, 41:167-176 (1984).

Stone, A.A. *Journal of Personality and Social Psychology*, Vol. 52, pp. 988-993, 1987.

Targ, R. and Puthoff, H. *Mind Reach: Scientists Look at Psychic Ability*, Delta Books, New York, 1977.

Targ, R. and Puthoff, H. "A Perceptual Channel for Information Transfer Over Kilometer Distances: Historical Perspective and Recent Research." *Proceedings of The IEEE*, Vol. 64, No. 3, March 1976.

Targ, R. and Harary, K. *The Mind Race*, Villard Books, New York, 1984.

Taub, E. "Self-regulation of human tissue temperature," Chapter 11, in *Biofeedback: Theory and Research*, Schwartz and Beatty (Eds.), Academic Press, Inc., New York, 1977, pp. 265-300.

Taub-Bynum, E. B. *The Family Unconscious. An Invisible Bond*, Theosophical Publishing House, Wheaton, Ill. 1984.

Turk, D. C. and Kerns, R. D. *Health, Illness and Families: A Life-Span Perspective*, J. Wiley & Sons, NY, 1985.

van Heerden, P.J. *The Foundation of Empirical Knowledge*, N.V. Uitgeverij Wistik-Wassenaar, The Netherlands, 1968.

Veith, I. (translator) *The Yellow Emperor's Classic of Internal Medicine*, University of California Press, 1949.

Warnes, H. and Finkelstein, A. "Dreams That Precede a Psychosomatic Illness," *J. Canadian Psychiatric Association*, 16:317-325 (1971).

Weinberg, S. *The First Three Minutes*, Bantam Books, New York, 1977.

Wickramasekera, I. "A model of people at high risk to develop chronic stress-related somatic symptoms: Some predictions." *Journal of Professional Psychology: Research and Practice*, V. 17, #5, 1986, p. 437-447.

Wickramasekera, I. ibid, 1986.

Wolman, B. (ed) *Handbook of Parapsychology*, Van Nostrand Reinhold Co., New York, 1977.

Woolsey, C. N. and Chang, T. H. "Activation of the cerebral cortex by antidromic volleys in the pyramidal tract. *Research Publication Association of Nervous and Mental Diseases*, 1948, 27:146.

Ziegler, A. "A Cardiac Infarction and a Dream as Synchronous Events," *Journal of Analytic Psychology*, 7:141-148, (1962).

Chapter 8

The Psychospiritual Dynamics of Forgiveness

Forgiveness is an attribute of the strong.

–Mahatma Gandhi

Forgive and you shall be forgiven.

–Jesus the Christ

To err is human, to forgive, Divine.

–A. Pope

Before Abraham was, I am.

–Jesus the Christ

THE INTIMATE DRAMA

It is the deathbed. Years have passed since the last time they spoke to each other. The pain felt so deep, the sense of betrayal brought on so much agony, that they both swore never to touch, see, or ever care about the other ever again. It was final, absolute, the break, the final break. One had gone down the road simply unthinkable to the other, changing the future and uprooting all they knew. It was done on purpose! A deep identity was violated! Distance healed what time soothed away, and eventually, an intellectual tolerance replaced the ragged anger and penetrating loss. Then the news of the older's impending death brought on the flood of deep images, memories, and regrets.

When the letters back and forth arrived and settled, the meeting was set not far away. Older now, and wiser through pain, they each in their own way acknowledge the event upon meeting. The carefully rehearsed self-control breaks down and the waves of emotion sweep through the body/mind like a tidal wave spilling over land. Anger, despair, and loss assimilate with sorrow, compassion, and seemingly bottomless emotion. The maelstrom changes all balances and former boundaries of meaning, insight, and intellect. Tears come. The body is drenched in heat, sweat.

Painted above we can see that forgiveness itself and the emotional act of forgiving someone is one of the most powerful emotional experiences known to the human psyche. It is a profound affective experience that interfaces with our vital, emotional, psychological, and psychic life. It arches into the noetic, or spiritual, dimension. Recall for yourself, either in a family or interpersonal situation, or even in the clinical setting, what occurs during the powerful experience of forgiveness. When the process of forgiveness is a serious one, it has the power to transform, to powerfully alter, the experience and the deeper personality of the person.

In the emotional process of forgiveness, there is usually a powerful sense, or image, of injury to one's own ego or to one's family that is involved. It is usually believed to have been done deliberately with little or no regard of how the other felt. A simple example is the one sketched out in archetypal fashion above in which someone may experience self-esteem or ego injury within a family or interpersonal context. However, it is not limited to experiences with intimate others. Think of the tragic situations that occur in war or other situations, in which we feel that we have been injured in some intimate way. There is no limit to examples in the everyday and clinical situation. However, when forgiveness is involved, the person to be forgiven has become an intimate and powerful aspect of the forgiving person's emotional, psychic, and psychological life. A *deep image* of the situation is retained by the mind of the person who experiences or perceives injury to themselves. In the process, the emotions of anger, depression, long-term resentment, and other painful feelings including the desire for revenge are experienced during the acute process *prior* to the act of forgiveness. I hope to demonstrate that there are emotions that arise during the actual process of forgiveness, and subsequent to that process, that have profound clinical implications. Accordingly, I would like to assert at the very beginning that this process of forgiveness is an almost fathomless one that touches our conscious and unconscious life, and interfaces intimately with our significant others. It should also be noted that the person who *accepts* forgiveness feels remorse, shame, guilt, depression, and anger, until finally there is redemption. He or she, in a sense, feels a debt. It is a debt or "uneven" situation that somehow must be paid on the deepest psychological level in order to "even out," to re-create wholeness, equilibrium and balance in the emotional, psychic, and noetic life.

The dictionary defines forgiveness as "giving up resentment against or the desire to punish, to stop being angry with; to pardon; to cancel a debt. To absolve." The word comes partially from the ancient word "to forego," which is to go past, to overlook, to neglect. It is a profound relinquishment of an intimate psychological condition. It is akin to the word "to forget." Both as people and clinicians, we see that forgiveness *releases* powerful affect and imagery from the person who is forgiving this or that other person. It is to this constellation of powerful affect and imagery involved in the process of forgiveness that I focus our attention.

COLLECTIVE FORGIVENESS

Forgiveness and its emotional concomitants is a world-wide cultural and psychological phenomenon, a universal human experience. All of us know that individuals, families, tribes, and even nations can collectively hold anger, resentment, and the imagery attendant to that process for generations and generations. We each understand the process of forgiveness in individuals, and to a lesser extent, we can understand the process of forgiveness that occurs in families. We are woefully inadequate, however, in understanding the process of forgiveness and transcendence when it occurs on a tribal or larger community and national level. It can be a history of strange contours and juxtapositions that stretch back for generations. Take, for example, the modern Holocaust of European Jews by the Germans. While the notion of collective guilt has been intellectually dismissed since 1945, the psychological and deep collective racial scars are acknowledged personally, politically, and socially by everybody, whether we want to admit it or not! In the modern Holocaust, the *Nazis,* German "tribes," selectively murdered the modern off-shoot of the ancient tribes of the *Nazarites* of Israel, presently called the *Ashkenazim.* We shall return to this presently because the story is older and more interconnected than we know.

On another scale, highly technological societies are increasingly inadvertently, but sometimes intentionally, *exterminating* indigenous tribal peoples in the search for raw materials and land for cattle. Species of animals and plants are being lost in *ecological holocausts* daily in the relentless march of our society toward increasing consumption. Many of our lifestyles directly contribute to this unprecedented situation.

For an individual, participation in this the process is an extremely intimate one in which the psyche of one person is deeply involved in the perceived act and shared history of another psyche. This other psyche, of course, can be a group of other psyches, as when one feels injured, hurt, or betrayed by a whole group of other people. I spoke earlier in the *Family Unconscious* of an intimate, shared, emotional field that develops and emerges in powerful, recurrent relationships between significant others. Identities are mutually shared, reinforced, and acted upon in such systems. It is the shared matrix in which the Child is sometimes Father to the man. This shared, interconnected matrix of the family unconscious is only one system that experiences the process of forgiveness. However, in any process of forgiveness, that same interconnectedness of psychological processes in seemingly different individuals is experienced. This interconnection and interrelatedness is a prominent reality, not only on the psychological level of the individual and the family system, but it is also cogent reality in the physical, somatic, and material world as well.

THE ASYLUM OF PAIN/ THE DYNAMICS OF RELEASE

The Spiritual Dynamics of the Body

What actually occurs in this mysterious, enigmatic process of forgiveness? We see this process in our personal daily lives, in therapy, in the tragic context of world affairs, including national and tribal war, and of course, in intimate family relationships. It is an intimate, subtle, and deeply moving experience.

In the context of ancient and modern Christianity, the process of forgiveness is seen to lead to one's own salvation because one is therein saved by being forgiven by a much greater other. Somewhere in the New Testament Christ says, "Judge not, and you will not be judged; condemn not, and you will not be condemned; forgive and you shall be forgiven . . . For the measure you give will be the measure you get back." The Christian is exhorted to forgive others and thereby *participate in something greater than themselves.* Martin Luther King (1963) firmly believed that the power of forgiveness lay in its inherent capacity to awaken the spiritual conscience of the other, who is believed to be one's oppressor. It is understood that the Christ, the gentle poet and avatar of Galilee, forgave those who "sinned against him" and therein awakened and aided their personal and collective salvation. The forgiving psyche identifies with and participates in the Christ consciousness. One learns to "forgive our debtors as our debtors forgive us." This appears to be a highly refined and eloquent statement of the timeless philosophy and *methodology* of non-attachment.

In the Yogic view of non-attachment, one experiences the world but does not identify with any particular experience in the world. This leads to "personal" salvation within that particular system. In the Buddhist system, there is also the deeply embedded notion of compassion as rooted in the universe. This compassion is experienced when one is profoundly non-attached to occurrences in that universe. This is said to lead to freedom from karma and samsaras which are understood to be our most subtle mental impressions from our present and preceding experiences as incarnated beings. We see that it is not only a process that affects our conscious life, but very importantly, affects our subtle mental operations that are largely unconscious. Our emotional and vital level is substantially affected. This emotional and vital level is deeply involved with our autonomic nervous system, the subtle root biology of our nature. This process of anger, resentment, forgiveness and compassion touches *all* levels of our being, our physical life, our emotional life, and our noetic and transcendental life.

It is well known that chronic deep anger body affects by way of subtle messages to the autonomic nervous system over time. Western psychoanalysis is acutely familiar with the unconscious dynamics of anger, repression, and resentment. Many serious diseases today are linked to long-standing, deep, emotional experiences of loss, resentment, chronic stress, and depression. The list includes headaches, Raynaud's disease, hypertension, arteriosclerosis, arrhythmias, angina pectoris, colitis, ulcers, asthma, and possibly cancer and many more (Pelletier, 1977).

In a real sense, the active emotional stance of feeling "unforgiving" affects the somatic life of the person. It appears to stimulate the brain to produce toxic biochemical substances that harm the heart and cardiovascular system, sustaining stress chemistry, if you will, and ultimately suppresses the immune system, that as we mentioned in the last chapter is implicated in our subtle bodily and psychic processes. When we finally open up, confide, release and forgive it has a positive, enhancing affect on our health and our immune system (Pennebacker, Kiecolt-Glaser, and Glaser 1988).

We have seen within the family unconscious system the effects of shared anger, resentment, and joys. These have a profound influence on personality development and the ways that we handle anger and anxiety as elucidated in previous chapters. In each of the clinical syndromes presented in this book, there were examples of attachment, of frantic clinging to images, ideas, and bodily tension states. Letting go of these tensions, both physiological and psychological, is an obvious aspect of therapy. It is another face of forgiveness.

Frozen Images

If we look at family and individual processes from a clinical perspective, the following dynamics appear to emerge. Very *intense* affect, idea, and imagery are seen in both the world of the one who needs forgiveness, and the one who must forgive another. It is very often a process that is seen in the mind of the one who needs to be forgiven, provided they accept that definition of the relationship on some implicit level. In that case, the person who needs to be forgiven very often feels a profound sense of debt, guilt, or depression. They seek to rebalance the imbalance, to "atone" for the situation, to again be "at-one-ment" again. The person who needs to forgive feels in disequilibrium or unbalanced in some primal relational way. Fantasies of revenge are usually orchestrated around re-balancing this disequilibrium. The "victim" often feels a collage of anger, blame, recrimination and helplessness to change things (Heider, 1958). This can be seen in the therapeutic situation in which one has the opportunity to observe these reciprocal relationships. Notice here that these images, affects, and ideas are almost always extremely painful. They appear as *frozen* memories of injustice and injury. I say frozen, not in the sense of static, but in the sense of dynamic, but unchanging. There is an image of the one who needs to be forgiven and the actual act or series of acts that must be forgiven. There is initially a great deal of resistance, sometimes over years and generations, to this process of forgiveness that involves profound emotional, vital, and noetic changes. These go past the conscious to the unconscious and beyond. This means it affects our physical bodies, our psychophysical syndromes, our emotional dispositions, and our transpersonal dimension. In the borderline, obsessive/compulsive, paranoid, and multiple personality types, and especially in the psychosomatic constellation, deeply entrenched patterns of imagery and affective-ideational fixation are found. The body is always implicated.

It is significant in this context that in certain forms of Tantric Yoga, there are techniques for the activation and release of intense affect with focused imagery. These usually involve activation of powerful affect and imagery that is focused on a certain pathway, or the methodology of a teacher. Psychophysically speaking, the sustained and intense imagery focused in certain aspects of the body will affect subtle changes in the psychobiology of the individual. Psychologically, however, I ask you to note that the process of forgiveness that encompasses all that I have spoken of so far, is an expansive, integrating, releasing flow of the life-force of the individual which has been *frozen* by these recurrent, painful images that bind the experience and the emotionality of the situation for that individual and system. This emotional dynamic of staying *frozen* serves to both keep the individuals at some distance from each other and also staying *within the framework* of the relationship! It sometimes even serves to ward off a sense of bottomless and self-dissolving grief. These images reach the content-root of the mind, where subtle memories, archetypal forces and samsaras dwell. This may be the Causal level of the mind. Profound degrees of energy and attention are released in this process.

I am emphasizing that there is a paradoxical identification with, and a transcendence of, the image/idea that has been held in the affective and cognitive field of the individual. When this occurs, there is an extremely powerful release of emotions. The emotions of anger, rage, and deep injury are usually the ones that are released. This leads to a non-contraction of the emotional field, which had been formerly held tightly bound by the images and affect of anger and injury. As this occurs, there is a mysterious and radical sense of freedom and non-attachment to that earlier constellation of images and affect, which may have been held for years, even generations. When this release occurs, there is the experience of euphoria and compassion that is deep and fulfilling. The world expands. For some individuals, depending upon their intuition and emotional coloration, they may experience a profound sense of peace and absence of suffering. This is a matter of personal style. What is central here is that the long, tightly held object/image of pain is *released* into and out of the former condition. There is a *dissolution* of the prior image and emotionality which leads to the experience of fathomless compassion and integration. We note here that the shared duality of forgiver/forgivee is transcended in a new, unitary consciousness. This consciousness recognizes its partial identification with "the other," their limitations and frailties and then moves beyond that. It transcends the pathology or subtle distinction between self and other found in Causal level dynamics. The *Nazi* is re-absorbed by the Ashkenazim; the racist by the "other." "The tongues of flame are enfolded into the crown knot of fire, and the fire and rose are One" (Eliot, 1943).

The process dissolves the earlier frozen, contracted, psychological condition that spans both conscious and the wider unconscious processes. This is based upon an intimate interrelatedness of relationship between and within individuals. This process changes perception and reaches into what has been called a spiritual, or noetic, dimension. Again, it transcends both the unconscious functioning and the conscious dimension in waves of experience. It evolves beyond the truncated psychology of vengeance (Searles, 1956). It touches that transcendental identity common to both psyches, and releases the light/intelligence/compassion dimension that is fervidly woven into the nature of the psychological and spiritual universe. This goes far, far beyond the frozen imagery of the injured individual unconscious.

Dialogue and Flow

You do not need to be a therapist to see that hatred, resentment, anger, and associated powerful affects have often been kept out of full consciousness and held in check by an image or series of images. These images are powerful and dynamic but also recurrent, and therein, in a certain sense, frozen or contracted. The "flow" of the life-force has been dammed in such situations. The unconscious and the door to the unconscious has been sealed, to a certain extent, by this forbidding image. In order for the process of forgiveness to occur, there must first of all be, on some level, a dialogue such that the channels and the web of interconnectedness may be made more supple. In other words, things and energy must be allowed to "flow through" as before. The very nature of dialogue involves mutuality, or shared positions.

There is an order in this process. It first requires an intellectual preparation and willingness to see through the present situation, imagery, and affective matrix of anger and resentment. The opening scene of this chapter is a painting of this. Subsequent to that there is the emotional approach or lead-up to the possibility of change itself. It is an extraordinarily difficult process, a rare process, and a process in which to a certain degree our deepest nature and habits are touched upon. It is a rare energy that transforms the individual. I also suggest that this radiant and deep transcendental energy is a primal aspect of our nature, and is intimately related to the healing process.

In the process of non-attachment, or "letting go," or forgiveness, the older configuration, or order, changes in some intimate way. The older or prior system has to *expand*, or rearrange itself in some way, in order to accommodate the change in the system. This change in the system is a change of images, shared identities, and transcendence of one-way projection of blame, anger, and loss. If this is not done and one's intense hatred of the other is not even recognized, persecutory delusions can arise with a split occurring between the "blameless" victim and the "evil oppressor" (Hunter, 1978; Close 1970). In a certain sense, therefore, the new system for its own health is made to go through a period of *disequilibrium* in order to reach a more stabilized state. The disequilibrium is manifested by intense, dynamic affect and imagery as formerly stated. This affect and energy, to some extent, is bound again by the new imagery that arises in order to put context and definition around the new system. The new images and ideas and the transcendental experience is drawn upon to restabilize, expand, and make more pliable the prior system of injury, hurt, and resentment. When forgiveness occurs, the life-force "flows through" the individuals and they are briefly no longer in divided conditions! The person who is in the process of forgiving someone or something releases a great deal of affect and recorded imagery of the prior situation. When this is done on the level of the family, or even the tribe, there is a collective transformation that occurs in the shared consciousness. This is much less understood. The process in the individual and the family is much more understood by contemporary psychology. In all of these, it is emphasized that great compassion ultimately arises at the end of the process of forgiveness. The transcendental life-force flows unobstructed again. Healing energy and non-contraction become the dominant mode of the individual psyche on both a conscious and unconscious level with respect to the prior constellation of images and affect that had been frozen in the process of anger, nonforgiveness, and attachment to that system of anger, mutually shared identities, and resentment. In a real sense, the new experience and insight generates a new wave envelope over the formally erratic episodes and understandings of the injured psyche.

In some cultural and religious contexts the person who is *to be* forgiven, and who *wants* to be forgiven or relieved of their debt will often try to experience pain of some sort, e.g., self-flagellation, etc., in order to expiate the image/sense of guilt or wrongness. This self-inflicted pain is also an attempt to consciously identify with the aggrieved or forgiving person's pain. Thus again both would enter into a new union or realm transcending the prior order or separation.

In the situation of self-forgiveness, all of the above occurs, except that the "other" is rather one's own behavior in former situations. The dialogue is either internal (intrapsychic) or held to be between oneself and one's creator, etc. In either case of self-forgiveness, all painful and pleasurable images and memories of the prior behavior and value-system that participated in the situation are surrendered. A new internal, free perception is engendered.

The person who forgives, during the actual profound process of forgiveness, is able to transcend the prior state and ultimately see an aspect of himself or herself in the other person. It may begin with small doubts interrupting the banquet of anger, revenge, and injury experiences, then move to shared identities and thoughts of reconciliation. Inner dialogue expands to wider and wider views. Eventually even more of the self is seen in the other. This is why it is ultimately a process and an act of compassion for the other person and for oneself. Forgiveness of others parallels forgiveness of self. The word compassion itself means sorrow for the sufferings or trouble of another person, including one's self. It is often accompanied by the urge to help and to be sympathetic to the other person's situation. In order to do so, in the situation involving two or more people one obviously has to feel deeply involved and yet not attached to that other person's perceived act. During this most intimate and affectively charged process, both the forgiver and the person who will be forgiven experience that shared transcendental reality. At the very time of the forgiving process, both the forgiver and the person who is being forgiven share a sea of healing energy that becomes a substratum of both of them. In this sense they are both *redefined* by this that flows through both of them. With the breaking up of the old system, a new identity and a new and more highly evolved equilibrium emerges. The ground of infinite compassion is touched upon which is extraordinarily intense to the body-mind of both. They are both redefined by that common experience.

The Further Reaches of Forgiveness

It is not at all unusual in this situation to see both overcome with profuse emotion, affect, suffering, and then release. Because of these strong energies and demands upon the systems of the individuals, it is difficult to sustain this particular kind of psychic energy. It is simply exhaustive to the body-mind in most conventional situations. This great energy, however, ultimately leads to a sense of bottomless *purification.* At its further ends, it leads directly to the transcendental experience of sustained ecstasy. One is, in a sense, born twice. Again, a deeper order is touched. This deeper order is, in many ways, the payoff, or the reward or fruit, of this transformative experience. This is the expression of greater wholeness, or harmony, or Maat.

In the process of forgiveness, we bring down into the world of suffering and pain the healing light of transcendental consciousness. We pierce the mirage of duality with its attendant processes of projection, splitting, denial, and frozen energy matrix. We regain a disowned aspect of our own self, our own nature. We briefly become identified with the free energy of the universe and the current of bliss and life-force. The painful imagery and experience is released into the immense sea of affective, compassionate, and collective imagery of our human experience. Since forgiveness and its process transcends the conscious and unconscious process, including the somatic and the dream life, it enters into what the ancient Yogis called the Causal Dimension. This is the dimension of profound peace and free energy in the universe.

In connection with the latter statement, there is a strong sense that both the waking and dream or unconscious image-affect of reality, that had previously been fixated or contracted around using these images to do so, is released back into the substratum of both of these. The *substratum* of both the waking and unconscious or dreaming state is again a Causal state in Yoga philosophy. The profound peace is similar to the profound peace that one experiences in deep sleep without dreaming. This is difficult for most of us to remember because it has no images associated with it. However, it is characterized by a state of profound peace and bliss. This occurs after the emotional orgasm of forgiveness. The prior memories and images of pain, injury, injustice and so on are released into the vast storehouse of the collective psyche. They are no longer the exclusive province of the conscious or unconscious mind of any individual. Perhaps they can be said to fall back into the Akashic records or the Alayavijnana of the Mahayana Buddhists, although these two references are usually associated with other processes.

Compassion is released in the renewed free flow of energy in the universe. This free-flowing intelligent energy is identical to the basic aliveness identified by the Buddhists, and the healing energy often identified by other practitioners of the healing arts. This experience is maximized by an attitude and a methodology of non-attachment to the process. This involves a paradoxical identification, and yet transcendence, of the experience. Again, the tranquil sense of purification is seen and felt, not only in the mind, but deeply in the body itself.

Notice the numerous motifs that appear in human history about great healers from time to time "taking on" the sins or bad karma of others, and in that process, helping them. This is obviously a profoundly selfless act. As mentioned earlier, in small tribal sects and religions, this can be seen in ritual self-flagellation. It can also be seen in some schools of monastic life with their excessive ascetic rituals and demands. However, it can also be seen as a process represented by an illuminated individual. It is often said that "Christ died for our sins." This is a collective and cosmological process of forgiveness and expiation. The noble Buddhist Bodhisattva vow is another example of selflessness and constant forgiveness leading to liberation or salvation. However, it is a salvation or liberation not only for human beings in the Buddhist perspective, but for all conscious creatures.

Finally, there is the magnificent example of the great healing propensity of the Avatar who brings the light down periodically into a dark and suffering world. This light of healing is brought down by the Avatar into the bowels and consciousness of the individual and collective sufferer. In this redemptive process, the used and conflicted world of the person is taken back and redeemed for something else. This something else is the deepest, primal condition of the being, the prior and limitless consciousness/light of the Self, before contraction into pain and suffering. The Avatar always appears in a period of conflict and sorrow in human history. The collective mind is, in a sense, far-from-equilibrium in its affairs. It is a painful collective fluctuation for the species, a species that seems painfully derailed from the evolutionary tract. The "mission" of the Avatar is to bring down the literal light into human consciousness and thereby keep evolution unfolding to higher and higher orders.

These periods of painful fluctuation appear to elicit, in a non-local way, the intervention of the Avatar whose power, grace, and insight helps lift the consciousness of those around them. In a peculiar sense, their dynamic, higher equilibrium attracts and "absorbs" the lower frequency, non-equilibrium disorders around them and either transmits them to a higher vibratory mode or at least restores balance and harmony. They take upon themselves "the sins" of others in the process of forgiveness and non-attachment.

Indeed, just as there are Black holes in the universe absorbing energy, and mini-white holes exuding energy, all oscillating in an interconnected way; and just as in biochemistry and the life sciences, higher and higher orders emerge in evolution from an inherent teleos in the universe, so is it with the enfolding, unfolding orders of intelligence and light in the human plane with the arising in cosmic evolution of the human Avatar incarnation. This incarnation is a higher light/intelligence and vibration arising and descending in humanity at certain crucial periods of need. Thus "true forgiveness" always partakes of a transcendental act, going beyond and integrating our previous condition and moving us toward something greater. It moves to a far more expansive, emotional, ideational, and noetic integration of our being. In the process, all these dimensions are altered.

TRANSFORMATIONS AND RESISTANCE STYLES TO A FREE-FLOWING HEALING AND LIFE-FORCE

Throughout this whole chronicle of life-force, energy, and personality predispositions, the styles of clinging to transience and the foam of ego have emerged from the limitless ocean of Self. Each style, with numerous crevices and odd contradictions, has developed methods to navigate this life-force, or current of living energy, if you will. At this juncture, I would like to focus more attention on those specific maneuvers that manifest in the syndromes that have been presented. How each clings, does not forego and therein profoundly forgives, but instead holds to the forms of psychophysical and mental/egoic contraction, will be the emphasis. By this way, in a certain sense, we will "arrive at the place from which we started and know it for the first time."

In the very beginning of this book, the borderline personality was characterized by constant *oscillation* around the perceived boundaries of his or her personality. In intimate and pseudo-intimate contact with others, the borderline personality is never really sure where his or her center or focus is. This individual feels alternately isolated from, and then fused with, the significant others in his or her life. This person is characterized by feeling alternately guilty and blameful, and then by a panicking attempt to escape. Escape then precedes a desired re-fusion. The life-field is constantly and tacitly consciously blurred in this personality style. In many ways, it is overly permeable in a non-stable way. Forgiveness and the free flow of energy naturally threatens the stability of this system. As a consequence, the acts and the process of forgiveness are a threat to the integrity and boundary of this system, for they involve an intimate and heart-felt contact with another, and possibly therein the dissolution and ego death of the borderline individual.

A "level" beyond the borderline personality, and a personality structure that appears to be even less stable in many ways although initially looking more stable, is the obsessive-compulsive personality style. As outlined previously, the obsessive-compulsive personality style is characterized by a *fixation* on the images and affects that serve to seal off anger, resentment, and rage in the unconscious process of this individual. This is true not only with intimate members of the individual's own system, especially one's system of family relationships characterized by family unconscious dynamics, but also with inanimate objects and institutional structures. In addition to that can be seen the defensive process of *denial* of real and imagined rage. This process of denial makes it extremely difficult for this individual to identify with others. In this way, the life-force and the flow of healing energy is constricted in an attempt to control and *compartmentalize* the process of the life-force. It has been my clinical observation in biofeedback and family therapy that this particular constellation, or style of dealing with the life-force, most often gives rise to somatic problems. In many ways, somatic problems are an attempt by this style to control, constrict, and compartmentalize affective feelings by putting them into the unconscious regions of the body. In situations where there is a great pressure of affective and ideational energy, this personality style can very often transmute its energy into hypomanic and, at times, compulsive behavior. Both hypomanic and compulsive behavior are different branches of what can be understood to be the obsessive-compulsive personality pattern. You can see in the obsessive-compulsive personality style, given the fixation and compartmentalization of energy, that it is extremely difficult to not only identify with others, but to open itself to the process of forgiveness which involves the free flow of intimate life-force energy. This also threatens the personality style in a different kind of way. The possibility of dissolution of the personality and the ego boundary is therefore a constant threat, and is dealt with in a peculiar way by the obsessive-compulsive personality constellation.

The next level seen that is beyond the obsessive-compulsive personality constellation, manifests the various forms of paranoid behavior. This level of adaptation has elements of the preceding level in its presentation, especially the loosened flood of ideas usually held in check by obsessive-compulsive defenses. This is the so-called hypomanic tendency. In all the different kinds of paranoid behavior, including paranoid personality, paranoid style and so forth, the processes of blame and guilt are *projected* away from the personality itself. This style is very much characterized by the phrase "where there is other, there is fear." As with the obsessive-compulsive style, in the paranoid style the rigid system of images and affects is held to very tightly. The life-force is seen to have turned against, or betrayed, the individual in this particular style. Another complication in this clinical picture is that as the "hero" of the world, the paranoid individual may indeed actually "save" aspects of the world and himself in some rare situations. However, as suggested before, the ego of this individual is not identified as the ego of the world. That aspect is seen as being distorted in the narcissistic personality. The ego of the paranoid personality is experienced in a particular way in which it is put into constant danger. The ego is not seen as embedded in the world process of the Self, but rather it is seen over and above and in counter-distinction to the world. Given the denial and the projection of guilt and blame, and the increasing fragmentation of the world to this individual, the personality style of the paranoid tends to overcompensate and create grandiose aspects of itself within the world context. In some cases, the flood of ideas pattern, or hypomania, occurs. It would appear that this grandiosity is in many ways a reflection of the implicitly true, but horribly failed, attempt of the

Avatar and Bodhisattva embedded, but not yet emerged, from our nature. In other words, the paranoid individual correctly intuits its need to sacrifice, forgive, or save the world, but substitutes its own fragile and transient ego for a true and profound identification of its deeper Self with the world. In many ways, the paranoid can be seen as a failed reflection of a true compassionate healer or Bohisattva or Avatar motif.

Finally, "beyond" the paranoid personality constellation, which appears to be a failed reflection of the true Avatar/Bodhisattva vision and realization, is that of the multiple personality. In other words, it appears that after the failed attempt to construct a reasonable picture of the world that takes into account not only the individual's ego but also its true and innate need to heal and save what it appears to see as the world, is the personality that is so fragmented, so conflicted and tormented, that none of these defenses are available to it. This is that splintered personality whose deepest defenses have been totally overwhelmed. This, of course, is the multiple personality. The process of forgiveness is totally beyond this personality style in most situations. The life-force has not only been subjected to intense pain and betrayal, but the life-force it actually experiences is rather terrifying. In many ways, panic rules this personality. There is no peace that is experienced in the world for this fragmented and unfortunate individual. Clearly, this is the most disturbed of the clinical syndromes presented in this study. In this situation, the universe certainly needs to be forgiven its colossal impact on the individual, not to mention those particular persons who have hurt this individual in the past and the present. This fragmentation and assault upon the person's defensive structures is so massive that it goes beyond the ego structures that are more common to the borderline, obsessive-compulsive, and paranoid style. The multiple personality has been so abused that multiple egos have been substituted for an integrated and composite individual. The life-force has been so fragmented, and branched off into so many different streams, that there is no core or central figure that is readily available. Intensive therapy, involving procedures that work on the profound levels of the personality, are absolutely necessary in order for this individual to benefit.

In each one of the major clinical pictures presented, there are different degrees and characterizations of the constriction and compartmentalization of the free-flowing life-force and healing energy. The borderline personality is primarily characterized by constant oscillation around boundaries with no sense of integrity. However, this individual is able to deal generally in the world, and even in interpersonal relationships. We all manifest some borderline tendencies in our most intimate relationships! These are always primarily characterized by rather blurred boundaries. For the borderline, the process of forgiveness never has any real resolution. In the obsessive-compulsive personality there is less oscillation but more fixation upon images in an attempt to constrict and hold on to the life-force. Compartmentalization and denial are used in an attempt to control this life-force, which at times even feels quite overwhelming. It can manifest hypomanic symptoms, with their flood of energetic ideas, and at the other end, compulsive behavior in an attempt to control and constrict the inevitable life-force. Beyond this, in some ways the paranoid personality is an even less-developed attempt to control and direct the life-force. The obsessive-compulsive defenses of fixation, denial, and compartmentalization, in a sense, have broken down and blame and guilt and other powerful emotions are projected out and away from this personality. The life-force has become increasingly more terrorizing to this individual. There is the genuine attempt to construct a world view by this personality that makes sense in the sense of saving it from various terrors and obstacles. However, this is a failed attempt, and in many ways the grandiosity is a distorted perception of the true and immeasurable Self of this individual. Finally, the multiple personality is so completely decimated and fragmented that the capacity to heal itself and to heal others has almost been totally obliterated. Panic rules this personality and the world process seems to be a disastrous one in which forgiveness is almost inconceivable.

Thus, all these personality styles are different levels of an attempt to deal with the inevitable transcendent and evolutionary life-force that is free-flowing, transcendent, and all-pervasive. Each represents, in its own way, a more debilitating attempt to control, perceive and live within this ever-flowing energy that moves from person to person, from life to life. To be sure, no one individual fits any particular style exactly but there are clear and consistent thematic influences of individuals across each one of these styles of psychic and living energy management. Each, however, is a variously failed attempt to live harmoniously with the free-flowing, healing life-force that is identical to transcendence, forgiveness, and peace. Each in its own way has missed the bottomless ecstasy of the Self. Yet this bottomless ecstasy, this luminous and transcendent reality, appears to be the archway and reach of evolution. It is the living inheritance of every human life born in the warm ooze and vortex of an ancient sea.

REFERENCES

Close, H. "Forgiveness and Responsibility: A Case Study," *Pastoral Psychology*, 2(205), 19-26, 1970.

Eliot, T.S. *Four Quartets*, Harcourt, Brace and World, New York, 1943.

Heider, F. *The Psychology of Interpersonal Relations*, Wiley, New York, 1958.

Hunter, R.C. "Forgiveness, Retaliation and Paranoid Reactions," *Canadian Psychiatric Association Journal*, 23, 167-173, 1978.

King, M.L. *Why We Can't Wait*, Signet, New York, 1963.

Pelletier, K. *Mind as Healer, Mind as Slayer*, Delta Books, New York, New York, 1977.

Pennebaker, J.W., Kiecolt-Glaser, J.K. and Glaser, R. "Disclosure of Traumas and Immune Function: Health Implications for Psychotherapy," *Journal of Consulting and Clinical Psychology*, 56(2), 239-245, 1988.

Searles, H. F. "The Psychodynamics of Vengefulness," *Psychiatry*, 19:31-40, 1956.

SECTION IV. METHODOLOGY: THE YOGA OF BLISS/LIGHT/EMPTINESS

We are inside truth and cannot get outside it.

–Maurice Merleau-Ponty

No thought or figure or any perception arising in the mind is, in itself, God. No thing, no body, no moment or place, in itself, is God. Rather, every moment, place, thing, body or state of mind inheres in God. Whatever arises should be recognized in God, not idolized as God. Then all conditions become Reminders that draw us into the ecstatic presumption of the Mysterious Presence of the Living One.

–Da Free John
Compulsory Dancing

Chapter 9

On Method

BACKGROUND AND THE LIFE-FORCE

> The Great Way is not difficult if you have no preferences.
>
> –Sengstan
> *Zen Faith Mind*

> This skill entails having one's attachment become the cause of experiencing great bliss and then using the mind of that great bliss to meditate upon the emptiness.
>
> –Geshe Gyatso
> *Clear Light of Bliss*

> Whatever may be the nature of these inward depths of consciousness, they are the very ground, both of the explicit content and of that content which is usually called implicit. Although this ground may not appear in ordinary consciousness, it may nevertheless be present in a certain way. Just as the vast "sea" of energy in space is present to our perception as a sense of emptiness or nothingness, so the vast "unconscious" background of explicit consciousness with all its implications is present in a similar way. That is to say, it may be *sensed* as an emptiness, a nothingness, within which the usual content of consciousness is only a vanishingly small set of facets.
>
> –David Bohm
> *Wholeness and the Implicate Order*

All that has gone before, our primeval mother, the arch of evolution, the play and unfolding of the personality syndromes, must all be subject to some form of observation. Otherwise, we are left with poetry, gesture, and speculation. It must be observed and capable of being reported to others. Therein a method or process of organizing data is required. All that has gone before can be obliged to demonstrate itself if a methodology can be made explicit. Freud adhered to this, Piaget did also, as did Mahler, Sullivan, and so many others on whose shoulders we now stand. In that frame of mind we open this final and, hopefully, well-mapped episode of our ancient mother's progeny and their arch through evolution.

This is a brief, yet crucial, chapter. As a method of working, it has been found helpful, but it is by no means exhaustive of the different methodologies that can develop in order to experience and understand the phenomena outlined in the preceding chapters. The central focus of the methodology is simply to facilitate the state or condition of psychophysical equanimity from which the other observations are made. It allows the observer to establish himself or herself in a position of equilibrium such that interferences or changes in this equilibrium are, themselves, the object of observation. This methodology is based primarily on technical considerations and, again, I fully realize that another method of practicing with this energetic field is quite possible. I will make reference to these other developments as the journey progresses. Disciplines can lead to success, but should also be able to point to mistakes in execution. Thereby they are able to satisfy one of the cannons of falsifiability in the domain of introspective and scientific investigation or subjective "proof." The present method, which exploits certain aspects of the current of life-energy in the body, can be used this way in the liberation of attention and energy and is subject to *direct observation* and *verification* by anyone who practices the method. Observation and verification are the heart of the scientific method.

This method, or way of working, is transpersonal in its operation. That is only to say that, while accepting and using the psychological systems that work with the physical-behavioral level of our being, that recognize the dynamic emotional-motivational dimension of our lives, and which embraces the higher mental functions of our existence, it also arches into the subtle, energetic, and occasionally psychic aspect of our nature. It does this from a consciously non-reductionist perspective. The procedures or practices outlined are gleaned and systematized in order to integrate the earlier psychological models and also, very importantly, to prepare the ground for other, "higher" processes to operate. It is confined primarily to technical procedures which, if diligently put into practice by a perceptive, alert practitioner, will yield observable results. It is not to be taken as a transformative path or approach. That is for other fully transformative disciplines. Rather the methodology is a series of psycho-physical and subtle experiments that the practitioner can test out in the laboratory of their own experience. As such, at a certain time the practitioner will then move on their own toward a fully transformative discipline. However, throughout the discussion of these methods, I will allude freely and in footnote to these other, more technical procedures and the directions toward which they point. The primary function of the fully presented practices is to free energy and various forms of attention in a way that can be observed, replicated, and tested.

In the first chapter, I spoke of a transcendental force or the will toward the Absolute, and the "current of living energy" that is the manifestation of this Absolute. Others have made similar observations about the current of living energy and have seen and experimented with it from many different perspectives. Every culture, every science that has arisen of a noetic or religious nature, has investigated this fundamental experience. In some of the most ancient of written texts, the Vedas and the Upanishads of India, this life-force and its numerous currents through the body are well outlined and mapped. Ch'i of the ancient Chinese is also another reference to this life-current that flows through the body. In Japan, of course, it is known as Ki. In both the Chinese Ch'i and the Japanese Ki, it is the foundation for the ancient medical practice of acupuncture. It is also the foundation for both medicine and the martial arts. The ancient Hebrews refer to it as Ruach, the Sufis refer to it as Baraka, the Gold Coast Africans, as Wong. There have been, of course, modern explorers and geographers of this energy field (Krippner and White, 1977).

At the turn of the present century it was Freud's libido theory that really breathed life into psychoanalysis. It moved the analysis of the human being out of philosophical speculation and into direct contact with a certain aspect of the life-force. Freud's original technique of "evenly suspended attention" made the observations of primary process, secondary elaboration, defense and counter-defense, transformation, sublimation, and the host of other psychic processes available to waking observation. His reductionist bias focused the data in a particular way. The original technique, however, is similar to certain meditational procedures found in Buddhist bare-attention or mindfulness. Unfortunately, much of this original genius has been lost by lesser practitioners (Epstein, 1984).

Anyway, whether we may agree or disagree with various aspects of Freud's theory, we cannot deny some of his basic observations, regardless of our particular opinion about how valuable they are. Later on, it was Wilhelm Reich (1971) who expanded the knowledge of the life-force or libido in Western psychology. He showed how this libido became entrapped, and ensnarled in its own defenses–defenses that manifested directly in the body as character armor. This character armor represents specific ways in which the body *contracts* or responds to threat and anxiety in the world that it experiences. These minute and eventually major muscle and other contractions arise from a certain contraction or egoic withdrawal from embracing the world. The developmental intricacies of this were outlined in Chapter 2. It is a contraction, or avoidance, or recoil and moving away from this all-pervasive life-force! It is all-pervasive simply because the life-force flows through more than human beings and animals. It is quite clear that the life-force in some function–in some manifestation–flows through everything that lives. This includes trees, grass, insects, birds, and innumerable other creatures that inhabit this planet. For many west African lineages the life-force and life is God.

Today we see in the work of Al Lowen in psychology/psychiatry, the more refined reflection of these egoic contractions from life in actual clinical practice. The various postures, positions, and chronic ways of holding energy and breathing patterns in the body are reflections of, and potentially protective to, the threatened ego.

Finally, in biofeedback and behavioral medicine therapy, using an electromyogram (EMG) or one of many other highly sensitive reflections of the activity of the automatic nervous system, I and others in our clinic have seen the minute ebb and flow contractions of the life-force with anxiety in the egoic perception of reality. This subtle perception of egoic contractions can be honed into very fine observational skills, such that if one places oneself in the observational position, so that when all disturbances of the condition of equanimity are registered dispassionately, one can come to subtly observe the minute flow of the life-force and our recoil or dance with it. "Be still and know that I am God."

One can begin to see how various personality styles deal with the subtle, yet all-pervasive, force in a certain manner. By placing oneself and becoming firmly established in that mode for significant periods of time, one can actually observe the play and unfolding pattern of each particular personality syndrome that has been elaborated in the preceding chapters. This is the method. It is to this end that certain procedures are used that take advantage of the specific pathway of this current of living energy through the body to present a method that has certain aspects that are relatively easily verified. As this is done, each conditional expression of the body-sense will arise. It may be the sense of the stomach, or hands, or sounds of different kinds. All are sensory modifications of the more primary experience of the body-sense itself arising. The body-sense is primary, the particular body-mind coloration or tonality is secondary, a modification of the current of living energy that is the substance of the various body-mind conditions. To help elucidate the process for subtle observation, a simple series of fundamental procedures will be elaborated within this context.

The modern rationalist and reductionist may object to this methodology as "scientific" because they have not personally seen or experienced it. Some even believe "life" can only be found by dissection. Yet this method of direct perception is common to the traditions of all humankind. Modern science as primarily a materialist, reductionist way of seeing the world is not without limits. Modern science itself is a *body* of knowledge. It assumes its own present limits of perception and experimentation to be the only path to truth or knowledge. The data of modern science confirms certain principles and then we assume that all the rest of reality fits the mode. Yet there is an embedded limit to this inductive method when it comes to generalization to all future and other conditions. Knowledge in the material realm is always expanding and the history of science is replete with situations that were later supplanted by different or more incorporative knowledge. It is the case in the history of physics, medicine, biochemistry, and psi. At the present time we are letting go our notions of fundamental "objects" bouncing off and interacting with other "objects," be they subatomic objects or psychological objects, as in the schools of object-relations psychology. We are moving closer to "fields" of interaction and mutual enfoldment/unfoldment in one interconnected whole movement. This, again, is the case in physics and family unconscious processes. Therein, the "body" of knowledge that comprises modern science must be expanded, otherwise it becomes merely the narcissism of the body of science caught in the limits of its own reflection.

THE NECESSITY OF PRACTICE

How can we experience this energy and follow its pathways through the body-mind?

Every branch of science must develop tools. The tools that are required for this particular kind of investigation involve at least the following three: *One*, observational skills. *Two*, an awareness of ego processes themselves, which means at times being in a position beyond or outside of conventional ego/world realities. That is to say, occasionally to be in a position to observe the ego itself, which means a rootedness of awareness in some other position of observation. While this is quite difficult to do, it can be done. It can be developed as a skill like any other skill. It is a position rooted in a certain basic aliveness, which one can identify with a primal receptivity, knowledge and faith in the vaster, seemingly unknowable reality. It is unknowable to the ego in the verbal sense, but it is not unknowable in itself. Primal receptivity and knowledge that arrives by this mode is, of necessity, intuitive. *Three*, this intuition, as we will describe it, is an intuition married to *energy* that is observable. Few of these observations can be made and then replicated without practice. It is, of course, possible to stumble upon various experiences in life that open one to this kind of experience, but these are haphazard and anecdotal. It is much more systematic to develop a working methodology that is specific to your particular style in order to increase the capacity for observation of this kind. This is especially important in a clinical situation.

I have spoken of energy. I have spoken of the current of living energy. This current of living energy can be located in the body by certain procedures and techniques that have been known to humanity since before the morning of antiquity. Modern day acupuncture and Yoga are only two of its representatives. Also, in the West, the recent exploration of the subtleties of the labile autonomic nervous system have provided much data that is *parallel* in many ways, but not identical to, some of the phenomena that are observed in Yoga.

Practice is absolutely necessary in order to progress from a kind of pseudo-neutral "objective" observation in the life-current to a sense of psychophysical equanimity. This condition of equanimity that will be cultivated is not identical to the "observing ego" of latter-day Freudian psychoanalysis.

The current of life-energy is, in a certain sense, pure or free. It is pure or free in the sense that it is not necessarily modified by various conditional experiences. It is the substratum of those conditions or states, but is not exhausted by those states and conditions. The life-force is all-pervasive, basic, and background. Out of its various constellations a positive, negative, or neutral valence arises. Various objects are perceived within this current of living energy. When the conditional experiences are gradually limited, this current of living energy encompasses the nature of bliss more than anything else that might be described in words. It is similar to the sense that the body-mind has when in deep sleep without dreaming. It is a living, radiant current that intuits emptiness, and yet is also luminous. That appears contradictory from an egoic perspective, but from the perspective of free living energy, it is not at all paradoxical. This tangible sense of current, or modulations of bliss, combined with a certain kind of luminous emptiness, or sensuousness, is near the Tantric Yoga tradition of Mahamudra. In the *Clear Light of Bliss*, a similar procedure is described. It is similar in the sense that it attempts to perfect the simultaneous union of great emptiness and bliss. It works specifically and directly with the currents of living energy in the body. I will directly demonstrate the affinity of the present methodology to this process as things unfold.

These procedures, which will be described presently, are specifically designed to put the body-mind into a physical and psychic state of balance, or equanimity. It is a form or translation of Maat, or order and balance, into the body-mind. In this state of equanimity, which can be measured by various external biofeedback measurements and other subjective measurements, minute observations of egoic body-mind contractions and expansions can be perceived from this perspective of the current of subtle living energy. This current of living energy is all-pervasive and yet constantly played-upon by the actions/reactions of conditional situations. This skill of observation can only come with practice in a regular systematic way. Again, like any other skill, it will develop. There is nothing mystical or esoteric about it! Allowing the egoic processes to occur, without prejudice, yet witnessing them from the perspective of the current of living energy, allows the arising of certain patterns when the ego is focused in the direction. Therein certain psychic and psychological states and personality patterns can be observed from this perspective and their patterns of energy confluence manifest. This method allows the practitioner/clinician to observe the different ways the life-current is dealt with and, therein, how the different syndromes and styles unfold and express themselves.

I want to emphasize that this particular procedure, which takes advantage of certain patterns of energy current in the body, goes a step beyond the "observing ego" of psychoanalysis. It is not a process of dissociation or regression in the service of something else. It is not either of these, for it identifies with something else quite different. It does not give way to self-hypnosis or the swoon of unconsciousness. This procedure gradually places the observer or experiencer in the position of open identification with the current of living energy, a current of living energy which reveals itself to have no boundaries and pervades all when one finally experiences it absolutely. The principle is one of overcoming contraction, of the literal expansion of the bound mind and ego to the infinite consciousness of bliss with no boundary. In the process, it avoids the extremes of body austerity/negativity, and total annihilation of the sensory world. Formless introspection reveals an ecstatic bliss innate in the structure of all conditional or passing forms. This bliss eventually emerges as anterior and prior to all arising conceptualization, day-to-day experiences and changes of cognitive, or other body-mind, state. Eventually, it perceives and assumes the ego itself to be a *localization* of this all-pervasive, living reality. One gradually moves toward free awareness itself, toward rootedness and basic aliveness, and sees all things, objects and emotions, etc., as modifications of this unstateable, nonverbally expressive THAT which enfolds, includes, and transcends all modifications of THAT. The various clinical syndromes are, in a very real sense, what different personality styles have done with this basic, all-pervasive and inclusive, free and intelligent, luminous energy.

THE LUMINOUS CURRENT AND THE FIVE FUNDAMENTAL PRACTICES

A single but definite procedure is as follows: experiment, find, and establish a physical posture of balance that allows you to eventually become physically quiet and a certain sense of relaxation to arise. A particular Yoga asana may be helpful but this may take a while if this is not already being practiced. However, whatever position you are in, it is absolutely crucial that the spine be relatively straight. This can be a particular Yoga position, or it can be sitting in a firm, comfortable, straight-backed chair. It is also helpful to have as few distractions as possible and to have the room relatively quiet and comfortable. It may take a long time to become so physically comfortable that you are not distracted externally. However, this very observation of the process of muscular realignment at various times is in itself a useful observation. The endpoint of all this, however, is to simply find a physical position that is comfortable and that can be maintained for a decent amount of time with little movement. I will now outline each simple practice and provide some empirical background as to why it is specifically helpful in technically handling the current of living energy that pervades the body-mind.

The First Practice

Pranayama, the science for the control of respiration and the subtle energies of the body and, therefore, eventually the subtle energies of the mind, is one of the practices that is very, very helpful. I have attempted to describe elsewhere how the conscious control of respiration leads to profound influences on the autonomic nervous system by way of the olfactory nerve, the vagus nerve, and the limbic system (Taub-Bynum, 1984). By control of the tenth cranial nerve, or the vagus nerve, conscious entry into the labile autonomic nervous system is opened (Rama, 1979).

The autonomic nervous system consists of two branches, the sympathetic and parasympathetic system. These two systems enervate all the organ systems of the body. Swami Rama, who worked at the Menninger Foundation for some time, demonstrated that radical control and influence over autonomic nervous system functions is possible. He not only stopped his heart for nearly half a minute at will with no dangerous side effects, but also was able to change the degrees of dominance in his brain waves from high beta all the way down to delta. Delta proliferation only occurs in deep sleep without dreaming, yet he was able to do this and retain consciousness. He also created a 10-degree temperature difference in his hand without movement. He attributed both of these to the science of pranayama, which he indicates is intimately related to the autonomic nervous system.

In his book on the ancient science of pranayama, Lysebeth (1983) demonstrated the effects of pranayama in a number of situations. He also made reference to the "immersion reflex." It is shown in this immersion reflex how great mammals in the ocean change their metabolism by changing their respiration. Children suddenly and tragically submerged in icy waters are known to dramatically and automatically do the same. This reflex is stimulated in certain Yogic breathing exercises. The metabolism is radically altered by these intelligent creatures by taking advantage of a psychophysiological reflex which exists in a rudimentary state in humans and which can clearly be developed. The interrelationship between oxygen and the brain is extraordinarily profound. While prana is certainly not oxygen, a manifestation of prana *is* oxygen. And as we all know, the condition of the brain has a profound effect on our perception of reality on all levels.

References have already been made to the effect of the olfactory nerve on the process of respiration and the limbic system. The nose can actually be thought of as a neurological organ. The first cranial nerve, the olfactory, has its nerve endings in the top of the mouth and the bottom of the nose. These are constantly being stimulated and sending messages to the limbic system, a system which supervenes all our primitive emotionality. Moreover, by stimulating nerve endings in the nostrils, which have a dominance cycle of approximately 1-1/2 to 2-1/2 hours, we can differentially influence the cerebral hemispheres in the brain in the process. Actually, it is a curious fact that the two nostrils have significantly different electrical potentials and are observed to effect the emotions and body/mind differently. By stimulating these nerve endings in the nostrils, you stimulate the reflex action in certain nervous centers in the spinal cord. These are particularly stimulated, it seems, in the medula oblongata, and it is thus possible to produce deep immediate reactions in all body functions. Remember, in the primeval times of our ancestral mother, we either lived or died depending on our sense of smell, for it alerted us to dangers or benefits in the environment. Today it is rarely used, except for food, and simple attraction or repulsion. However, it is a powerful evolutionary possibility that is obliquely used but always in potentia.

This amazing sensitivity of the neurological apparatus operating through the brain to experience and interpret external reality is powerful. We profoundly affect the respiratory system by learning how to control this, and through respiration we offer the process of the life-current and perception itself. For this very reason, as part of the methodology, slow deep diaphragmatic breathing is extraordinarily useful. This is not deep chest or thoracic breathing, which tends to strengthen and reinforce the panic response. Rather, deep, vulnerable diaphragmatic breathing is done in which the peristalsis of the GI tract is stimulated, all the organs in the body are subtly massaged, the lungs are used to their full capacity and the whole system works much more efficiently. Children, and all other creatures when they are relaxed, breathe diaphragmatically. When a child is frightened, the breathing goes up into the thoracic cavity. It is panic breathing, it is stress chemistry, it is an aberration in the field of equanimity. Thus, diaphragmatic breathing is a foundation practice. It is the first fundamental practice.

The practitioner/clinician will also notice a natural, gentle closing and uplifting of the anal sphincter with the full exhalation phase of this breath. This movement of the anal sphincter, when exercised and amplified, is called the Mulabanda technique or root-lock in the Kundalini Yoga tradition. The practitioner/clinician will also notice a gentle pull to the pit of the stomach and a small closing of the neck in the throat area. These are called Uddiyana and Jalandhara, respectively, when streamlined and coordinated with other breathing procedures. These three locks, or bandhas, are embedded in, and naturally arise from, the full diaphragmatic breath. When disciplined, they harness and *conduct* the life-force or current of living energy through the biopsychic axis of the spine.[1] The whole autonomic nervous system is profoundly engaged. After a long period of time, and this includes months and months, a certain physical state is achieved where relaxation and a relatively erect spine can be maintained. As this is done the process and the procedures of that very simple pranayama come into effect. These procedures have a long and useful career in clinical treatment of numerous disorders. It restores a necessary balance (Arpita, 1982). These all begin with very slow, deep diaphragmatic breathing.

The Second Practice

After some time, the next procedure follows. It simply consists of alternate nostril breathing in order to balance off any disturbances that may arise in the labile autonomic nervous system. Recent research has tended to confirm the observations of the ancient Swara yogis that breathing in specific ways activated certain areas of the

---

1. The spine is one of the earliest structures to emerge in human development. By the twenty-eighth hour after conception the ectoderm has already begun to invaginate into the interior of the cluster of early fetal cells to form a long tube. Most critically, this neural tube eventually develops into the spinal cord. The end of the tube (the neural crest mid-point), brain, and cells along its length evolve into melanocytes and all of the endocrine glands, e.g., pineal, pituitary, adrenal, hypothalamus, thyroid, parathyroid, pancreas, and other glands found in the stomach, GI tract and lungs. These melanocytes are sensitive to light! S. Grof in *Beyond the Brain* (p. 387) has noted that when clinically using the opposite of slow diaphragmatic breathing, what is called the hyperventilation process (Fried, 1987), that tight muscle bands or armor develop in patients in the areas of the body associated with the autonomic nervous system plexes, where some of these glands are located, and also where the chakras of Yoga are said to be. It is not at all difficult to see a connection between these melanocyte/light sensitive areas, the ANS plexus and chakras, and the path of Kundalini as it rises through the body-mind!

brain (Khalsa, 1984). It has been shown by experimentation that the hemispheres of the brain also go through a period of dominance between the right and left hemisphere (Klein and Armitage, 1979). This period cycles roughly every 90 to 120 minutes. It has also been shown that certain deep forced breathing and diaphragmatic breathing can create a certain nostril dominance which stimulates particular areas of the brain. In other words, after diaphragmatic breathing, when alternate nostril breathing is done, we can help significantly deepen the state of body-mind equanimity by taking advantage of this life-current manipulation. The physical state of equanimity is now deepened by diaphragmatic breathing and then alternate nostril breathing to further deepen the subtle mental aspect that contributes to the overall sense of body-mind equanimity. This is the second fundamental practice.

Alternate nostril breathing is extremely simple. In a relaxed state, with the spine relatively straight, simply begin to breathe diaphragmatically. Do this for at least five minutes. Now place the right thumb up against the right nostril and simply exhale completely and then inhale fully through the left nostril until the lungs are full. At that point, simply move the forefinger of the hand over and close the left nostril and exhale through the right nostril. Exhale completely so that there is a slight sensation of a pull between the pit of the stomach and the anal sphincter area. At that point, simply inhale completely again through the right nostril that is open while keeping the left one closed with the forefinger. At that point, when the lungs are full, switch nostrils by placing the right thumb again on the right nostril and exhale out completely through the left nostril. This constitutes one full cycle. If you will simply, slowly, and deliberately do fifteen rounds of this with the breath deep and even, it is extraordinarily difficult not to experience a profound state of relaxation. I encourage you to take advantage of these basic procedures to deepen the capacity for observation from the position of intuition married to observable energy. With prolonged practice, up to thirty full cycles can be done without loss of body orientation of various kinds.

The Third Practice

Next in the procedure is a very simple, yet very effective, technique. It is the third fundamental practice. It involves focusing the mind in a way that increases its subtlety and yet deepens its intensity. The analogy here is to a laser. In the room that you may be sitting in as you read this, if there is a light overhead or in the room, it is radiating luminous frequencies in a certain band width that produces light that is visible. However, if the total energy that is coming through the light were narrowly focused through a specific frequency, we have what is called a laser. Well, by analogy, if the mind can be focused in its attention in a specific way and not scattered, it becomes a very powerful tool. This is what the application of sushumna can do. Therefore, after one has committed a substantial amount of time and energy, such that there is a physical state of profound relaxation, a steady and even practice of diaphragmatic breathing, and an ease with the process of alternate nostril breathing, sushumna is to be applied. This is the third fundamental practice.

By focusing at the end of the alternate nostril breathing cycle on a certain spot in the body, there is deepening of the range of this specific mode of observation. The sushumna is the central axis of the body and corresponds to the spinal cord or the spinal column. By focusing one's attention after alternate nostril breathing on the spot at the bottom of the nose, the top of the lip, the place where the nostrils flow evenly with alternating warm and cool sensations, there is a profound deepening of the capacity to enter into purely the state of psychophysical equanimity. Instead of the various specific conditions or modifications of the body-mind arising, the substratum or energetic position is opened. It is diffuse, yet clearly experienced.

After this is done, one may, of course, decide to focus on another area of the body depending on one's needs and personal development. This guidance may come from reading, from a personal teacher of various kinds, from an inner experience, or a number of different ways. Be open to that. However, it is important what area one focuses on. I am referring, of course, to the chakra system. The chakras are experienced as energy vortexes, or centers, in the subtle body. They are highly associated with the various plexuses of the autonomic nervous system and are harnessed in various schools of Yoga and meditation. They are seven in major number, from base to crown of the spine. These are represented on the modern medical caduceus where the serpents criss-cross. Whether they are stimulated one by one as in Raja Yoga, or coursed around and up the spine as in Kriya Yoga, or any other method combined with pranayamas and other disciplines, they are a powerful source of psychic and other energies embedded in the human body-mind. The advanced practitioner has experimented with his/her own tendencies and therein helps to clarify the particular path for themselves (Rama, 1982). However, for purely technical reasons, it is extremely helpful initially to follow this present procedure and then end with one's attention focused primarily at the top of the lip and the bottom of the nose.

Initially, the use of the eye muscles to direct the focus of attention at this spot is exceedingly helpful. Later, as the current is more clearly discerned, the eye muscles are less needed to keep attention at this spot. One can later even more powerfully amplify the other area of the body that is being focused on if one focuses on those other areas of the body *through* the "lens" of the focus of the bottom of the nose, top of the lip![2]

The reason for this is quite old and yet quite simple. It is first of all an ancient technique followed and written down in text by the tenth century Yogi, Goraknath. It had been around for centuries in the Indus Valley before that. It is also mentioned in numerous other Yoga texts. However, other than simply tradition, there are other reasons. First of all, in Yoga theory and practice, the ida and pingala nadis, or subtle channels of life-energy, terminate, after coursing through the body upward and around it, at that spot at the bottom of the nose, top of the lip! By focusing one's attention there, one stimulates this root of primal energy from the endpoint to the beginning point. In actual practice, one may note that focusing at the base of the nose, top of the lip tends to stimulate other areas of the body.

2. Common to not only Hatha and Raja Yoga, but also Kundalini Yoga is a procedure called Shambhavi Mudra. Here the mind is inwardly fixed on a plexus or chakra while the outer gaze rests on this spot with eyes half-closed. A sense of luminosity arises with practice. Each plexus or energy vortex has a characteristic movement or vibrational mode, all being variations of light. The mystics Plotinus, Boehme, Philo Judaeus and many others have described their experiences of this luminous current or intelligent radiance (*Hatha Yoga Pradipika*, translated by Hans-Ulrich Rieker, pp. 164-175). Still others regard the Shambhavi Mudra to rest its inner gaze on the space between and above the eyes. This area is the Ajna chakra, where the pineal gland, a gland sensitive to light, is located (Muktananda, *The Play of Consciousness*, 1978; Motoyama, (*Theories of the Chakras*, 1981).

It is not at all unusual to directly experience the awakening of significant amounts of subtle living energy at this point and also to experience, at the base of the spine, a certain stimulation or warmth. This is referred to as pranothana. This experience may take on many forms and there are definite extremely powerful technologies for amplifying this into Kundalini awakening. That is not our interest here for a number of reasons. I simply want to call your attention to this as a methodology that will accentuate the manifestation of the current of living energy, at which point, one clinically observes that from a certain perspective of equanimity specific syndromes and psychological processes tend to arise. This technique is also mentioned in the Shandiya Upanishad and the Shri Jabala Darshana Upanishad, where it is outlined that the current of living energy can be recognized experientially at the spot between the bottom of the nose and the top of the lip where the nostrils constantly are enervated by an alternating current. By focusing one's attention on this current, one can deepen one's control of the process or directionality of this energy. If this is done successfully, it begins to experientially make sense that "if therefore thine eye be single, thy whole body shall be full of light" (Matthew 6:19-23).

Eventually the practitioner/clinician can "locate" this current of energy in the midst of everyday life. Constant application of sushumna helps the mind overcome the tendency to flow outward, and instead to begin to flow inward. This will also tend to mix the sense of bliss with the current of everyday matters. There is an affinity here to the Tibetan practice of "blending the nature of the Clear Light with the path during the day time." Eventually, all these matters begin to arise in, or unfold out of, bliss as a vast background. This is the conscious and unconscious cultivation of equanimity on all levels, not only in the waking state. One becomes firmly established in the luminous current of living energy. This delicious work of "locating" the luminous current in the midst of everyday matters begins to transform the perceptual process in many different and interesting ways. It amounts to the gospel of bliss in some practitioners although it in itself is not a final practice. There arises a tendency to identify the self-sense with this blissful covering. This eventually must be overcome in discipline, but provides a guidepost for one's development in the meantime. Technically speaking alone, it is a valuable experiment that will demonstrate the tangible experience and process of the current of living energy that is blissful and seems to arise itself out of a sensuous emptiness.

It is extremely helpful to note that in acupuncture theory research there is a strong indication that the ida and pingala nadis of Yoga correspond intimately to the second lines of the urinary bladder in acupuncture theory (Motoyama, 1981). By alternate nostril breathing, these two nadis are forced to send the primal energy up the primal nadi, or channel, which is the sushumna. Again, the sushumna corresponds to the spine as we know it.

Now, in Chinese medical history and theory there is a major "extraordinary" meridian that is known as the governor vessel meridian. It is thought to be present from the earliest of human embryonic times. From Motoyama's research, this meridian seems to correspond extremely closely to the sushumna, or spine. Its function in Chinese acupuncture theory is the overall coordination of the six yang meridians. It is said to start at the top of the coccyx, that is at the root of the spine, and course up the center of the back to the top of the head and terminate in the upper lip. This parallels the path that the awakened Kundalini is sometimes known to partially take except that the Kundalini's loop then proceeds further down into the stomach (Sannella, 1978). It is said that Ki energy is stored in this meridian like water in a lake. The flow of Ki, therefore, through the twelve ordinary meridians are likened to different kinds of rivers by Motoyama, which distribute vital energy to the various organs and tissues. It is thought that in the event of an energy imbalance or insufficient Ki in a particular organ or part of the body due to various diseases or malfunctions, that the energy stored in this extraordinary governor vessel meridian is mobilized to supplement the flow in the related ordinary meridians. Much, but not all, of Yoga practice is dedicated to moving this energy upward from the base of the spine to other centers, or to the crown center itself. That, again, is not our aim here. Our aim is simply to take advantage of the fact that energy can be *recognized* and *amplified* in certain areas of the body and is therein open to direct observation by the reader if the reader will commit time and energy in order to develop certain observational skills. These, obviously and hopefully, could be used in other forms of practice.

As mentioned earlier in the treatise called *The Clear Light of Bliss* by the Tibetan Lama, Geshe Gyatso, this subtle yet luminous energy can be realized and channeled intelligently through the body by one's own observational skills, discipline, and evolution. This is very important in the present methodology because, as stated earlier, we do not want to simply rely on an abstract concept. It must be directly felt, directly experienced, directly observable, in order to be useful and scientific. That is why we are taking advantage of certain lines of energy in the body that are more easily recognizable than others. Let us return to practice.

The Fourth Practice

The first practice involved slow, deep diaphragmatic breathing, in a comfortable position, the second, alternate nostril breathing. The third practice was the application of sushumna which was to gently focus attention to that spot at the bottom of the nose, top of the lip. The fourth fundamental practice involves sensory control and withdrawal from external referents. This is similar to pratayhara in Yoga practice and sensory deprivation experiments. However, control is maintained and consciousness deepened. It involves the use of subtle and neural pathways in the brain.

You may recall that in the chapter on the psychosomatic web, where a holonomic model of psychobehavioral processes was presented, the precentral gyrus or brain fold of the sensory-motor cortex was discussed. This sensory-motor fold has all the organs and voluntary areas of the body projected and located on its lens or surface, from toe to lip! See Figure 7.2, Chapter 7.

The neurocortex is the physical mediator of consciousness, integrating body, emotions, and cognitions into an intelligent system. The neurosurgeon can stimulate the body by stimulating the brain. In the current practice here, we start at the other end by increasing the specific awareness of the body area in order to awaken and stimulate that area in the brain. This not only deepens relaxation and clears the neuronal pathways to the brain, but also stimulates the configuration of the motor homunculus or body representation along the line of the precentral gyrus. The flow of subtle and neural stimulation through this "circuit" tends to create a spontaneous dissociation of consciousness from the sensory and motor channels of experience *without* loss of consciousness. The somatopsychic energies are stimulated but not turned out externally and lost. They are retained and opened to observation. Perception undergoes a radical and pleasurable shift.

Now in order to maximize this curious fact, it is important to build on what was cultivated in the previous three practices. Thus, continue to fully inhale and exhale diaphragmatically; execute simple alternate nostril breathing for twenty full cycles, and then breathe only diaphragmatically. Then apply sushumna for a few minutes. When this is done and attention is gently kept at the "lens" of the bottom of the nose, top of the lip, focus the mind's imagery internally on the following sequence with a *full*, slow breath cycle on each area. You may wish to repeat a relaxing phrase or sound at each point to cut down on distractions. The main thing is to give each point a *full, un-rushed* breathing cycle.

1. Big toe right foot
2. Second toe right foot
3. Third toe right foot
4. Fourth toe right foot
5. Small toe right foot
6. Achilles heel right foot
7. Ankle right foot
8. Calf of right leg
9. Knee of right leg
10. Thigh of right leg
11. Hip of right leg
12. Lower right side of body
13. Mid right side of body
14. Upper right side of body
15. Armpit of right arm
16. Shoulder of right arm
17. Elbow of right arm
18. Wrist of right arm
19. Back of palm right hand
20. Center of palm right hand
21. Small finger right hand
22. Ring finger left hand
23. Middle finger right hand

24. Index finger right hand
25. Thumb finger right hand
26. Big toe left foot
27. Second toe left foot
28. Mid toe left foot
29. Fourth toe left foot
30. Small toe left foot
31. Achilles heel left foot
32. Ankle left foot
33. Calf of left leg
34. Knee of left leg
35. Thigh of left leg
36. Hip of left leg
37. Lower left side of body
38. Mid left side of body
39. Upper left side of body
40. Armpit of left arm
41. Shoulder of left arm
42. Elbow of left arm
43. Wrist of left hand
44. Back of palm left hand
45. Center of palm left hand
46. Small finger left hand
47. Ring finger left hand
48. Middle finger left hand
49. Index finger left hand
50. Thumb finger left hand

Now, while still keeping the "lens" at the tip of lip, bottom of the nose, focus sequentially with the same full, deep breathing on:

51. Base of spine/perineum
52. Genitals
53. Navel
54. Heart
55. Throat
56. Between the eyebrows
57. Top of head

then continue slowly, with full, slow, and deep breathing to:

58. Upper right side of face
59. Upper left side of face
60. Right eye
61. Left eye
62. Right cheek
63. Left cheek
64. Nose
65. Top of lip, bottom of nose
66. Low lip
67. Mouth and jaw
68. Tongue
69. Lower base or root of the tongue
70. Top of lip, bottom of nose

We begin at the big toe and foot because the ki/ch'i or acupuncture energies also enter the system there as sometimes does the luminous current of the Kundalini energy (Sannella, 1978; Motoyama, 1978; 1979; 1981; Veith, 1972). The hands, face, and mouth are also given more detailed coverage because of their correspondingly larger represented area in the brain's precentral gyrus due to evolutionary development. Throughout this whole process, consciousness has been sustained! The body-mind is now imbued with a diffuse sense of bliss and equanimity.

The breath is deep, slow, and even. In order to deepen the state of primal energy, receptivity, and basic aliveness even more, it is helpful to do the following. Periodically during the deep diaphragmatic breathing, with the focus at the base of the nostrils, it is helpful to deepen and focus on the *exhalation* phase of the breath. Sometimes exhalation is twice the length of inhalation. The exhalation phase emphasizes the parasympathetic aspect and function of the autonomic nervous system. It will open the pores of the skin and increase heat. This focus will tend to feel expansive and loosen the hold of ego/muscular contraction and boundary experience. This is particularly the case when *full attention* is poured or surrendered into the slow exhalation.

When completed, this practice will eventually gently affect and influence the first functional unit of our multileveled or triume brain, the reticular activating system. The reticular activating system serves to keep a certain energetic level or tone in the brain and also activates and inhibits all sensory and motor functions, most likely by way of the well-developed descending fibers of the reticular formation (Luria, 1973). The frontal and prefrontal lobes where complex and generative activity are focused have dense and multiple connections to all other areas of our brain.

Occasionally a sense of disorientation "within" the body is experienced. This is merely the release of energy and attention from usually frozen or fixated states of attention, both conscious and unconscious. Technically, this release of energy and attention called pranothana is normal, healthy, and necessary, even though it may feel strange initially (Krpalvanand, 1977). As a consequence, it will call into play, in subtle fashion, the tendency toward reactive egoic and muscular contraction when the exact sequence of the fourth practice is followed. The consciousness principle seems to rotate in the body. This must be experienced and experimented with in order to be verified.

In the successful application of the practice, the current of bliss is progressively liberated from the constricting patterns of the sensorimotor and cognitive frames of reference. Dwelling for periods in this current leads gradually to a sense of non-locality in the origin of bliss. From this opened perspective, the observer more easily sees the contracted patterns that the body/mind uses to structure and navigate reality, e.g., repression, denial, anxiety, the defense mechanisms, etc. These patterns are the same patterns as those that operate in the dream world, only less fluidly so. This insight or realization is exceedingly helpful as the observer moves from the waking state through the dream state and attempts to enter the Causal state where often the "objects" of perception begin to appear empty.[3]

The Fifth Practice

From this position of cultivated equanimity and lucid detachment, begin to *observe* the images, memories, and drifting associations that

---

3. When the objects or phenomena of observation are revealed to be experientially "empty" or unsubstantial, this may be because of: (a) The function of Hebb's notion of a brain/neural habituation process; (b) The action of the reticular activating system seeking new stimulation; (c) The Buddhist notion that all phenomena are empty; (d) All of the above, since they do not contradict each other!

arise from your subconscious process. After doing this for a sufficient amount of time, simply return to steady, even, diaphragmatic breathing, focusing on the root of the nose. The inhalation and exhalation being equal again, repeat the observations. Doing this simple practice and remaining *awake* leads to a slow but definite and radical change in the position of observation. This is the fifth fundamental practice, the one that makes the *observation* of clinical syndromes available as they unfold against the seamless current of living energy.

OBSERVATIONS

What are some of these observations? One of the first that the clinician may see is the subtle pervasive reactive fear that people express with deepening somatic and psychological relaxation. The fear of "letting go" of tension is related to the fear of loss. They then increase obsessive ideas and experience the impulse toward affect controlling compulsive behavior. I have seen this many times. This fear of relaxation occurs for many in the general population (Heide, 1985).

Beyond that, however, into deep muscle relaxation experiences, the practitioner/clinician can intimately witness the coordinations between body tension and psychological expressions. As these body tension areas are focused on, body tonicity decreases progressively and proprioceptive feedback also decreases. The neuromuscular system speaks. Various associations to specific body areas arise from intrapsychic, family memory and deep collective reservoirs. The method now practiced, based on the condition of equanimity, allows one to study this subtle neuromuscular tension and its concomitant ideational or mental forms. The mind naturally focuses inward, but do not be too absorbed in inwardness. Harness the capacity to witness all phenomena as simply arising on subtle levels without prejudice.[4]

At times, the practitioner may experience partial body dissociation

4. This is really a mastery of the process of attention. Attention, in purely psychophysiological terms, is currently understood to be the expression of three separate but interacting neural systems. For an excellent review, see Pribram and McGuinness (1975) "Arousal, Activation and Effort in the Control of Attention." The article does not address the psychospiritual dynamics of attention turned back upon itself, but is clinically quite useful.

or a sense of immobility. It will pass. There may be muscle tics, and somatic localizations of body armor, etc. The method allows one to observe the mind and personality styles and syndromes in germ form that arise in various attempts to deal with these situations. As attention is brought back to the focal point of the lip/nose, *all* the arising perceptions *dissolve* back into the current of living energy. The witness eventually perceives and experiences all phenomenal appearances as arising out of and then falling back into this boundaryless living energy. This process of the dissolution of phenomena, be the phenomena physical, mental, or energetic, and then the perpetual arising again of phenomena in this current is the result of the practice of this method. The thoughts and respiratory system naturally slow down in this process. A certain withdrawal of normal attention, or pratyahara, from its external sensory focus spontaneously occurs. The subjective experience of lucidity and intelligence, fused with intuition and energy or light, increases.

The Tibetan Tantric tradition describes the space between the slowing, discrete thoughts as variations of the Clear Light. Between the death of one thought and the birth of another is the primordial condition of mind called the Mother or Fundamental Clear Light. This Clear Light also dawns at times in the dream state. Various methods are employed to re-cognize or dwell more fully in this condition (Evans-Wentz, 1958). This Clear Light is the essence of the Voidness or emptiness. This light and energy and voidness are fused. There are many levels and gradations in this experience as thoughts become discrete. In the process the *fifth* fundamental practice naturally emerges. The observer witnesses the rise and fall of the various constellations and possibilities for ordering and dealing with the current of living energy. In a sense, one is looking into the interior of one's own psychic immune system and witnessing in germ form the potential processes of the syndromes and personality styles in their energetic expression.

All that has so far been spoken of has tended to be focused on the "subtle" and energetic aspects of the process. There is a tendency here toward "inner" experience. This fosters a split between inner and outer. The next area, therefore, is the "other" side or aspect of this process. It is the consciousness change that occurs. First, let us summarize.

The clinician/practitioner applies the five fundamental practices of this methodology, which are: (1) relaxed body posture, straight spine, and deep, slow, rhythmic diaphragmatic breathing to the point where one feels not only that one is breathing, but also that one is being breathed; (2) alternate nostril breathing for a continuous period, such that one subjectively feels the spinal column to be the central channel of bio-energy and consciousness; (3) the application of sushumna such that the Ki energy is stimulated at the top of the lip, bottom of the nose, and a tangible sense of the life-current is experienced in a blissful way. The experience is deepened when attention is completely surrendered into the exhalation. This is intuition married to a tangible sense of energy; (4) slow conscious stimulation of the somatopsychic route through the precentral gyrus of the brain. This leads to sensorimotor stimulation and withdrawal without loss of consciousness. A tangible position of balance and equanimity married to energy is cultivated. (5) observation of associations, images, body-tension zones and memories as they become entangled in the various syndrome and personality styles. *Each style and syndrome has characteristic ways of handling the flow of the life-current which have been given different diagnostic names.* The position or perspective is from that of psychophysical equanimity.

As this method becomes easier with practice, certain changes in consciousness itself occur. The mind slows down and the thought-mesh becomes more porous. One can approach the subtle fiber of thought with another tool. As energy and attention are freed by the methodology, the current of living energy becomes more tangible. It becomes more and more the vast "sea of energy" that envelops the tacit world of unconscious and unrecognized world processes. The breath continues to slow as does the train of thought.

At this stage the ego or "I" sense is directly experienced as a process with no boundaries. Thoughts drift in and out, as do all other associations and relations. The ego or "I" sense is directly felt to be an open field or process of experience, not an "object" or entity. The greater the free *tension* in the body/mind, the greater the force of *attention.*

The "I" sense slowly undergoes a shift in primary identification. Bateson pointed out that this is one of the great problems of modern science. He said that in the process or act of knowing, our epistemology and our ontology will merge. They will merge because in the act of knowing, the subject, or knower, fuses with the object of knowing in a common ground. There needs to be a transformational grammar of the identity matrix in order to move from one perspective to another. That is provided by, paradoxically, the current of living energy.

In its "field" of experience, the current is initially recognized primarily in the unconscious regions, so to speak, where the primary processes mode of *intense* emotions, themes, and personal memories are involved. The current has moved to the more *subtle* regions, however, when the thought-grid or movie screen is thin, light, and initially unfamiliar with newer images, intuition and bliss. This is a fine but important differentiation to make in practice. Primary process regression is not the same as dawning transpersonal experience.

As energy and attention are freed, the pool of free energy is conscious. It can go, so to speak, into this frame or that frame, etc. However, the current or reservoir of free energy is available and tangibly conscious. As that reservoir becomes fuller or deeper through practice, it takes on a decidedly blissful color. Its nature, boundary, and expression is blissful. This pool of blissful energy and attention is *conducted* through the body/mind by the disciplined, slow diaphragmatic breath. On occasion the experience of bliss will not be associated with any body/mind condition at all. It will simply be free energy and free attention, living and conscious. Experiences arise in it, a kind of Copernican revolution, you could say.

You may have already noticed in the practice of these procedures that "objects" only appear when "I" exists. When the mind's non-local field of consciousness contracts from the undivided whole and all pervasive reality, an "object" arises, much as matter arises from the greater background field of energy. As the Shivasutras say "Chiti Herself, descending from the plane of pure consciousness, becomes the mind by contracting in accordance with the object perceived." This observation is not confined to only meditative introspective traditions. At the level of diffuse or limitless boundary in the sub-atomic world, the physicist Capra (1982) has pointed out that ". . . properties of particles are determined by principles closely related to the methods of observation . . . observed patterns of matter are reflections of patterns of mind." Bohm's (1951) classic textbook on quantum theory offered a number of perceptive analogies between thought processes and subtle quantum processes. The list is quite long from both scientific approaches, one internal and the other external. Thus the cultivation of bliss, both intellectually and psychophysically, is immeasurably helpful in developing a consciousness capable of focusing or meditating on that seamless emptiness out of which all objects and forms unfold. It can then be extended or located in other contexts.

With the increase in bliss in this condition, the practitioner/clinician can notice a certain affinity to other body/mind experiences. One is the brief condition of body/mind bliss right *after* a deep, full, unconflicted sexual orgasm. There are no special or constituted thoughts in the mind. Deep orgasm oblates the mind briefly and allows bliss to arise. It is open, expansive. Eventually, thoughts feel as real and objective as external nature. The body feels deeply relaxed into a sensual current or process of experience. The boundaries are warm and tenuous. In a certain sense, the experience is one of sensuous emptiness! Not nothingness, emptiness.[5] The current of living energy here is both sensuously empty and luminously conscious with only a few thoughts. The adept lover or practitioner/clinician can also come to know a dim sense of this long before orgasm and therein deepen the condition and explore a certain level of bliss. While all that is helpful, *the primary reason for generating the great bliss condition is to fuse with it in meditation.*

By cultivating the condition of body/mind equanimity on all levels, not only the waking level, the condition of bliss becomes more apparent. This is energy intuition married to attention. It occurs naturally in deep sleep without dreaming. Yet because of the lack of images and words to weave memory, there is only a tangible sense of it. After deep orgasm, this bliss is also briefly experienced again. This method, however, is tricky.

5. A long digression into the correct view of emptiness would take us far afield. The interested reader is referred to (1) Lati and Denma Locho Rinbochay and Zahler and Hopkins *Meditative States in Tibetan Buddhism: The Concentrations and Formless Absorptions* (1982); (2) G. K. Gyatso *Clear Light of Bliss* (1983); (3) *The Diamond Sutra* where we see "form is emptiness, emptiness form."

It is easier to cultivate the bliss body from steady practice of psychophysical equanimity and the simple fundamental practices outlined here. When bliss is deep enough, the "I" sense relaxes into it naturally. The current of living energy flows through a boundaryless process as the "I" sense repeatedly emerges and submerges in the flux. This pool of free energy and attention is paradoxically one of bliss/intuition/energy. As the "I" process repeats this, it recognizes itself arising from an unmanifest realm. It is experienced as a localization of events, feelings, memories, and ideas in a vast non-local sea of free energy/intuition/light and bliss. This is reflected in the rise and fall of the sense of "other" in experience. The "other" is always an expression of mind, and too often merely an expression of ego. The non-existence of the "other" experience increases and the notion of continuous extension and duration increases. It becomes self-luminous, this intuition/intelligence. The aphorism of Patanjali reflects this process succinctly when it states "the mind is not self-luminous since it can be seen as an object." An aspect of the "I" sense is always unmanifest and it intuitively feels the unmanifest to also be the source of the current of living energy. All is directly experienced as arising from it, all passing back into it. It is the zero-point energy[6] where all manifest energy and form is enfolded and therein unmanifest. The "I" sense in its former expression as phenomena is slowly but eventually radically *outshined* in the unutterable bliss/intuition/energy backdrop or sea.

---

6. Zero-point energy refers in physics to the primary sea of energy, of which particle and wave are projections or abstractions and, would appear to be virtually *limitless* as compared to the rest of material reality, and also, paradoxically, a void or emptiness (Bohm, *Causality and Chance in Modern Physics*, 1957, p. 163-164).

7. At this point, the clinician/practitioner must choose which way to go. Many paths or options are open; the way of knowing by Raja Yoga, an experimental-scientific approach; the way of devotional energy of Bakti Yoga; the way of fine discrimination, of Jnana or Buddhist practices perhaps; perhaps of Kundalini the primal power; perhaps the way of not knowing itself, of Divine Ignorance or Sahaj Samadhi. Observe your own tendencies, then choose. Eventually a personal teacher will appear. This process of teachers appearing when the student is ready is a manifestation of this non-local agency. The teacher who "appears" for the student corresponds to the student's level of development. A similar non-local process may be seen between individuals who later become intimate. Their needs meet at corresponding levels of adaptation. The former, however, is a child of expansion, teleology; the latter a child merely of equilibrium.

This method exhausts the possibilities of *subtle* experience that can be brought through the body-mind structure. Beyond it intuition and consciousness co-mingle in ways that make no sense at all to the normal mode of perception. It is totally unfamiliar from moment to moment and yet is not disorganization or chaos or dissociation.[7] In the process up to this point, all the major psychological styles and syndromes can be seen to operate. Beyond it there is no body-mind structure that can be called upon to guide the practitioner/clinician other than a formal psychospiritual path and teacher.

It is the territory that is prior to the body/mind and all manifest nature.[8]

RECAPITULATION, LUCID DREAMS, AND BEYOND

Let me now briefly recapitulate. This method draws from the conditions embedded in the physical and subtle structures of the body/mind and enhances them for creating the ground experience of psychophysical equanimity. This leads to an increase in free energy and attention from which position the "I" sense as process, not object or entity, arises. This can be experimented with, replicated, and proved empirically and experientially to the observing person. Care must be taken not to fall into the swoon of unconsciousness. Focusing on the current of sensation becomes more subtle until it becomes the current of bliss. By witnessing everything that occurs mentally as a modification of this current of living energy, one becomes rooted in the pure non-verbal current of "basic aliveness." More and more progressively "the awakened mind is not fixed anywhere nor does it exclusively abide." At this point, a

8. In the method of Divine Ignorance or the Sahaj Samadhi school of Da Free John, the *full* liberation of attention and energy frees the individual principle of consciousness to reside in the locus of the right side of the heart, such that the radical intuition of Transcendental consciousness can fulfill itself and achieve agency in the body/mind of the manifest being. In a real sense, $E = mc^2$ is the transformational matrix of the matter-energy aspect of our nature. The non-local theater, however, encompasses this matrix and also opens beyond this matrix. Our body/mind aspect is a particular manifestation of the non-local, transcendental reality whose own theater manifests different laws and purposes in the seamless flux that gives rise to matter and energy, space and time. The latter unfold out of that emptiness into our local universe at 10^{-33} cm, 10^{-44} sec.

point that may take years to reach after daily diligent practice, from this point, the serious practitioner may move toward the following:

1. Intuit the physical/mental "I" sense to be a condensation or localization of energy/intelligence with no apparent boundary or limit to its background. In other words, the center of the conventional self becomes a localization of a non-local Self.

2. Observe the subtle body contractions *and* the mental associations and feelings from the perspective of basic aliveness with no prejudice.

3. Feel into the body the subtle current of living energy that appears to condense into a black hole of narcissism when the gravity of thought and ownership feeling increases. Observe the basic aliveness of the universe of the body and the universe outside the body, free of tension lines, fear and reactivity. Simple, unprejudiced receptivity. Assume that everything is okay. It may be necessary at times to intensify focus, while at other times it will be necessary to lessen this intensity. In either case, subtle and careful attention must be taken not to allow oneself to fall into the swoon of unconsciousness. This in and of itself is a very delicate art of balance. It is akin to keeping one's balance atop a fountain that is constantly spewing water and the specific shape of the water is constantly in flux. This stabilization, this equanimity, can again be greatly increased by a focusing of the attention at that point at the top of the lip and the bottom of the nose. Slow and deep diaphragmatic breathing, that has already been outlined, is also extremely helpful at this point. Breathing air into the deep recesses of the lungs is always healthy anyway.

When this is done in combination with the above description of the alternate nostril breathing, the focus of attention at a certain spot that corresponds to certain acupuncture meridians and the other fundamental practices, the current of living energy is brought under gradual control. When focused on, there is a simultaneous union of the intuition of luminous emptiness and space with that of an intelligent, blissful living energy. This becomes an observable, clinical reality.

Finally, after all of the above is done, and this takes some patience and some time, the *final* step is undertaken. That step, after a sense of equanimity and body-mind peace is attained in a very practical way, one slips into the following. Compassionately and humorously release the tacit assumption and body/mind sense that the current of living energy actually originates in you! Simply fall back into this current of living energy and see all as arising in and out of it. It becomes prior to, and more inclusive than you. You arise phenomenally in it. The usual "I" sense becomes a foreground while the ground out of which the "I" sense arises becomes a blissful, paradoxically empty background. The witness progressively identifies with the background and therein studies to locate other "higher" disciplines than the present one that will better and more idiosyncratically help cultivate this. The experience of boundaries will greatly expand and change. At certain points, both waking and dreaming, an extraordinary luminosity unfolds.

From this position of a directly experienced and felt current of living energy, watch the constellations of affect, thoughts, subtle body-mind contractions in the face of these thoughts and images, and other changes in the equilibrium of the system. There will be continuous small, minute changes. However, despite these minute changes and metamorphoses, a general pattern of styles will emerge in this context. These styles emerge as characteristic ways of dealing with the life current. Various personality and motivational styles will arise and form a constellation around particular ways of handling this current of living energy.

One need not be in this state perpetually. Freud was not unconscious when he re-discovered aspects of the unconscious process. However, he periodically did have to experience the processes of the unconscious without reflection. For Freud, the unconscious broke through occasionally, and on its own, but was also opened by using specific procedures. Here the all inclusive unmanifest realm breaks through into waking, dreaming, and sleeping consciousness by way of transient intuitions of oneness, lucid dreams and clear light dreams/experiences respectively. It is the fleeting, spontaneous breakthrough of the prior being, the condition that is also identical to the radiant transcendental being or light-intelligence. We are asking the reader and clinician to identify *primarily* with the current of living energy and only *secondarily* with the thoughts, affects, and constellations of emotional energies and body-mind reactions that occur and are observed. This conducts the energy through the whole system and avoids it becoming locked in the waking state only. It will eventually affect your dream life in blissful, pleasurable imagery and subsequently, you will be able to "locate" it in the midst of other events. You will notice that this occurs in these four examples taken from a brief period of my records:

> Lucid Dream 1. (10/18/84) Last night, after some events of the day that involved my attempting to contact two different people to convene about lucid dreams and serial dreams, I had a lucid dream . . . In the dream I was flying over the UMass campus when I casually realized that I was flying and that *therefore* this was a dream! Then I remained consciously calm and continued to fly. I flew higher and then decided to fly as high up to the sun as I could. I remained lucid for a good while and then attempted to "meditate" in the dream. I was a little disappointed that I could not "open" the higher door after two attempts. Then the dream faded.

> Lucid Dream 2. (10/19/84) . . . I had awakened from an early morning flying dream. This time, however, I went straight from waking back into the dream (Yoga Nidra practice). . . . In the next flying dream I consciously looked toward the crown chakra at the top of the head and seemed to pull myself in a soaring motion upward. I was aware that there were no other backdrop dream images this time. This was a little new. Suddenly I felt a cracking-nerve sensation in my head and spine. I realized that my body was in the fetal position and stopped the conscious meditation on upwardness out of some fear of hurting myself. At this point I lost lucidity.

The next two examples show how, with a little discipline over time, that the process can be "located" in contexts beyond this initial one. It is a form of "generalization" I suppose, but the dynamics are somewhat different from those we usually associate with the principles of behavioral generalization. Also, as a matter of technique, try to refrain from involuntary orgasm despite the extremely pleasurable sensations of this state. If you do, then eventually the mind will become stable, intense, and oblated by light and one can thereby more easily fuse both the blissful sense, which increases, and the paradoxical emptiness/light experience:

> Ecstasy-Light Dream 3. (3/3/84) . . . In the dream I was dreaming! In the deepest dream I became aware of a warm, blurred point of light. The light "felt" very compassionate, non-verbally intelligent and directed "at" me. I awoke from that dream and wanted to tell others especially how only dimly aware we are of the human potential. I was tearful about this because the dim light was felt to be everyone's and was also experienced by me to be ecstatic or full of subtle ecstasy. I could feel the ecstasy and it felt familiar, like in other "clear light" dreams I've experienced.
>
> Then I awoke into regular waking awareness *and* was aware of keeping the original ecstasy of the dim light with me. There was a clear sense of the *continuity* of the light experience *into* the waking state, albeit much less intensely. I spoke to Alyse about this over breakfast.

This next somewhat lengthy example shows how the current can easily flow through or manifest in several states of consciousness and yet maintain its identity. It is merely a matter of sustained practice and acquiring learnable observational skills:

> (10/22/85) Kathmandu, Nepal. A long luminous and strange night! The new Diamond Hotel where we stayed had us on the ground floor, next to an alleyway. All night one could hear foot-traffic, children crying, people clearing their throats of phlegm, dogs and some other animal sounds I couldn't really identify. [We had to move for one night from our other nice hotel, the Ambassador, because of scheduling problems.] As a result I couldn't sleep and initially occupied my mind with images gathered earlier that day of dead squashed rats in the back alley roads, dismembered black cows and severed lamb heads on tables in the marketplace. This wasn't taking me nearer to sleep in our dark room! It was *10 p.m.*, and so I decided at least to relax my body and give some measure of peace to my waking consciousness.

I began to recite various mantras . . . [the luminous current] was gracefully active. In the darkness I began to *synchronize* my breathing with specific and also "spontaneous" phrases and mantras e.g., AUM, "surrender into God." Each was done for a good length of time. I know because I twice got up to use the bathroom. . . .

I returned to bed [singles] and began the mantras again [after assuring myself] that no disease infested rat could slip into the room. My concentration deepened after awhile as I synchronized the slowed breath with the phrases "surrender into God" and "AUM." I felt that somewhat familiar slippage sensation and knew I was gliding into sleep. I focused my attention/imagery on myself as a large bird whose big slow wings would carry him into flight. With a sluggish sense and a lot of calm effort I glided up into the air [in the dream]. I went higher and higher, fully aware that I was using Yoga Nidra techniques to enter into a successful lucid dream. This continued for only a brief while, perhaps 5 minutes, and I was drawn out of it by a heavy scratching noise on the window or outside bathroom wall. I was laying on my right side.

I then went back to the mantra of AUM with deep, slow, spiraling inward-sense concentration. I had the conceptual awareness that anyone who did this needs to feel that ego surrender or dissolution was into a benign sphere or domain. I then switched back to the "spontaneous" mantra "surrender into God." This continued for a good half hour as I used it to steady my technical concentration [Dharana in Patanjali's system].

Quite suddenly, but not sharply, I felt a distinct sense of light or luminous movement arise from the heart/chest region. I was laying on my back this time after being on my right side for the Yoga Nidra practice. Laying on my back is unusual for me because in the past it often creates nightmares and brief dissociation experiences that are unpleasant. This isn't always the case, but often is so.

So I lay on my back and watched as this luminous current of energy (white and amorphous and pleasurable/blissful) moved up and out of the heart region. It widened from its more narrow opening or source as it coursed up the spinal column. My eyes were drawn upward.

My ego initially was surprised, then became alarmed. At that instant, as my lower body from below the heart downward began to become cold and rigid, I thought to call out to Alyse [in the other bed]. I was clearly wide awake, not dreaming. Then, since I had some prior brief experience with this dissociation at least in the past and knew this was not a cerebral hemorrhage (a nasty fantasy I've used to scare myself with before), I consciously decided "not to resist," but to relax into it. This all transpired consciously and quickly.

The luminous current then spread even more as it flowed up the spinal line into my neck, lower brain, and enveloped my whole head. My lower body had gone cold and then lost sensation. My upper body, above the heart, seemed to dissolve in this luminous, intensely pleasurable/blissful current. Cognition became blurred as a sense of body-mind boundless light ecstasy pervaded me. "I" seemed to be engulfed by "It." The "I-It" differentiation was no longer in actuality. The pleasure was radically *more* intense than a hashish-inspired sexual orgasm and the "boundless environment" was closest to the few clear-light dreams I have had.

At the moment the current seemed to stabilize in its luminosity I suddenly achieved self-consciousness again. I said "not here," referring to the lousy place of the Blue Diamond hotel. It then gradually decreased and faded back down to the slim, luminous current . . . along the spine that I am familiar with on a daily basis. I did not want a full opening in such a cheap place and knew that the current could be raised again under more favorable circumstances.

Body feeling and control returned. I then lay there and made sure I was awake and would remember in *detail* the sequence of events that lead to the experience [for my journal]. Technically and psychospiritually I reviewed the whole process. . . . At no time did I lose consciousness, but the form or texture or character of the mode of consciousness radically altered. My eyes [. . .] were drawn upward from the level at the nose . . .

> up to the eyebrows and crown area. This felt like an involuntary process . . .

Lucid dreaming is an ancient practice long known to the Tibetan lamas, Kemetic Egyptian mystery schools of the upper Nile and numerous other psychospiritual disciplines. Recently it has been subject to extensive laboratory study and can be learned with diligent practice, motivation, and skill (LaBerge, 1985). It is one of the many useful experiences that arise as other conditions are met in the emergence of the noetic consciousness.

As we can see in this particular condition of cultivated equanimity the general patterns which we outlined in the early chapters have been seen to consistently arise. The current of living energy can therein be engaged in an experimental way at the level of consciousness or being itself. In so doing, one is able to go beyond the conventional pursuits of science that engage primarily in a descriptive analysis of phenomena exterior to consciousness or reality itself. In other words, the basic aliveness of the universe is directly and intuitively experienced. Of necessity this means at times an outshining by the experience of the ways to describe that experience. However, eventually an *intuitive language* will arise from being able to take advantage of this process. Eventually the source out of which this current of living energy itself arises becomes tacitly and intuitively known. At this point the clinician/practitioner has become good friends not only with the unconscious mind, but has also had prolonged intimate contact with and dwelled in the current of living energy. At such a point an appropriate Yoga or path to liberation becomes obvious. Therein the clinician/practitioner can select a path or method conducive to his or her style and tendencies or make an appropriate referral to others. These many paths are varied and found in some degree of development in all the major and perennial traditions.

The body-energy methods of Hatha are selected by some after distilling the traditions. The cool abstraction and absorption of the intellectual schools of the Vedantists, the Mahayanists, the Zen teachings and others appeal to some intuitively, leaving others untouched. There are many many more examples, not all derived from these Eastern traditions. The Kemetic Egyptians evolved similar traditions to respond to the particular tendencies of their students. They had three levels of initiation in the mystery schools of the houses of light; the neophyte or initiate, the intellect or nous, and the "sons of light." These schools had a profound and millennial influence in the ancient world and were to deeply impact the foundation of later Greek civilization, both in science and religion (James, 1976; Finch, 1992). Thus every culture, every face of humankind has seen itself reflected in every tradition from Ancient Egypt to the Tibetans of today. This is how we are all bound to each other, locally and otherwise. Therefore "The Great Way is not difficult if you have no preferences." Listen to your heart, without prejudice, without mind. The current of living energy is a fountain that arises spontaneously as bliss. See and feel into it in all states of mind: waking, dreaming, and the void/energy/bliss of deep sleep. When all things, objects, and events arise and dissolve in it, the way unique to you opens. It opens to that beyond the body/mind and all manifest nature.[9]

THE LATER UNFOLDMENT

At the beginning of this chapter it was emphasized that this transpersonal view, or perspective, has its own limits. It arches midway between contemporary psychology and the older, more inclusive transformative disciplines. The work of the methodology I have presented is empirically testable by observation and experimentation with one's own experience and corroboration with others. All along I have pointed to what unfolds beyond the five fundamental practices that are designed to elucidate the play of the various syndromes with the life-force. These fundamental practices,

---

9. The method or Yoga of the sound current, called the Surat Shabd Yoga, is still another development of this current of living energy. After the appropriate pranayamas, the practitioner applies Nauamukhi Mudra, which closes all the nine gates of entry into the body. A series of sounds is heard in the central axis or sushumna. By stages, it courses through the body on progressively more subtle levels until it rises through the heart, throat, and eyebrow center out beyond the manifest body/mind. It is an advanced practice requiring a personal teacher. (Rieker, *Hatha Yoga Pradipika*, pp. 176-188; Motoyama, *Theories of the Chakras*, pp. 105-129; Singh, *The Crown of Life: A Study in Yoga*, pp. 142-186).

not those others I have mentioned briefly in footnote and reference, will take the practitioner to those levels usually described as subtle or psychic. We have only fleetingly mentioned what lies beyond. Each level or plane beyond is accompanied by its own problems and gorges into which one might fall. The level of psychic unfoldment is replete with the potholes of pseudo-realization, most often expressed in excessive attachment to natural, healthy, spontaneously occurring psi episodes and psychic phenomena. Beyond its potential use in healing, the psychic and subtle offer the practitioner ways to delude themselves that they have entered the domain of unutterable light and intelligence. These potholes also include ego-inflation, tundra, sokrlung, pseudo-Nirvana and dissociation. Each discipline or path has pitfalls especially associated with its trajectory. Psychological disturbance can be mis-labeled spiritual insight, as occurs sometimes in the mixed state of the "spiritual emergency." The ego has simply replaced noble aspiration for lofty fantasy. All kinds of trance states and related phenomena emerge and need to be examined with a personal teacher of a chosen transformative discipline. Sometimes the clear mind of tranquil abiding can be mistaken for radiant emptiness or Shunyata. Sometimes pranotthana is mistaken for Kundalini or else Kundalini is prematurely awakened and out of control. These deeper, more archetypal aspects of our unfolding process arise and require a clear understanding of their real, somewhat obscuring nature. It is a natural phase.

Beyond this is the Causal level which has only been briefly mentioned. Here one "confronts" the subtle self-sense or rarified differentiation of self and other. Its signature is the intuition of relationship itself. There is still a sense of experienced difference between the manifest "I" and the unmanifest, non-local ground of consciousness itself. The paradoxical nature of the life-force as both luminously intelligent and "empty" is played out here, until there is an integration of this subtle distinction. "Make the slightest distinction and heaven and earth are set infinitely apart." This most subtle differentiation of self and other, or manifest and unmanifest, is by way of a subtle addiction to bliss itself. However, if one can learn to consciously recognize and generate bliss, then one can proceed to carefully use that consciousness pervaded by great bliss to meditate on the luminous, intelligent emptiness that enfolds all forms and objects.

Technically speaking, one has turned attention back upon itself using some technique or discipline and reversed the outward flow of consciousness. The inward flow alters perception such that instead of each *next* to each, each is *in* each. The primal apprehension is, to extend the useful but limited holonomic analogy, that all is in each and each is in all. It is the interpretation of consciousness, the quantum interconnectedness, the dependent origination of the Buddhists.

My own bias on this particular issue is to use this model of subtle contraction upon the self-essence and the tangible current of living energy that has threaded through this entire portrait of syndromes. There are other ways, of course, to label and navigate this level of the radical disappearance of all phenomena into noumena. Form flows from the formless source and that source is identical to the transcendental condition. Using the structures of post-formal cognitive operations as a staging, preparatory mode for what lies beyond and still includes it, one moves from subtle contraction upon bliss as the self-essence to the witness of all ideas, events, and conditions including the modifications of the bliss sheath of fine discrimination as modifications of the radiant transcendental Self. It is the perspective that participates in the disposition that

> no thought or figure or any perception arising in the mind is, itself God . . . Rather every moment, place, thing, body or state of mind inheres in God . . . then all conditions become reminders that draw us into the ecstatic presumption of the mysterious presence of the Living One.

SUMMARY

Above, I have presented one particular method of amplifying the experience of body-mind balance or equanimity. It is a method that makes use of the union of great bliss and emptiness with sustained intuition and the observation of a current of living energy in the body. This is done by taking advantage of the energetic constellation of the body/mind. It eventually leads not only to the sense of equanimity and fine, highly polished observations of the process of egoic contraction, but it also leads to subtler and subtler mental states. The gradual loosening and freeing of attention from habitual associations, memories, and body-mind reactions, leads eventually to the ability to focus progressively on the non-local, boundaryless source out of which the current of living energy arises. Thus, it is necessary at the very end of the process, as I have pointed out above, to be able to fall back totally within the current of living energy and to drop the modern "logical assumption" that this energy originates within the boundaries and body/mind of the person who is focusing on it. This allows for the energy to fall back to its very source condition. As one moves in and out of this process, it allows for the observation of thought and thought-affect styles that are most noticeable in the culture of a person's individual thoughts. One has associations and thoughts not only to what is available to one's individual unconscious, but also to one's family unconscious and collective unconscious. It is only necessary to periodically experience this state in order to gain a great deal of information and wealth from it. While it may be a "subtle problem,"[10] that a person become addicted to the experience of bliss itself, it is possible to bypass this. As Sankaracarya (1978) observes:

> 209 Nor is the blissful sheath the Supreme Self, because it is endowed with changeful attributes, is a modification of the Praketi (objective nature), is the effect of past good deeds, and imbedded in the other sheaths which are modifications.

This practice in its mature form need not remain a purely "fifth stage"[11] practice, but may actually lead the person to the source of all of these experiences when they transcend the fine discrimination of the mind. By taking advantage of certain energies immediately

10. In some introspective traditions the body/mind is divided into gross, subtle, causal and supercausal states, each unfolded out of the others before it toward manifestation. The subtle refers to the energetic dimension of life. The body is the gross or most manifest and the mind is the least and is embedded in the causal. The supercausal refers to that beyond mind. It is Turyia or the fourth state.

11. This refers to the exclusive focus on the subtle physiology of the body/mind conditioned by the nervous system. It is not yet fully free attention. It is full awareness of the life-current, however, and this life-current is also not dissociated from oneself or the circumstances of everyday life. (Free John, *The Enlightenment of the Whole Body*, 1978).

available, one can greatly increase and observe one's progress. It also allows for an observational position that can be replicated not only within oneself, but to other individuals in the system of one's life.

At the end of this sitting, when the body-mind equanimity is well established, when the general sense of bliss and energy that is directly experienced are unified, there is a natural automatic and inevitable loss of the experience of conventional boundaries. The very "basic aliveness" of the universe clearly is not delimited by the boundaries of one's own individuality, regardless of how that individuality is defined in terms of body, or mental boundary. The particular constellations of thought and energies and ways of handling the body/mind can be seen to fall into various constellations or clinical syndromes. The actual practice of the above simple exercises several times a day over a period of time will substantially increase the clinician's observing skills. It will also manifest how the different constellations of reactivity, or clinical syndromes arise, interact and reflect each other in various ways and yet are thematically distinct from each other in specific aspects. Through all of them, they are a way of handling the current of living energy and the boundary disturbances that arise in this process. Beyond these clinical, energetic, and subtle navigations, the practitioner must learn to master the discipline of attention itself. One needs to persist in the chosen practice until all structures of mind dissipate in boundless radiance and ecstasy. Do that and thereby, even while waking, never be seduced by the illusion of objects, death, and separation again. Eventually every vortex and ripple in the current and stream opens beyond itself into the unutterable ocean that is intelligence and light.

REFERENCES

Arpita, "The Role of Breathing in Current Clinical Interventions," *Research Bulletin*, E.N. Dana Laboratory, Himalayan Inst., Honesdale, PA, 1982.

Bohm, D. *Causality and Chance in Modern Physics*, Routledge and Kegan Paul, London and Boston, 1957.

Bohm, D. *Quantum Theory*, Prentice-Hall, New York, 1951.

Capra, F. *The Turning Point: Science, Society and the Rising Culture*, Simon and Schuster, New York, 1982.

Epstein, M. D. "On the neglect of evenly suspended attention," *Journal of Transpersonal Psychology*, Vol. 16, No. 2, 1984, pp. 193-205.

Evans-Wentz, W. Y. (Ed.) *Tibetan Yoga and Secret Doctrines*, Oxford University Press, London and New York, 1958, pp. 222-232.

Finch, C. S. *Echoes of the Old Darkland*, Khenti Inc. Decatur, GA, 1992.

Free-John, D. *The Enlightenment of the Whole Body*, Dawn Horse Press, Middletown, CA, 1978.

Grof, S. *Beyond the Brain: Birth, Death and Transcendence in Psychotherapy*, SUNY, NY, 1985.

Gyatso, L. *Clear Light of Bliss*, Wisdom Publications, London, England, 1983.

Heide, F. J. "Relaxation: The storm before the calm," *Psychology Today*, Vol. 19, No. 4, April 1985, pp. 18-19.

James, G. G. M. *Stolen Legacy*, Julian Richardson, San Francisco, 1976.

Khalsa, D. S. "Rhythms and Reality: The Dynamics of the Mind," *Psychology Today*, September 1984, pp. 72-73.

Klein, R. A. and Armitage, R. *Science*, Vol. 204, 22 June 1979.

Krippner, S. and White, J. (eds.) *Future Science: Life Energies and the Physics of the Paranormal*, Garden City, New York: Anchor Books, 1977, pp. 550-555.

Krpalvanand, S. *Science of Meditation*, New Karnodaya Press, Bombay India, 1977.

LaBerge, S. *Lucid Dreaming: The Power of Being Awake and Aware in Your Dreams*, J. P. Tarcher, Los Angeles, 1985.

Luria, A. R. *The Working Brain: An Introduction to Neuropsychology*, Basic Books, Inc., New York, 1973, pp. 58-60, 86.

Lysebeth, A. V. *Pranayama: The Yoga of Breathing*, Universe Paperbacks, London/Boston/Sydney, 1983.

Motoyama, H. "PK influence on the meridians and psi-energy," *International Journal for Religion and Para-Psychology*, Vol. 5, No. 2, July 1979.

Motoyama, H. "A biophysical elucidation of the meridian and Ki-energy" ibid.

Motoyama, H. "The ejection of energy from the chakra of Yoga and Meridian points of acupuncture." *International Journal for Religion and Parapsychology*, 1978.

Motoyama, H. *Theories of the Chakras: Bridge to Higher Consciousness*, Theosophical Publishing House, Wheaton, IL, 1981.

Muktananda, S. *Play of Consciousness (Chitshakti Vilas)*, Harper and Row, New York, 1978.

Pribram, K. H. and McGuinness, D. "Arousal, Activation and Effort in the Control of Attention," *Psychological Review*, Vol. 82, No. 2, 1975, pp. 116-149.

Rama, S., Ballentine, R., and Hymes, A. *Science of Breath*, Himalayan Publishers, Honesdale, Pennsylvania, 1979.

Rama, S. *Choosing a Path*, Himalayan Publishers, Honesdale, Pennsylvania, 1982.

Reich, W. *Character Analysis*. Farrar, Strauss and Giroux, New York, (1949), 1971 (Part 3, section 13, sub-part 9).

Reiker, H-U. *The Yoga of Light: Hatha Yoga Pradipika of Swami Svatmarama*, (Trans. by E. Becherer), The Dawn Horse Press, Middletown, CA, 1971.

Rinbochay, L., Rinbochay, D. L., Zahler L. and Hopkins, J. *Meditative States in*

Tibetan Buddhism: The Concentrations and Formless Absorptions, Wisdom Publications, London, 1983.

Sankaracarya, S. *Crest-Jewel of Discrimination*, Advaita Ashrama, Mayavati, India, 1978.

Sannella, L. *Kundalini-Psychosis or Transcendence*, H. S. Dakin Co., San Francisco, CA, 1978.

Singh, K. *The Crown of Life: A Study in Yoga*, Ruhani Satsang, Delhi, India, 1973.

Taub-Bynum, E.B. *The Family Unconscious: An Invisible Bond*, Theosophical Publishing House, Wheaton, IL, 1984.

Veith, I. (translator) *The Yellow Emperor's Classic of Internal Medicine*, Univ. of Calif. Press, 1972.

Epilogue: On Identity, Ecstasy, and Light

> As we live through thousands of dreams in our present life, so is our present life only one of many thousands of such lives which we enter from the other more real life . . . and then return to after death. Our life is but one of the dreams of that more real life, and so it is endlessly, until the very last one, the very real life,–the life of God.
>
> –Leo Tolstoy

All is light. Light, the substratum, the tissue and primordial identity of all that exists. All that exists is a relative of light. Above the range of the eye ride constellations of light and energy in vast unfolding networks of collision and expanse. Below the microscopic lens into the sub-atomic spaces all is radiance, interconnectedness and force. Indeed all is light. This is the deeper heart of science, this is also the root of spirituality, both unfolded and developing from a higher, enfolded order.

From the dawn of the human adventure spanning the full length of cognitive, physical, emotional, and noetic development, intelligence and teleology have been seen as *immanent* in the structure of the organism, its actions in the world and surely even in matter itself. We must non-apologetically bring this gentle light into the mechanical dream of modern science. For enfolded in matter is energy, light itself, the radical alchemy of $E = mc^2$ and beyond.

Intelligence, prior even to language, operates on this unconsciously and physically at first. Through the early sensorimotor era and maturing cognitive stages it flows on up through those higher structures of post-formal operations that eventually allow thought to become so supple, so lucid and clear, that the literal light that supports and infuses it is slowly recognized in its natural state again.

It is an open secret in every heart that light is intelligence and the fountainhead of purpose. That ancient mother, that later kin of "Lucy," intuited this but was ages away from clear reflection. The Vedas refined reflection and grew into this as did all the mystery schools from Africa to dateless China. That all this world of matter and form is literally light is now the common perspective of contemporary science. In this moment-to-moment ocean of possibilities and fleeting experience all the mellifluous and terrifying forms of light arise and disappear.

The life-force that pervades and animates all that lives is also deeply embedded in us. This universe is not a dead vacuum tube ruled by chance and improbable occasions as the dogma of materialist science would have us believe. Materialists can no more isolate and locate the life-force in a test tube or dissecting table than they can locate their own "I" anywhere specifically in the brain, body, or known universe. Mystery and science feed on each other and the growth of one does not in the least diminish the other.

The life-force was seen throughout this chronicle to animate and enervate the intimate life of each of us. It was not an abstraction, but rather a living, breathing reality. It flows through us in a current unique to each and yet is open to observation, experimentation, that necessary replication and then eventual communication. It was the tangible, daily reality to that ancient one; it is an identifiable reality for us if we will listen and work with sensitive tools. It is the most natural healing of our alienation from light, our estrangement from infinity.

Each personality style, each syndrome that was presented, was seen as a unique and thematic way of living with and in this tangible current, a current we have suggested to be a reflection of an embedded evolutionary current, intimately associated with the unfoldment of the neuromelanin nerve tract that is our inheritance since the earliest of embryonic times. This living current was known in antediluvian times. It will be the source of wonder and mystery and scientific fascination in ages to come. Should some massive climatic and ecological holocaust end the reign of our *homo sapiens sapiens* species, then surely some new form, some new trans sapiens, some new homo noetis will rediscover this evolutionary tract and develop even further. Neurobiology points in this direction! This unfolding life-force is an expression of nature and the evolutionary drama itself, immanent and transcendental all at once. It is purposeful. Its identity that is even expressible at all will always be closest to our most adventurous conception of light. Yet it will always be more than can be expressed and manifest, and as such must always most fully reside not simply in the unconscious, but in that all inclusive unmanifest realm enfolding all space, time, mentation and their derivative forms.

The stones of a river bed, the ragged sides of its banks, will direct the current's flow and support the life of fish, trees, and meadow or forest that feed on it. The life-rich current of water, however, is what makes it a river, that keeps nature multiplying in complexity along the evolutionary arch. Dry the river and the life eventually goes. Each bed of stones and contours in the personality styles and syndromes we explored turned the necessary river this way and that, made it stagnant or kept it flowing and resplendent with life. That river is the current of living energy. Its atoms and particles are aspects of light. It comes from light, plays in light, and returns to light. It is a form of light itself.

Since we become what we meditate on, it is wondrously obvious that in all things, in all events, in order to unfold our future in evolution we must meditate on light. Every object and form inheres in light. All manner of occurrences unfold out of light.

Think about it. Peer into the ancient chamber of your own heart. Has not *every* profound experience, waking, dreaming or sleeping, enormously expanded the "I" sense, pervaded it with a sense of truth and eternity? Unspeakable, yet scientific and mysteriously arising, our ultimate identity is realized in ecstasy and light!

It is no accident, no random coincidence of history, that every great religion, every mystery school, drew the initiate's attention toward light itself. It is deeply embedded in the metaphysics of those almost forgotten methodologies and is now the obvious substratum and matrix of reality for modern science. The Buddhist at death and deepest meditation enters the Clear-Light; the pious Hindu at death and dhyana goes through the body-mind and all manifest nature into the light beyond expression; the Christian at death and near-death (NDE) confronts the blinding white light of Christ, the radiant Avatar of Galilee. Each major tradition describes a different way of "returning" to earthly existence or some other realm of light, vibration, and "mental" existence or "bardo" unless, yes unless, they have entered that unspeakable domain beyond all verbal and mental definition. Unless, as they say, one has entered into the life of Light or God or the Absolute. Each interprets this "light" according to the tradition they issue from. The point is that they all refer strikingly to this light or luminous, creative source and Condition, a light that the greatest theorems of modern science proclaim to be the substratum and primordial identity of all that exists.

It is curious that also at death or in the near-death experience (NDE) the mind sees "members" of its relatives and deceased family members. We reportedly *see* and *feel* how our lives and the lives of all our significant others are enfolded into each other and how our actions implicate and interweave with the actions of others. This is that other earthly form of what we call "quantum interconnectedness" in science and "dependent origination" in philosophy. We are implicitly each a part of each other and at our best can emerge into a "communion of subjects." This may actually be the deeper levels of the great family unconscious dimension of the mind arising in energetic form and stretching back over generations. These "others" are reached or experienced in their *real* yet energetic form, not their dense material frame.

When mind is less localized with the body, as in death or NDE, and these family unconscious members arise, the functional structures of the mind begins to flow more freely in the non-local/holonomic sea of consciousness itself. Those family unconscious figures that do arise to us are due to our resonate affinity to them in life. Mind seems to invert and turn in upon itself as the field of enfolded family relationship becomes manifest to the "I."

Perhaps as the mind is freed of its physical constraints, it releases its phenomenal constructs and lens that functionally focuses the moment-to-moment world process and turns unerringly back upon its primordial condition and source. It either fearfully succumbs to, or ecstatically surrenders into, the ego's perennial nightmare and fully dissolves into the creative light and intelligent matrix of all matter, energy, and form. Beyond verbal and mental qualification in it arise all shifting, functional illusions of birth, death, space-time, name and form.

In the future, the great laboratory will be the body-mind, in which the most sublime science of humanity, the science of the life-force and its trajectory into the generative order of intelligence and consciousness itself, will occupy much of our time. Where else better to study $E = mc^2$ in the universe than in our own bodies, respiration, and intimate thoughts? They reflect the external universe more than we imagine. Indeed it is even possible that other life-forms have gone beyond our post-formal operations in their mental and life-force methodologies. It is all in the study of light. It is the evolutionary way that arches beyond man and the limits of the earth.

The intuition of that ancient one by shores and forgotten lakes matures and is no longer bound by name or fortune or frame. As she reflected herself in the mirrors of those waters and eventually learned to sail them to and fro, we, her progeny, go further and see ourselves reflected in and translated by the ocean of light. She opens fully now, in her progeny, to what is greater and beyond her fused association with matter, life, and form. Luminosity replaces ideation, ecstasy the existential storm. She-who-has-no-name awakens into the light beyond the dream.

Appendix: Suggested Further Readings

These references carry the explorations of areas mentioned in the text into deeper detail and provide a greater sea of data for the interested reader.

1. The Life-Force and the Kundalini Process

Chinmoy, S. *Kundalini: The Mother Power*, Agni Press, Jamaica, NY, 1974.

Colton A. R. *Kundalini West*, ARC Publishing Co., Glendale, CA, 1978.

Greenwell, B. *Energies of Transformation: A Guide to the Kundalini Process*, Shakti River Press, Cupertino, CA, 1990.

Krishna, G. *Kundalini: The Evolutionary Energy in Man*, Shambhala Publications, Inc., Boulder, CO and London, 1971.

_______ . *The Biological Basis of Religion and Genius*, Harper and Row, New York, (1972), 1971.

_______ . *Kundalini: The Secret of Yoga*, F.I.N.D. Research Trust, Ontario, Canada, 1972.

_______ . *The Wonder of the Brain*, F.I.N.D. Research Trust, Ontario, Canada, 1987.

Motoyama, H. *Theories of the Chakras: Bridge to Higher Consciousness*, Quest Books, Wheaton, IL, 1981.

Muktananda, S. *Kundalini: The Secret of Life*, SYDA Foundation, South Fallsburg, NY, 1979.

Narayananada, S. *The Primal Power in Man or the Kundalini Shakti*, N.U. Yoga Trust & Ashrama, Gylling, Denmark, 1979.

Radha, S. S. *Kundalini Yoga for the West*, Shambhala Publications, Inc. Boulder, CO, 1978.

Rieker, H-U. *The Yoga of Light: Hatha Yoga Pradipika*, (Trans. by E. Becherer), The Dawn Horse Press, Middletown, CA, 1971.

Sannella, L. *The Kundalini Experience: Psychosis or Transcendence*, Integral Publishing, Lower Lake, CA., 1987.

Scott, M. *Kundalini in the Physical World*, Arkana, London, 1983.

Silburn, L. *Kundalini: Energy of the Depths*, S.U.N.Y., 1988.

Sivananda, S. *Kundalini Yoga*, Divine Life Society, Shivanandanagan, India, 1980.

White, J. (Editor). *Kundalini, Evolution and Enlightenment*, Anchor Books, Garden City, NY, 1979.

Woodroffe, J. (Arthur Avalon). *The Serpent Power: The Secrets of Tantic and Shaktic Yoga*, Dover Publications, New York, 1974.

2. Physics and the Philosophy of Science

Bohm, D. *Wholeness and The Implicate Order*, Routledge and Kegan Paul, London, Boston, 1980.

_______ . *Causality and Chance in Modern Physics*, Routledge and Kegan Paul, London and Boston, 1957.

_______ . *Unfolding Meaning*, ARC (Routledge and Kegan Paul), London and Boston, 1987.

Bohm, D. and Peat, D. F. *Science, Order and Creativity*, Bantam Books, Toronto, London, New York, 1987.

Capra, F. *The Tao of Physics*, Bantam Books, New York, 1976.

Davies, P. *Superforce: The Search for a Grand Unified Theory of Nature*, Simon and Schuster, NY, 1984.

Heisenberg, W. *Physics and Philosophy: The Revolution in Modern Science*, Harper and Row, New York, 1962.

Herbert, N. *Quantum Reality: Beyond the New Physics*, Anchor Books, Garden City, NY, 1987.

Jantsch, E. *The Self-Organizing Universe*, Pergamon Press, Oxford, New York, Toronto, Paris, Frankfurt, 1980.

Kane, J. W. and Sternheim, M. O. *Physics*, John Wiley & Sons, NY, 1978.

Kaufman, W. J. (editors). *Particles and Fields: Readings from Scientific American*, W. H. Freeman & Co., San Francisco, 1980.

Prigogine, I. and Stengers, I. *Order Out of Chaos* Bantam Books, Toronto, New York, London, Sydney, 1984.

Scott, W. T. *Erwin Schrodinger: An Introduction to His Writings*, University of Massachusetts Press, Amherst, MA, 1967.

White, J. and Krippner, S. *Future Science: Life Energies and the Physics of Paranormal Phenomena*, Anchor Books, Garden City, NY, 1977.

3. Neuropsychology, Medicine, and Behavioral Medicine

Dossey, L. *Space, Time and Medicine*, Shambhala, Boulder, CO and London, 1982.

Gatz, A. J. *Clinical Neuroanatomy and Neurophysiology*, F. A. Davis Co., Philadelphia, (4th ed.), 1970.

Locke, S. and Colligan, D. *The Healer Within: The New Medicine of Mind and Body*, New American Library, New York and Scarborough, Ontario, 1986.

Luria, A. R. *The Working Brain: An Introduction to Neuropsychology*, Basic Books, Inc., New York, 1973.

Pribram, K. H. *Languages of the Brain: Experimental Paradoxes and Principles in Neuropsychology*, Brandon House, Inc., New York, 1971.

_______ . *Brain and Perception: Holonomy and Structure in Figural Processing*, Lawrence Erlbaum Associates, Hillsdale, NJ, 1991.

Rumelhart, D. E. and McClelland, J. (Eds.). *Parallel Distributed Processing* (2 vols.), MIT Press, Cambridge, MA, 1986.

Selye, H. *The Stress of Life*, McGraw Hill Book Co, (1956), 1976.

4. Cognitive and Emotional Development

Alexander, C. N. and Langer, E. J. (Eds.) *Higher Stages of Human Development*, MIU Press (Oxford University Press), Fairfield, IA, 1992.

Baldwin, A. L. *Theories of Child Development*, John Wiley & Sons, Inc., New York, London, Sydney, 1967.

Commons, M., Richards, F. and Armon, C. (Editors) *Beyond Formal Operations: Later Adolescent and Adult Cognitive Development*, Praeger Publishers, New York, 1984.

Erikson, E. H. *Childhood and Society*, W. W. Norton & Co., New York, (1950), 1963.

Langer, J. *Theories of Development*, Holt, Rinehart and Winston, Inc., New York, 1969.

Mussen, P. H. (Editor). *Carmichael's Manual of Child Psychology*, John Wiley & Sons, Inc., New York, London, Sydney, Vol. II, 1970.

Piaget, J. *The Origins of Intelligence in Children*, W. W. Norton, New York, (1952), 1963.

5. Evolutionary Development of Humanity

Ardrey, R. *African Genesis*, Dell Publishing Co., New York, 1967.

Darwin, C. *The Illustrated Origin of the Species*, (intro. by R. E. Leakey), Hill and Wang, New York, 1979.

Johanson, D. J. and Edey, M. A. *Lucy: The Beginnings of Human Evolution*, Simon and Schuster, New York, 1981.

Kessler, E. *Women: An Anthropological View*, Holt, Rinehart and Winston New York, 1976.

Leakey, R. E. and Lewin, R. *People of the Lake*, Avon Books, New York, 1979.

_______ . *Origins: The Emergence and Evolution of Our Species and its Possible Future*, E. P. Dutton, New York, 1977.

Pilbeam, D. R. *The Ascent of Man*, Macmillan, New York, 1972.

6. Mahamudra Lineages

Dowman, K. (Trans.). *Masters of Mahamudra: Songs and Histories of the 84 Buddhist Siddhas*, S.U.N.Y., 1985.

Garma, C. C. H. (Trans.). *Six Yogas of Naropa and Teachings on Mahamudra*, Snow Lion Publications, Ithaca, NY, 1963.

Gyaltsen, K. K. and Rogers, K. *The Garland of Mahamudra Practices*, Snow Lion Publications, Ithaca, NY, 1986.

Gyatso, G. K. *Clear Light of Bliss: Mahamudra in Vajrayana Buddhism*, Wisdom Publications, London, 1982.

Namgyal, T. T. *Mahamudra: The Quintessence of Mind and Meditation*, (Trans. by L. P. Lhalungpa), Shambhala, Boston & London, 1986.

Wang-ch'ug, Dor-jo (the 9th Karmapa). *The Mahamudra: Eliminating the Darkness of Ignorance*, Library of Tibetan Works and Archives, Dharmsala, Himachal Pradesh, India (1978), 1981.

7. African Roots of Civilization

Asante, M. K. *Afrocentricity*, Africa World Press, Trenton, NJ, 1989.

ben-Jochannan, Y. *Africa: Mother of Western Civilization*, Alkebu-Lan Books Assoc., NY, 1971.

_______ . *Black Man of the Nile and His Family*, Alkebu-Lan Books Assoc., NY, 1971.

Bernal, M. *Black Athena: The Fabrication of Ancient Greece, 1785 to 1985*, Rutgers University Press, Rutgers, NJ, 1986.

Churchward, A. *The Signs and Symbols of Primordial Man*, Greenwood Press, Westport, CT, 1978.

Coppens, Y., Howell, F., et al. *Earliest Man and Environments in the Lake Rudolf Basin*, University of Chicago Press, 1976.

Davidson, B. *Africa in History*, Macmillan Publishing Co., New York, 1968.

Diop, A. C. *The African Origin of Civilization* (trans. by M. Cook), Lawrence Hill and Co., Westport, CT, (1955), 1974.

_______ . *Precolonial Black Africa*, Africa World Press, Trenton, NJ, 1989.

Fairservis, W. A. *The Ancient Kingdoms of the Nile and the Doomed Monuments of Nubia*, Thomas Crowell, Co., New York, 1962.

Georg, E. *The Adventure of Mankind*, E. P. Dutton, NY, 1931.

Jackson J. G. *Introduction to African Civilizations*, Citadel Press, Secaucus, NJ, 1970.

James, G. G. M. *Stolen Legacy*, United Brothers Communications Systems, (1954), 1989.

Massey, G. *A Book of the Beginnings* (2 vols.), Williams and Norgate, London, 1881.

Seignobos, C. *History of Ancient Civilization*, Fisher Unwin, London, 1910.

Volney, C. F. *The Ruins of Empires*, Peter Eckler, New York, 1890.

Williams, C. *The Destruction of Black Civilization*, Third World Press, Chicago, IL, 1987.

Subject Index

Author Index